The Art is Long

*

PRIMARY TEXTS ON MEDICINE AND THE HUMANITIES

Edition 1.0

Edited by Alexis M. Butzner, PhD

The Art is Long: Primary Texts on Medicine and the Humanities
© 2021 by Alexis M. Butzner

ISBN-13: 978-1-943536-93-1

All rights reserved. Edition 1.0 2021.
No part of this book may be reproduced or transmitted in any form or by any means, electronic or mechanical, including photocopying, recording, or by any information storage and retrieval system, without permission in writing from the publisher.

Chemeketa Press
Chemeketa Community College
4000 Lancaster Dr NE
Salem, Oregon 97305
collegepress@chemeketa.edu
chemeketapress.org

Cover design by Katie Hildebrant
Interior design by Abbey Gaterud

References to website URLs were accurate at the time of writing. Neither the author nor Chemeketa Press is responsible for URLs that have changed or expired since the manuscript was prepared.

Printed in the United States of America.

LAND ACKNOWLEDGMENT

Chemeketa Press is located on the land of the Kalapuya, who today are represented by the Confederated Tribes of the Grand Ronde and the Confederated Tribes of the Siletz Indians, whose relationship with this land continues to this day. We offer gratitude for the land itself, for those who have stewarded it for generations, and for the opportunity to study, learn, work, and be in community on this land. We acknowledge that our College's history, like many others, is fundamentally tied to the first colonial developments in the Willamette Valley in Oregon. Finally, we respectfully acknowledge and honor past, present, and future Indigenous students of Chemeketa Community College.

Contents

Introduction: The Long Art	Alexis M. Butzner, PhD	1

Selections

Sushruta's Compendium (Sushruta Samhita)	Sushruta	13
The History of the Peloponnesian War	Thucydides	20
The Hippocratic Corpus	Various Authors	26
On the Nature of Things (De rerum natura)	Lucretius	31
Letters to Lucilius on Sickness and Death	Seneca	37
On the Natural Faculties (De naturalibus facultatibus)	Galen	41
A Treatise of the Small-Pox and Measles (Kitab al-Judari wa al-Hasbah)	Rhazes [Abū Bakr Muhammad ibn Zakarīyā Rāzī]	47
Causes and Cures (Causae et curae)	Hildegard von Bingen	57
The Salernitan Regimen of Health (Regimen sanitatis Salernitanum)	Unknown	59
On Wounds and Fractures	Guy de Chauliac	67
The Book of Margery Kempe	Margery Kempe	69
Syphilis: or, the French Disease (Syphilis sive morbus gallicus)	Girolamo Fracastoro	75
The Castle of Health	Sir Thomas Elyot	84
The Herbal, or General History of Plants	John Gerard	87
Seven Defenses (Sieben Defensiones)	Paracelsus	90
The Compendium of Materia Medica (Bencao Gangmu)	Li Shizhen	96
A Litany in Time of Plague	Thomas Nashe	100
A Brief Discourse of a Disease Called the Suffocation of the Mother	Edward Jorden	103
Devotions upon Emergent Occasions	John Donne	109
Poems on Sickness and Death	John Donne	122

On the Art of Surgery and Universal Antidotes	Ambroise Paré	125
Theories of Circulation and Reproduction	William Harvey	133
The Midwives Book	Jane Sharp	143
On Animalcules	Antonie van Leeuwenhoek	148
Upon the Sight of an Anatomy	Nahum Tate	153
The Sham Doctor	Joseph Addison	157
On Smallpox Inoculation	Lady Mary Wortley Montagu	163
Historical Account of the Smallpox Inoculated in New England	Zabdiel Boylston	167
After the Small Pox	Mary Jones	172
Domestic Medicine	William Buchan	174
On the Dissection of a Body	Anonymous	178
A Letter to a Lady on the Mode of Conducting Herself during Pregnancy	Sarah Brown	181
An Inquiry into the Causes and Effects of the Variolæ Vaccinæ	Edward Jenner	187
Medical Ethics	Thomas Percival	194
On Mediate Auscultation	René Laënnec	200
Sketches in Bedlam; Or, Characteristic Traits of Insanity	By a Constant Observer	204
The History of Mary Prince, a West Indian Slave	Mary Prince	211
To the Siamese Twins	Hannah Flagg Gould	222
The Masque of the Red Death	Edgar Allan Poe	225
Lecture on the First Surgical Operations under Ether	Crawford Williamson Long	232
Notes on Nursing	Florence Nightingale	235
In Hospital	William Ernest Henley	242
Selected Poems	Emily Dickinson	246
Memoirs of a Civil War Nurse	Emily Elizabeth Parsons	249
American Nervousness: Its Causes and Consequences	George Miller Beard	258

Specimen Days	Walt Whitman	262
Notes from Sick Rooms	Julia Stephen	272
A Book of Medical Discourses: In Two Parts	Rebecca Lee Crumpler	277
Neurasthenia	Agnes Mary Frances Robinson	285
The Yellow Wallpaper	Charlotte Perkins Gilman	287
Books and Men	William Osler	306
On Psychosexual Development	Sigmund Freud	313
Selected Works	Ohiyesa/Charles Alexander Eastman	318
"Out, Out—"	Robert Frost	328
On the Asylum Road	Charlotte Mary Mew	330
Mental Cases	Wilfred Owen	332
The Repression of War Experience	W. H. R. Rivers	334
The Repression of War Experience	Siegfried Sassoon	344
A Country Doctor	Franz Kafka	347
Complaint	William Carlos Williams	354
WPA Ex-Slaves Narrative Project	Federal Writers Project	356

Themes

MANUS DEI: FAITH AND MEDICINE — 365

Sutrasthanam: Sushruta's Compendium	Sushruta	367
Biblical and Apocryphal Sources	Various authors	369
Airmed and the Divine Knowledge of Healing Herbs	Unknown	373
Erra, the Plague God	Unknown	375
Pythian Odes III—For Hieron of Syracuse	Pindar	377

WHAT YOU SEE: ASSUMPTION, ANXIETY, AND THE APPEARANCE OF HEALTH — 383

Of a Monstrous Child	Michel de Montaigne	385
Of Monsters and Prodigies	Ambroise Paré	388
On Reproduction and Generation	Paracelsus	392

Mary Toft's Extraordinary Delivery	Nathaniel Saint-André & John Howard	396
Phrenology: Topographies of the Skull	John Taylor	400
Vaught's Practical Character Reader	Louis Allen Vaught	403
The Physiognomy of Insanity	Hugh Welch Diamond John Conolly	408

LIFE IN TIMES OF PLAGUE: DEPICTING THE BLACK DEATH — 413

The Decameron	Giovanni Boccaccio	415
An Order of the Lords…	City of Oxford	424
Diary of Samuel Pepys	Samuel Pepys	427
A Journal of the Plague Year	Daniel Defoe	439

DOING BATTLE: HEALTH AND MEDICINE ON THE FRONT LINES — 455

The Iliad	Homer	457
Photography from the American Civil War	Various Artists	460
Reminiscences of My Life in Camp with the 33d United States Colored Troops	Susie King Taylor	462
The Wound-Dresser	Walt Whitman	466
Images of World War I	Various Artists	471
Food Propaganda: Making Nutrition Patriotic	Various Artists	473

ACKNOWLEDGMENTS	479
INDEX	480

Introduction: The Long Art

ALEXIS M. BUTZNER, PHD

"Life is short, the art is long." So begins *Aphorisms*, a collection of around four hundred briefly stated medical principles attributed to the ancient Greek physician Hippocrates, who some consider the father of medicine. The art he refers to here is that of medicine. The sentiment suggests that the art of medicine is ongoing and that learning it takes more time than one short life will allow. This aphorism is often applied beyond medicine, however, to suggest, more simply, that art of all kinds endures beyond the individual lives that craft it. Applied to the collection you now hold in your hands, the aphorism acts as a reminder of both these ideas. The long timeline of the art of medicine, and of the process of learning it, is reflected in artistic products that have been passed along through the centuries.

Critical Backdrop

The works in this collection run the gamut from science to poetry to philosophy to autobiography. Many of the texts may appear difficult and foreign to us now; they contain both important principles and ones that feel laughable, sometimes even horrifying. Nonetheless, they are all worth taking seriously as documents of their own moments in time. The selected works offer a series of earnest attempts to make sense of the human body and condition. They offer stories of how we got to now. Science, medicine, art, literature, philosophy, history: these do not follow an unbroken line of progress. They are fundamentally human endeavors, which means they can be ambitious, and foolhardy, and imprinted with the foibles of their practitioners.

And humanity is a cornerstone of this collection.

This collection aims to trace some of the intellectual history illustrated in works concerned with medicine, health, and sickness. That history includes key moments in medical science and theory, of course, but also requires that we listen to the voices of those who witness, experience, and fear sickness, and those who strive for health. The selections in this volume tend to emphasize the human element. Among these works are stories of discovery, experiment, and invention; notions of what makes a good caretaker or practice; and experiences of or with illness.

In recent decades, the disciplines of medical humanities and health humanities have begun to explore the overlap and interconnection between traditional, science-based approaches to health and other disciplines, such as the arts, literature, philosophy, and music. These fields arose in the late twentieth century in response to increased emphasis on the technological and economic elements of medical study over the human element. Those working in these disciplines identified that the relationship between practitioners and patients was strained by an understanding of science and health that had too narrowly focused on specific body parts and the pathologies that impacted them, rather than on the whole person. Medical and health humanities, then, seek in part to restore a clearer sense of the connections between the scientific and the humane. As a sign of the importance of these connections, medical and health humanities have emerged as a course of study at colleges and universities, with programs at both the undergraduate and graduate level, as well as incorporation into the curriculum for some medical professionals. Renewed interest in these intersections between medicine and culture forms the critical backdrop of this collection.

Inclusion

Medical and health humanities recognize that medicine, and those who practice it, should not be walled off into a fortress of science and technology without reference to and connection with the humans who create and are impacted by that science and technology. The humanities can build empathy and strengthen intellectual reasoning and critical thinking, which are intrinsically useful skills in all settings and are particularly important for the work that practitioners and caretakers do. So, thanks in part to the rise of these fields, we have started to reconsider how overlaps between the disciplines, as well as their relative independent strengths, can help improve the empathy, critical thinking, and communication skills so important to caretaking. We are also beginning to recognize how the study of humanities can help each and every one of us be smarter, more self-aware, and more connected to the world in useful ways.

The intent of this book is to take that backdrop, and the recognition that our physical, mental, and emotional health are central to our lives and our world, and offer a collection that can spark inquiry and observation for teachers, students, and other interested readers. It is meant, first, to be a classroom edition, making texts accessible to readers while also leaving room open for exploration and interpretation. To this end, each text is accompanied by a brief introduction and contextualizing or explanatory footnotes.

This anthology presents, alongside major canonical works, an array of underrepresented voices and texts. The writing of medicine and the literary canon itself has, historically, marginalized many voices. This is partly because much of the material that has, in recent centuries, been deemed most important by Western practitioners and readers reflects Western traditions. In matters of health and sickness, the emphasis has been on Western medicine, the approach taken by much of modern medical science and research. It relies on the treatment of symptoms and diseases using so-called conventional treatments that target those issues, such as pharmaceuticals and therapeutics, surgery, and radiation.

Western medicine's approach has, of course, produced great gains for human health, but it does not represent the whole picture. It is often contrasted with traditional or alternative medicine, which takes a wide range of forms, many of which are thousands of years old and consider the whole body as opposed to focusing on a disease or body part. Traditional medicine also tends to use a broader mix of treatment types in order to promote health in that whole person. Although traditional and alternative medicines are still widely used around the world, they have long been viewed by many Western practitioners as mere superstition, and derided as folk medicine or belief. The prioritizing of modern medical science over all other approaches has meant that a great deal of human knowledge and endeavor has been underrepresented in Western culture. In response, this collection actively seeks to amplify relevant, diverse voices that have been heard less frequently.

This volume begins outside the confines of Western medicine, with one of the ancient, foundational texts of Ayurvedic medicine; it ends its individual selections with first-person health narratives of formerly enslaved African Americans, collected as part of the Work Project Administration's Slave Narrative Project. In between, a significant portion of the volume is dedicated to featuring the works and words of women and people of color.

Historical Scope

Similarly, this volume focuses on a much longer historical timeline than most existing anthologies; an attempt has been made to provide a broad survey of periods, from antiquity to the early twentieth century. We all benefit from the marvels of modern medicine, but fewer of us know the foundations on which those marvels have been built.

The first chronological category in this volume is ancient medicine (ca. third century BCE through fifth century CE), a body of work that includes some of the oldest recorded medical texts. Some of these offer principles that are still in use today. The period established the description of hundreds of illnesses and their treatments. It also gives us the first oaths of medical ethics, which contain principles practitioners still abide by, as well as a comprehensive system of medicine based in observation and experience. That system, with its belief in the necessary balance of four humors in the body, would be the dominant medical theory for some 1,400 years, and would remain influential until the germ theory of disease gained full acceptance in the nineteenth century.

The medieval period (ca. fifth through fifteenth centuries), far from being a dark age, was filled with medical advancements, including the invention of eyeglasses, the founding of the first pharmacies (though pharmacy as a practice was itself much older), and the development of medical study in university settings. This era also brought about the first use of quarantine as a measure for controlling the spread of epidemics, as well as substantial changes in legislation and regulations relating to public sanitation and health. Translations and the printing press made medical knowledge from around the world more accessible, and developments in the use of antiseptic and anesthetic substances, surgery and anatomy laid important foundations for future discovery.

The early modern period (ca. 1500–1750) brought further advancements. The scientific method became a formalized approach to inquiry. Alchemy, the forerunner to modern chemistry, offered chemical approaches to treating disease; colonialism brought important medicinal substances from the Americas back to Europe; and science solved the mystery of how blood circulates in the body. Major mechanical inventions include the first hinged prosthetic limbs, and microscopes that made it possible to view bacteria and sperm for the first time. In medical texts, anatomical descriptions and illustrations developed the level of detail and much of the style that is recognizable to us today. The early eighteenth century brought the introduction of inoculations against smallpox to Europe, part of the journey to modern vaccination. All of this—and there is much more—comes before the explosion of new technologies and discoveries that took shape from the late eighteenth century onward.

This approach necessarily limits the depth to which any period can be represented, but the trade-off is, hopefully, a recognition of the universality and continuity of the human relationship to health and medicine. No single region in the world, no single group of people experiences health and sickness as less important or less relevant to their culture and people. Thus it is with medicine: there is no single moment when *medicine* starts, or when it starts mattering more to those who practice it, or when it suddenly becomes more apparent in a number of cultural products. These works, taken together, show us a small glimpse into the vast ways in which these concerns of health and sickness matter to us all, and always have.

Genesis of the Collection

The seed of this volume was planted during my own undergraduate and graduate education, where I discovered a deep love of archival work and a growing interest in the history of science and medicine, and how they interact with literary texts. It grew into formal academic work, and then into my classrooms, where I discovered that these old primary texts weren't just my own hobbyhorse. My students also often found the texts fascinating, and they humored me long enough to see the value of looking at the primary sources themselves. Out of classroom conversations, the exciting insights and connections in their work, and the search for new texts to answer their questions and deepen our collective understanding, grew the anthology itself.

This book comes at a particularly apt moment. Over the course of the development of this book, the world was stricken with the novel coronavirus SARS-CoV-2 (which causes the disease called COVID-19), a pandemic that has had devastating impacts on every facet of our lives. Suddenly, many more people are thinking about our history with infectious disease. The influenza outbreak of 1918 and the HIV/AIDS crisis are the nearest analogue pandemics, but the centuries-long scourge of the Black Death has also loomed large. And even for those who aren't thinking of plagues past, the human connection with our health has started to show more clearly, as it always does in times of health crises, in our cultural output. Media, art, and writing have all been affected by this global infection, reminding us once again of how our physical, emotional, and mental health are reflected in our art.

How to Read this Book

Anthologies are often read in fits and starts and are not necessarily designed to be read in order from the first to the last page. That is certainly true for this anthology. The breadth of works is wide, not just in terms of time period, but also in theme, genre, and approach. After all, no single lens can show the full scope of sickness, of health, and of medicine and its many approaches. These selections are necessarily limited by the size of the volume. There are, however, through lines, and ways of approaching the texts that can draw those out. The individual selections are laid out in chronological order, from antiquity to the early twentieth century. To read from start to finish could illustrate some of the ways that health-oriented texts develop over time. A reader taking this approach might ask the following questions:

- How do the modes of writing and thinking about health change from century to century?
- How do particular beliefs about the body or disease impact the creators of these works?
- How do later works connect with (or break from) earlier ones in terms of approach or concerns?

Chronology is not the only thread weaving the works together, however. No work in the volume stands entirely alone, and it is possible to approach this volume through the pairing of texts. Readers interested in autopathography (a first-person illness narrative) might look to read Margery Kempe, John Donne, and Mary Prince alongside one another. Similarly, ethics, mental health, and narratives of medical discoveries, among others, may be found here. Readers can also consider works by genre, including poetry and many different kinds of prose: letters, lectures, histories, short fiction, academic writing, and more. Considering the range of genres, readers might ask themselves:

- How does the genre or main issue affect the way material is presented by its creator?
- How do different genres impact how a work might be received by its audience (both when it was written, and now)?
- How do works dealing with discoveries and advances in medical science incorporate the human (or humane) experience?

For those readers interested in thematic considerations, this volume contains four themed sections at the end that examine several threads that bind health-oriented texts:

- "Manus Dei: Faith and Medicine" reminds us that the separation of medical science and religious belief is a relatively recent phenomenon by bringing together a collection of works that see the two as bound together.
- "What You See: Assumption, Anxiety, and the Appearance of Health" takes up the problems of tying physical appearance to assumptions about health and behavior, either through things we can see, such as the shape of the head, or things we can't see, at least not with the naked eye, such as the development occurring in the womb.
- "Life in Times of Plague: Depicting the Black Death" focuses on

works composed during the Black Death, or bubonic plague, and offers a brief look into the vast array of works produced in times of epidemic, which often prompt tremendous outpourings of literary and artistic works alongside the attempts to grapple medically with disease.
* "Doing Battle: Health and Medicine on the Front Lines" considers just some of the ways that health-related matters have intersected specifically with the clashes and combat of war.

Note on the Texts

Several editorial choices have been made in order to help make these works accessible to more readers, and in particular to serve as an edition that can be of use for students. This means that the texts are presented with the readers in mind. The intent of the editorial guidance is not to hold their hands, but to enable navigation and spark interest.

This anthology aims to present reliable selections that recreate a moment in their individual history as texts in context. Although the volume relies upon works that are in the public domain, texts are not uncritically reproduced. Where possible, either the earliest reliable edition or a reliable edition reflecting a key moment in the textual history has been chosen.

A brief introduction accompanies each text and situates it in its context, whether historical, literary, scientific, or all three, and texts are supplemented with footnotes. In providing these footnotes, the goal is to provide clarification and context with minimal editorial interpretations. Another goal is to avoid overwhelming the text with notes: an over-explained text can suggest to readers that no further investigation is needed, and glossing every allusion or unfamiliar word robs teachers and students of opportunities for intellectual exercise. It's also, quite simply, exhausting to read a page with more footnote than text.

In general, then, the footnotes take the following forms: in difficult texts, challenging clauses or phrases are glossed or translated; when words have archaic or specialized meanings that wouldn't be immediately noticed in a basic dictionary search, those individual words are glossed;

where reasonable, and with as much brevity as possible, explanation of allusions, context, and other clarifying information are provided.

For texts not originally in English, the anthology either follows a key English translation (as in A. A. Brill's translations of Freud) or another reliable translation, or has been translated for the anthology. For original translations from Middle English, the translation aims to retain as much of the original vocabulary and character as possible while improving readability. For translations from a different language, such as German or Latin, translations aim to be as fluid as possible without loss of original sense and meaning. Titles of translated works are provided in English with the original title following in brackets, when available.

In editing individual texts, the guiding principle is to preserve as much of a work's original character as possible. However, since readability is a goal, individual texts are silently regularized for modern audiences. This means, in particular, that archaic graphemes (letter forms) are converted to their modern counterparts or uses (f to s; v to u; vv to w; i to j), and outdated typography practices (like mixed italic and roman fonts) and orthography (archaic or irregular spellings) are also silently emended. In rare cases, such elements as unexpected line breaks and missing punctuation are adjusted for clarity or to correct obvious errors.

Working Together

This collection challenges the notion that science is objective, the humanities are not, and thus the two are not compatible. As the works included in this book show, they are more than compatible. In fact, they are and have always been inextricably linked. The history of anatomy is tied to art history; science has its roots in philosophy (and for centuries was called natural philosophy); records of diseases and their spread are found widely in history, poetry, and literary prose. The humanities are also a source—perhaps one of the main sources—for understanding the human condition and human experience, in health and in sickness. The long arts of medicine and the humanities, ultimately, work hand in hand.

Selections

Sushruta's Compendium
(*Sushruta Samhita*)*

SUSHRUTA

(Indian, ca. sixth century BCE)

Sushruta Samhita translates literally as "Sushruta's Compendium." It was composed at some point during the sixth century BCE by the Indian physician Sushruta, who was renowned as a physician and is called by some the father of surgery. His compendium is a foundational text of ancient Ayurvedic medicine, one of the oldest systems of health in the world. Ayurveda means "knowledge of life" in Sanskrit and is still widely practiced in its modern form, although Western practitioners have labeled it an alternative medicine. The Ayurvedic system understands health to rely upon a harmonious balance of three Doshas (*vata*, *pitta*, and *kapha*). These Doshas govern the functions, movement, and growth of the body. As you read, consider these excerpts' descriptions of the various branches of Ayurvedic medicine, its theory of disease, and the practices and oaths required of new students.

---

* Reprinted from *An English Translation of* The Sushruta Samhita, *Based on Original Sanskrit Text*, 3 vols. trans. and ed. Kaviraj Kunja Lal Bhishagratna (Calcutta, 1907), 1: 2–5, 10–14, 16–19. Internet Archive.

[On the Origin and Types of Ayurveda]

The Áyurveda (which forms the subject of our present discourse), originally formed one of the subsections of the Atharva Veda;[1] and even before the creation of mankind, the self-begotten Brahmá[2] strung it together into a hundred thousand couplets (Shlokas[3]), divided into a thousand chapters. But then he thought of the small duration of human life on earth, and the failing character of the human memory, and found it prudent to divide the whole of Áyurveda into eight different branches such as, the Salya-Tantram, the Sálákya-Tantram, the Káya-Chikitsá, the Bhuta-Vidyá, the Kaumár-Bhritya, the Agada-Tantram, the Rasáyana-Tantram and the Vájeekarana-Tantram. Now about the characteristic features of each of these branches of the Science of Áyurveda:

The Salya-Tantram[4]—The scope of this branch of the Medical Science is to remove (from an ulcer) any extraneous substance such as, fragments of hay, particles of stone, dust, iron or bone; splinters, nails, hair, clotted blood, or condensed pus (as the case may be), or to draw out of the uterus a dead fetus, or to bring about safe parturitions in cases of false presentation, and to deal with the principle and mode of using and handling surgical instruments in general, and with the application of fire (cautery) and alkaline (caustic) substances, together with the diagnosis and treatment of ulcers. The Shálákya-Tantram[5]—embraces as its object the treatment of those diseases which are restricted to the upward (lit: region above the clavicles) fissures or cavities of the body, such as the ears, the eyes, the cavity of the mouth, the nostrils, etc.

---

1 *Atharva Veda*: One of the four Vedas, which are major books of Hindu scripture, and the one most dedicated to practices of daily life.
2 *Brahmá*: In Hinduism, the creator god.
3 *Shlokas*: Literally, songs; a *shloka* is a traditional verse form in Sanskrit, composed of two lines of sixteen syllables each.
4 *Salya-Tantram*: *Salya* refers to a sharp, painful object; the Salya-Tantram is the practice of removing factors causing pain.
5 *Shalakya-Tantram*: *Shalakya* refers to a small, sharp instrument, such as a needle or a tool, used in surgery; Kaviraj Kunja Lal Bhishagratna, the translator of this edition (the first in English), asserts that the branch is named for the instrument because of its frequent use in treating conditions of the head and neck.

The Káya Chikitsá (General diseases)[6]—treats of diseases, which, instead of being simply restricted to any specific organ, or to any particular part of the body, affect the entire system, as Fever, Dysentery, Hemoptysis,[7] Insanity, Hysteria, Leprosy, unnatural discharges from the urethra, etc.

The Bhuta-Vidyá (Demoniacal diseases)—lays down incantations and modes of exorcising evil spirits and making offerings to the gods, demons, Gandharvas, Yakshas, Rakshas[8], etc. for cures of diseases originating from their malignant influences.

The Kaumára-Bhritya (Management of children)—deals with the nursing and healthy bringing up of infants, with purification and bettering of mothers' milk, found deficient in any of its characteristic traits, and also with cures for diseases peculiar to infant life and due to the use of vitiated mother's milk or to the influences of malignant stars and spirits.

The Agada-Tantram (Toxicology)—deals with bites from snakes, spiders, and venomous worms, and their characteristic symptoms and antidotes. It has also for its object the elimination of poison whether animal, vegetable, or chemical (resulting from incompatible combinations) from the system of a man, overwhelmed with its effects.

The Rasáyana-Tantram (Science of Rejuvenation)—has for its specific object the prolongation of human life, and the invigoration of memory and the vital organs of man. It deals with recipes which enable a man to retain his manhood or youthful vigor up to a good old age, and which generally serve to make the human system invulnerable to disease and decay.

The Vájeekarana-Tantram (Science of Aphrodisiacs)—treats of measures by which the semen of a man naturally scanty or deficient in quality becomes shorn of its defects; or is purified, if deranged by the vitiated humors of the body (such as wind, etc.); or is invigorated and increased in quantity (if pure and healthy); or acquires its healthy and

---

6 *Káya Chikitsá*: Literally, this refers to medical treatments of the body, so it is best understood as generalized medicine.
7 *Hemoptysis*: Coughing up blood.
8 *Gandharvas, Yakshas, Rakshas*: Classes of supernatural entities in Hindu mythology.

normal consistence (if thinned and enfeebled by indiscretions of youth). [In short, it deals with things which increase the pleasures of youth and make a man doubly endearing to a woman].

*

Thus the entire science of Áyurveda is classified into the eight preceding branches. Now tell me, which of them is to be taught and to which of you? Said the disciples:—"Instruct us all, O Lord, in the science of surgery (Shalya) and let that be the chief subject of our study." To which replied the holy Dhanvantari: "Be it so." Then the disciples again said:— "We are all of one mind in the matter, O Lord, that Sushruta shall be our spokesman and ask you questions conformably to the general trend of our purpose. All of us will attentively hear what you will be pleased to discourse to Sushruta, [and that will save you the trouble of teaching us individually]". To which replied the venerable sage—"Be it so. Now listen, Sushruta, my dear child. The object or utility of the science which forms the subject of our present discussion, may be grouped under two distinct sub-heads such as (1) the cure of diseased persons, and (2) the preservation of health in those who are not afflicted with any sort of bodily distempers."

[On the Definition and Nature of Disease]

Disease: Its Definition:—The Purusha (man)[9] is the receptacle of any particular disease, and that which proves a source of torment or pain to him, is denominated as a disease. There are four different types of disease such as, Traumatic or of extraneous origin (Ágantuka), Bodily (Shárira), Mental (Mánasa) and Natural (Svábhávika). A disease due to

---

9   *The Purusha*: The text elsewhere defines this as a "self-conscious organic individual" composed of "the soul and the five primary material principles" [earth, water, fire, air, and sky (or ether)] (9). Translator Bhishagratna further notes that Purusha, so defined, seems to signal that the body rather than the "Self or Ego" (which is, per the translator, "above all human concerns") is thus the purview of Ayurvedic medicine.

an extraneous blow or hurt is called Ágantuka. Diseases due to irregularities in food or drink, or incidental to a deranged state of the blood, or of the bodily humors acting either singly or in concert, are called Shárira. Excessive anger, grief, fear, joy, despondency, envy, misery, pride, greed, lust, desire, malice, etc. are included within the category of mental (Mánasa) distempers; whereas hunger, thirst, decrepitude, imbecility, death, sleep, etc. are called the natural (Svábhávika) derangements of the body. The Mind and the Body are the seats of the abovesaid distempers according as they are restricted to either of them, or affect both of them in unison.

Samshodhanam (Cleansing),[10] and **Samshamanam** (Pacification of the deranged or agitated bodily humors giving rise to the disease), and the regimen of diet and conduct are the four factors which should be duly employed in order to successfully cope with a disease....

Physicians should look upon these four factors of food, conduct, earth and time, as the accumulators, aggravators and pacifiers of the deranged bodily humors and of the disease resulting therefrom in man. Diseases due to causes which are extraneous to the body may affect the mind or the body. When it would affect the body in the shape of any traumatic disease (such as an inflammation due to a blow or sword cut), it should be treated medicinally like the rest of the physical maladies, while the remedy should consist in the enjoyment of pleasurable sounds, touch, sights, taste or smell where the mind would be found to be the seat of the distemper....

The term Purusha should be interpreted to include within its meaning the combination of its five material components, and all things resulting therefrom, such as the limbs and members of the body, as well as the skin, the flesh, the blood, the veins and the nerves, etc. The term Disease signifies all distempers incidental to the several or combined actions of the three deranged bodily humors and blood. The term Medicine signifies drugs and their virtues, tastes, potency, inherent efficacy (Prabháva) and reactionary properties (Vipáka). Appliances

---

10 Translator Bhishagratna notes that this cleansing takes two forms: external (by way of surgical methods or topical treatments) and internal (by way of purgatives like emetics, enemas and bloodletting).

(kriyá) denotes such processes as, surgical operations, injections, emulsive measures, lubrications, etc. The term Time signifies all opportune moments for medical appliances.

[On the Initiation of a Student into Ayurvedic Study]

Now we shall discuss the Chapter which deals with the rites of formal initiation of a pupil into the science of Medicine (Shishyopanayaniya-madhyáyam).

Such an initiation should be imparted to a student, belonging to one of the three twice-born castes such as, the Bráhmana, the Kshatriya, and the Vaishya,[11] and who should be of tender years, born of a good family, possessed of, a desire to learn, strength, energy of action, contentment, character, self-control, a good retentive memory, intellect, courage, purity of mind and body, and a simple and clear comprehension, command a clear insight into the things studied, and should be found to have been further graced with the necessary qualifications of thin lips, thin teeth and thin tongue, and possessed of a straight nose, large, honest, intelligent eyes, with a benign contour of the mouth, and a contented frame of mind, being pleasant in his speech and dealings, and usually painstaking in his efforts. A man possessed of contrary attributes should not be admitted into the sacred precincts of medicine....

Then having thrice circumambulated the sacrificial fire, and having invoked the firegod to bear testimony to the fact, the preceptor should address the initiated disciple as follows:—"Thou shalt renounce lust, anger, greed, ignorance, vanity, egotistic feelings, envy, harshness, niggardliness, falsehood, idleness, nay all acts that soil the good name of a man. In proper season thou shalt pair thy nails and clip thy hair and put on the sacred cloth, dyed brownish yellow, and love the life of a truthful,

---

11 *The Brahmana, the Kshatriya, and the Vaishya*: Hinduism classified society into four Varnas (or castes); The Brahmana was the class of scholars, teachers, and priests; the Kshatriya was the class of leaders and warriors; and the Vaishya was the agricultural class. Left out of medical study entirely were the Shudra (the labor class) and the Avarna, or those outside of the caste system.

self-controlled anchorite and be obedient and respectful towards thy preceptor. In sleep, in rest, or while moving about—while at meals or in study, and in all acts thou shalt be guided by my directions. Thou shalt do what is pleasant and beneficial to me, otherwise thou shalt incur sin and all thy study and knowledge shall fail to bear their wished for fruit, and thou shalt gain no fame. If I, on the other hand, treat thee unjustly even with thy perfect obedience and in full conformity to the terms agreed upon, may I incur equal sin with thee, and may all my knowledge prove futile, and never have any scope or display. Thou shalt help with thy professional skill and knowledge, and Bráhmanas, thy elders, preceptors and friends, the indigent, the honest, the anchorites, the helpless and those who shall come to thee (from a distance), or those who shall live close by, as well as thy relations and kinsmen [to the best of thy knowledge and ability], and thou shalt give them medicine [without charging for it any remuneration whatever], and God will bless thee for that. Thou shalt not treat medicinally a professional hunter, a fowler, a habitual sinner, or him who has been degraded in life; and even by doing so thou shalt acquire friends, fame, piety, wealth and all wished for objects in life and thy knowledge shall gain publicity.

The History of the Peloponnesian War*

THUCYDIDES
(Greek, ca. 460–400 BCE)

The historian Thucydides's *The History of the Peloponnesian War* (ca. 431 BCE) recounts twenty-one of the actual conflict's twenty-eight years (431–404 BCE), and his style has influenced the genre of historical writing ever since. The work discusses the so-called Plague of Athens, which struck the city in 430 BCE and wiped out roughly one-quarter of its inhabitants. Thucydides's work has been praised not just as history but also as medical narrative and as literature. It's unclear the extent to which Thucydides paints a complete picture of the epidemic, for which scholars have never determined a precise cause. As you read, consider his attempt to trace a devastating disease's path and its impact on those in that path.

---

* Reprinted from Thucydides, *The History of the Peloponnesian War*, trans. Richard Crawley (London: Longmans, Green, 1874), chap. 7, 129–34, Internet Classics Archive.

[The Plague at Athens]

In the first days of summer the Lacedaemonians[1] and their allies, with two-thirds of their forces as before, invaded Attica, under the command of Archidamus, son of Zeuxidamus, King of Lacedaemon, and sat down and laid waste the country.[2] Not many days after their arrival in Attica the plague[3] first began to show itself among the Athenians. It was said that it had broken out in many places previously in the neighborhood of Lemnos and elsewhere; but a pestilence of such extent and mortality was nowhere remembered. Neither were the physicians at first of any service, ignorant as they were of the proper way to treat it, but they died themselves the most thickly, as they visited the sick most often; nor did any human art succeed any better. Supplications in the temples, divinations, and so forth were found equally futile, till the overwhelming nature of the disaster at last put a stop to them altogether. It first began, it is said, in the parts of Ethiopia above Egypt, and thence descended into Egypt and Libya and into most of the King's country. Suddenly falling upon Athens, it first attacked the population in Piraeus—which was the occasion of their saying that the Peloponnesians had poisoned the reservoirs, there being as yet no wells there—and afterwards appeared in the upper city, when the deaths became much more frequent. All speculation as to its origin and its causes, if causes can be found adequate to produce so great a disturbance, I leave to other writers, whether lay or professional;[4] for myself, I shall simply set down its nature, and explain the symptoms by which perhaps it may be recognized by the student, if it should ever

---

1   *Lacedaemonians*: Inhabitants of the region of Greece that included the city of Sparta.
2   *Laid waste the country*: A reference to the Peloponnesian War (431–405 BCE), fought between Athens and Sparta.
3   *Plague*: Although most translations use the term "plague," some translators have opted for "less limiting" terms to avoid conclusively linking the epidemic to bubonic plague Helen King and Jo Brown, "Thucydides and the Plague," in *A Handbook to the Reception of Thucydides*, eds. Christin Lee and Neville Morley (Hoboken, NJ: Wiley, 2014), 452.
4   The speculation Thucydides mentions here has yet to be resolved. Although bubonic plague has been considered, a wide range of other causes have also been suggested, including (but not limited to) smallpox, typhus, influenza, and strains of viral hemorrhagic fever.

break out again. This I can the better do, as I had the disease myself, and watched its operation in the case of others. That year then is admitted to have been otherwise unprecedentedly free from sickness; and such few cases as occurred all determined in this. As a rule, however, there was no ostensible cause; but people in good health were all of a sudden attacked by violent heats in the head, and redness and inflammation in the eyes, the inward parts, such as the throat or tongue, becoming bloody and emitting an unnatural and fetid breath. These symptoms were followed by sneezing and hoarseness, after which the pain soon reached the chest, and produced a hard cough. When it fixed in the stomach, it upset it; and discharges of bile of every kind named by physicians ensued, accompanied by very great distress. In most cases also an ineffectual retching followed, producing violent spasms, which in some cases ceased soon after, in others much later. Externally the body was not very hot to the touch, nor pale in its appearance, but reddish, livid, and breaking out into small pustules and ulcers. But internally it burned so that the patient could not bear to have on him clothing or linen even of the very lightest description; or indeed to be otherwise than stark naked. What they would have liked best would have been to throw themselves into cold water; as indeed was done by some of the neglected sick, who plunged into the rain-tanks in their agonies of unquenchable thirst; though it made no difference whether they drank little or much. Besides this, the miserable feeling of not being able to rest or sleep never ceased to torment them. The body meanwhile did not waste away so long as the distemper was at its height, but held out to a marvel against its ravages; so that when they succumbed, as in most cases, on the seventh or eighth day to the internal inflammation, they had still some strength in them. But if they passed this stage, and the disease descended further into the bowels, inducing a violent ulceration there accompanied by severe diarrhea, this brought on a weakness which was generally fatal. For the disorder first settled in the head, ran its course from thence through the whole of the body, and, even where it did not prove mortal, it still left its mark on the extremities; for it settled in the privy parts, the fingers and the toes, and many escaped with the loss of these, some too with that of their eyes. Others again were seized with an entire loss of memory on their first recovery, and did not know either themselves or their friends.

But while the nature of the distemper was such as to baffle all description, and its attacks almost too grievous for human nature to endure, it was still in the following circumstance that its difference from all ordinary disorders was most clearly shown. All the birds and beasts that prey upon human bodies, either abstained from touching them (though there were many lying unburied), or died after tasting them. In proof of this, it was noticed that birds of this kind actually disappeared; they were not about the bodies, or indeed to be seen at all. But of course the effects which I have mentioned could best be studied in a domestic animal like the dog.

Such then, if we pass over the varieties of particular cases which were many and peculiar, were the general features of the distemper. Meanwhile the town enjoyed an immunity from all the ordinary disorders; or if any case occurred, it ended in this. Some died in neglect, others in the midst of every attention. No remedy was found that could be used as a specific; for what did good in one case, did harm in another. Strong and weak constitutions proved equally incapable of resistance, all alike being swept away, although dieted with the utmost precaution. By far the most terrible feature in the malady was the dejection which ensued when any one felt himself sickening, for the despair into which they instantly fell took away their power of resistance, and left them a much easier prey to the disorder; besides which, there was the awful spectacle of men dying like sheep, through having caught the infection in nursing each other. This caused the greatest mortality. On the one hand, if they were afraid to visit each other, they perished from neglect; indeed many houses were emptied of their inmates for want of a nurse: on the other, if they ventured to do so, death was the consequence. This was especially the case with such as made any pretensions to goodness: honor made them unsparing of themselves in their attendance in their friends' houses, where even the members of the family were at last worn out by the moans of the dying, and succumbed to the force of the disaster. Yet it was with those who had recovered from the disease that the sick and the dying found most compassion. These knew what it was from experience, and had now no fear for themselves; for the same man was never attacked twice—never at least fatally. And such persons not only received the congratulations of others, but themselves also, in the elation of the moment, half entertained the vain hope that they were for the future safe from any disease whatsoever.

An aggravation of the existing calamity was the influx from the country into the city, and this was especially felt by the new arrivals. As there were no houses to receive them, they had to be lodged at the hot season of the year in stifling cabins, where the mortality raged without restraint. The bodies of dying men lay one upon another, and half-dead creatures reeled about the streets and gathered round all the fountains in their longing for water. The sacred places also in which they had quartered themselves were full of corpses of persons that had died there, just as they were; for as the disaster passed all bounds, men, not knowing what was to become of them, became utterly careless of everything, whether sacred or profane. All the burial rites before in use were entirely upset, and they buried the bodies as best they could. Many from want of the proper appliances, through so many of their friends having died already, had recourse to the most shameless sepultures:[5] sometimes getting the start of those who had raised a pile, they threw their own dead body upon the stranger's pyre and ignited it; sometimes they tossed the corpse which they were carrying on the top of another that was burning, and so went off. Nor was this the only form of lawless extravagance which owed its origin to the plague. Men now coolly ventured on what they had formerly done in a corner, and not just as they pleased, seeing the rapid transitions produced by persons in prosperity suddenly dying and those who before had nothing succeeding to their property. So they resolved to spend quickly and enjoy themselves, regarding their lives and riches as alike things of a day. Perseverance in what men called honor was popular with none, it was so uncertain whether they would be spared to attain the object; but it was settled that present enjoyment, and all that contributed to it, was both honorable and useful. Fear of gods or law of man there was none to restrain them. As for the first, they judged it to be just the same whether they worshiped them or not, as they saw all alike perishing; and for the last, no one expected to live to

---

5   *Sepultures*: Burials. Thucydides refers here to people failing or refusing to adhere to traditional burial customs, which included careful preparation of the body and either burial or individual cremation.

be brought to trial for his offenses, but each felt that a far severer sentence had been already passed upon them all and hung ever over their heads, and before this fell it was only reasonable to enjoy life a little.

Such was the nature of the calamity, and heavily did it weigh on the Athenians; death raging within the city and devastation without. Among other things which they remembered in their distress was, very naturally, the following verse which the old men said had long ago been uttered:

"A Dorian war shall come and with it death." So a dispute arose as to whether dearth and not death had not been the word in the verse; but at the present juncture, it was of course decided in favor of the latter; for the people made their recollection fit in with their sufferings. I fancy, however, that if another Dorian war should ever afterwards come upon us, and a dearth should happen to accompany it, the verse will probably be read accordingly. The oracle also which had been given to the Lacedaemonians was now remembered by those who knew of it. When the god was asked whether they should go to war, he answered that if they put their might into it, victory would be theirs, and that he would himself be with them. With this oracle events were supposed to tally. For the plague broke out as soon as the Peloponnesians invaded Attica, and never entering Peloponnese (not at least to an extent worth noticing), committed its worst ravages at Athens, and next to Athens, at the most populous of the other towns. Such was the history of the plague.

The Hippocratic Corpus*

VARIOUS AUTHORS
(Greek, compiled ca. fourth century BCE)

Hippocrates of Cos (ca. 460–ca. 375 BCE) was a Greek physician who some now call the father of medicine. His legacy includes a collection of around sixty texts known as the Hippocratic corpus. This collection was written over the course of the fifth and fourth centuries BCE by a range of mostly unidentified authors—the debate about how many Hippocrates wrote himself continues. Below are excerpts from the Corpus. As you read, consider how "The Law" approaches the status of medicine and its requirements for those who wish to study it. In the "The Oath," which has, through various translations and revisions, come down to us as "the Hippocratic oath," consider the ethical foundations being laid. And in "On the Nature of Man,"[1] which is here presented in the form of an epitome, or abstract, rather than a full translation, consider the Hippocratic description of the theory of the four humors, which would come to be a dominant system of medicine in the second century CE and remain influential well into the nineteenth century.

---

1 The author of "On the Nature of Man" has been identified as Polybus, a student and son-in-law of Hippocrates himself.

---

* "The Oath" and "The Law" reprinted from *The genuine works of Hippocrates*, trans. Francis Adams (New York: W. Wood, 1886), 278–80, 283–85. "On the Nature of Man" reprinted from *The Writings of Hippocrates and Galen, Epitomised from the Original Latin Translations,* trans. John Redman Coxe (Philadelphia: Lindsay and Blackiston, 1846), 150–51, 153. Internet Classics Archive.

The Oath

I swear by Apollo the physician, and Aesculapius, and Health, and All-heal,[2] and all the gods and goddesses, that, according to my ability and judgment, I will keep this Oath and this stipulation—to reckon him who taught me this Art equally dear to me as my parents, to share my substance with him, and relieve his necessities if required; to look upon his offspring in the same footing as my own brothers, and to teach them this art, if they shall wish to learn it, without fee or stipulation; and that by precept, lecture, and every other mode of instruction, I will impart a knowledge of the Art to my own sons, and those of my teachers, and to disciples bound by a stipulation and oath according to the law of medicine, but to none others. I will follow that system of regimen which, according to my ability and judgment, I consider for the benefit of my patients, and abstain from whatever is deleterious and mischievous. I will give no deadly medicine to any one if asked, nor suggest any such counsel; and in like manner I will not give to a woman a pessary to produce abortion.[3] With purity and with holiness I will pass my life and practice my Art. I will not cut persons laboring under the stone, but will leave this to be done by men who are practitioners of this work.[4] Into whatever houses I enter, I will go into them for the benefit of the sick, and will abstain from every voluntary act of mischief and corruption; and, further from the seduction of females or males, of freemen and slaves. Whatever, in connection with my professional practice or not, in connection with it,

---

2   *Aesclepius*: The son of Apollo and god of medicine who was the father of five daughters, all associated with medicine. The author mentions Health, or Hygieia (goddess of hygiene) and All-heal, or Panacea (goddess of universal remedy).

3   Hippocrates only forbids one of several known abortion methods. While some legal restrictions on terminating pregnancy existed at the time, the practice was legally allowed and medically condoned. In other texts, Hippocrates offers some approved methods. Hippocrates rejected the use of the pessary—essentially a rigid block infused with herbs and/or chemicals inserted directly into the vagina to induce abortion—because of its potential to cause serious infection in the pregnant woman.

4   For centuries, physicians and surgeons were very different professions, and they had little overlap in training and practice, though they would share some knowledge. Here, the author promises not to perform lithotomy, which is surgery to remove calculi (stones) from kidneys, bladders, or gallbladders.

I see or hear, in the life of men, which ought not to be spoken of abroad, I will not divulge, as reckoning that all such should be kept secret. While I continue to keep this Oath unviolated, may it be granted to me to enjoy life and the practice of the art, respected by all men, in all times! But should I trespass and violate this Oath, may the reverse be my lot!

The Law

Medicine is of all the Arts the most noble; but, not withstanding, owing to the ignorance of those who practice it, and of those who, inconsiderately, form a judgment of them, it is at present far behind all the other arts. Their mistake appears to me to arise principally from this, that in the cities there is no punishment connected with the practice of medicine (and with it alone) except disgrace, and that does not hurt those who are familiar with it. Such persons are like the figures which are introduced in tragedies, for as they have the shape, and dress, and personal appearance of an actor, but are not actors, so also physicians are many in title but very few in reality.

Whoever is to acquire a competent knowledge of medicine, ought to be possessed of the following advantages: a natural disposition; instruction; a favorable position for the study; early tuition; love of labor; leisure. First of all, a natural talent is required; for, when Nature opposes, everything else is in vain; but when Nature leads the way to what is most excellent, instruction in the art takes place, which the student must try to appropriate to himself by reflection, becoming an early pupil in a place well adapted for instruction. He must also bring to the task a love of labor and perseverance, so that the instruction taking root may bring forth proper and abundant fruits.

Instruction in medicine is like the culture of the productions of the earth. For our natural disposition is, as it were, the soil; the tenets of our teacher are, as it were, the seed; instruction in youth is like the planting of the seed in the ground at the proper season; the place where the instruction is communicated is like the food imparted to vegetables by the atmosphere; diligent study is like the cultivation of the fields; and it is time which imparts strength to all things and brings them to maturity.

Having brought all these requisites to the study of medicine, and having acquired a true knowledge of it, we shall thus, in traveling through the cities, be esteemed physicians not only in name but in reality. But inexperience is a bad treasure, and a bad fund to those who possess it, whether in opinion or reality, being devoid of self-reliance and contentedness, and the nurse both of timidity and audacity. For timidity betrays a want of powers, and audacity a want of skill. There are, indeed, two things, knowledge and opinion, of which the one makes its possessor really to know, the other to be ignorant.

Those things which are sacred, are to be imparted only to sacred persons; and it is not lawful to import them to the profane until they have been initiated in the mysteries of the science.

On the Nature of Man

Now the body of man contains blood, pituita, and two kinds of bile—yellow and black;[5] and his nature is such that it is through them that he enjoys health, or suffers from disease. He enjoys the former when each is in due proportion of quantity and force, but especially when properly commingled. Disease takes place if either is in excess or deficient, or if not duly united. For when separate, not only the part in which there is deficiency must be affected, but the part to which it goes being surcharged, will experience pain and uneasiness. When more than a mere superfluity is discharged from the system, the void occasioned thereby is productive of pain; but if this void is caused by the separation of the humors in one part, and being carried by metastasis to another, the pain is twofold, viz.: that induced by the vacuity of the part it leaves, and the repletion of that to which it is conveyed. I have stated that I would show, that those things of which man is composed remain always the same, both from their nature, and their true intent. Now I say that blood, pituita, and yellow and black bile are invariable the same and at all times

---

5   *Pituita*: Typically translated as "phlegm," which would become most common in the English-language discussion of the four humors. Yellow bile is also known as choler, and black bile is known as melancholy.

so considered, since none of those terms are at all equivocal, or liable to any obscurity; and moreover, the things themselves are in their nature entirely distinct—for pituita in no respect resembles blood, nor does blood resemble bile, nor bile pituita....

The human body has, therefore, constantly, all the above humors; but they increase or diminish, each according to the season, as it may be conformable or otherwise to their nature respectively. As, throughout the year, there is always present both heat and cold, dryness and moisture, and as nothing in nature could for an instant exist without their presence; if one alone was wanting, universal destruction would be the result; for the same law that subserved the creation of all things, is equally required for their preservation. It is the same with man; if one of those things that are essential to his constitution, were destroyed, he could not possibly exist.

On the Nature of Things
(*De rerum natura*)*

LUCRETIUS
(Roman, ca. 94–55 BCE)

Titus Lucretius Carus's life is largely a mystery: only one contemporary account of the poet and philosopher exists, in a letter by Cicero.[1] Lucretius's one surviving work written in 50 BCE is a long didactic (educational) poem of Epicurean philosophy and Natural Philosophy, an early term for science. Epicureanism sought happiness through the absence of pain and anxiety, and it offered a detailed theory of knowledge and nature. Lucretius's work takes on some of these concerns, covering theories of physics (including early notions of atoms), the nature of the human soul, and cosmic and natural phenomena. Though popular in its own time, the poem was lost for several centuries. It was rediscovered by Renaissance humanist scholar Poggio Bracciolini in a German monastery in 1417. As you read these excerpts, drawn from William Ellery Leonard's influential 1916 translation, consider the description of the relationship between the body and the mind, as well as the work's understanding of plagues and disease.

1   The most enduring biography of the author, by Jerome, is short, fairly unreliable, and claims that Lucretius was driven mad by a love potion, wrote only during brief moments of lucidity, and eventually committed suicide before completing *On the Nature of Things*.

---

* Reprinted from Lucretius, *De Rerum Natura*, trans. William Ellery Leonard (New York: E. P. Dutton, 1916), 109–12, 293–95. Perseus Digital Library.

Book III

Then, too, we see, that, just as body takes
Monstrous diseases and the dreadful pain,
So mind its bitter cares, the grief, the fear;
Wherefore it tallies that the mind no less
Partaker is of death; for pain and disease
Are both artificers of death,—as well [5]
We've learned by the passing of many a man ere now.[2]
Nay, too, in diseases of body, often the mind
Wanders afield; for 'tis beside itself,
And crazed it speaks, or many a time it sinks,
With eyelids closing and a drooping nod, [10]
In heavy drowse, on to eternal sleep;
From whence nor hears it any voices more,
Nor able is to know the faces here
Of those about him standing with wet cheeks
Who vainly call him back to light and life. [15]
Wherefore mind too, confess we must, dissolves,
Seeing, indeed, contagions of disease
Enter into the same....
And, since we mark the mind itself is cured,
Like the sick body, and restored can be [20]
By medicine, this is forewarning to
That mortal lives the mind. For proper it is
That whosoe'er begins and undertakes
To alter the mind, or meditates to change
Any another nature soever, should add [25]
New parts, or readjust the order given,
Or from the sum remove at least a bit.
But what's immortal willeth for itself
Its parts be nor increased, nor rearranged,

---

2 Lucretius argues, in book III, that the human mind and spirit are composed of physical matter, like the body, and that they are therefore also mortal and subject to the experience of sickness (like the body). In this excerpt, he explores this idea.

Nor any bit soever flow away: [30]
For change of anything from out its bounds
Means instant death of that which was before.
Ergo, the mind, whether in sickness fallen,
Or by the medicine restored, gives signs,
As I have taught, of its mortality. [35]
So surely will a fact of truth make head
'Gainst errors' theories all, and so shut off
All refuge from the adversary, and rout
Error by two-edged confutation.
And since the mind is of a man one part, [40]
Which in one fixed place remains, like ears,
And eyes, and every sense which pilots life;
And just as hand, or eye, or nose, apart,
Severed from us, can neither feel nor be,
But in the least of time is left to rot, [45]
Thus mind alone can never be, without
The body and the man himself, which seems,
As 'twere the vessel of the same—or aught
Whate'er thou'lt feign as yet more closely joined:
Since body cleaves to mind by surest bonds. [50]
Again, the body's and the mind's live powers
Only in union prosper and enjoy;
For neither can nature of mind, alone of itself
Sans body, give the vital motions forth;
Nor, then, can body, wanting soul, endure [55]
And use the senses.

Book VI

Now, of diseases what the law, and whence
The Influence of bane upgathering can
Upon the race of man and herds of cattle
Kindle a devastation fraught with death,

I will unfold.[3] And, first, I've taught above [5]
That seeds there be of many things to us
Life-giving, and that, contrariwise, there must
Fly many round bringing disease and death.[4]
When these have, haply, chanced to collect
And to derange the atmosphere of earth, [10]
The air becometh baneful. And, lo, all
That Influence of bane, that pestilence,
Or from Beyond down through our atmosphere,
Like clouds and mists, descends, or else collects
From earth herself and rises, when, a-soak [15]
And beat by rains unseasonable and suns,
Our earth hath then contracted stench and rot.[5]
Seest thou not, also, that whoso arrive
In region far from fatherland and home
Are by the strangeness of the clime and waters [20]
Distempered?—since conditions vary much.
For in what else may we suppose the clime
Among the Britons to differ from Egypt's own
(Where totters awry the axis of the world),[6]
Or in what else to differ Pontic clime [25]

---

3   The final part of this poem takes on the Athenian plague of 431 BCE. Lucretius's description is based entirely on the account provided by the historian Thucydides; see "The Plague at Athens," pp. 20–25). This excerpt immediately precedes that description, and offers Lucretius' theory of the nature and spread of disease.

4   *That seeds there be of many things*: Lucretius follows the philosophical theory of atomism, which held that the universe is composed of "atoms" (a Greek word meaning "uncuttable"). Unlike our modern understanding of atoms, these came in many shapes and sizes, bounced around (non-atom space was the "void"), and clustered and combined to make the substances that form our world. Lucretius never uses the Greek term "atom" in his work—here, the reference is to the "seeds" of things.

5   Lucretius describes the theory of miasma, which held that "bad" or foul-smelling air—such as from rotting vegetation or bodies, excrement, or molds—caused disease, and spread those diseases through poisonous mists and vapors. This model was a major epidemiological theory until well into the nineteenth century, when the germ theory of disease became dominant.

6   *Where totters awry the axis of the world*: Possibly a reference to axial precession, in which the axis of the earth rotates in a full circuit every 26,000 years (and "totters").

From Gades'[7] and from climes adown the south,
On to black generations of strong men
With sun-baked skins? Even as we thus do see
Four climes diverse under the four main-winds
And under the four main-regions of the sky, [30]
So, too, are seen the color and face of men
Vastly to disagree, and fixed diseases
To seize the generations, kind by kind:
There is the elephant-disease[8] which down
In midmost Egypt, hard by streams of Nile, [35]
Engendered is—and never otherwhere.
In Attica the feet are oft attacked,[9]
And in Achaean lands the eyes.[10] And so
The divers spots to divers parts and limbs
Are noxious; 'tis a variable air [40]
That causes this.[11] Thus when an atmosphere,
Alien by chance to us, begins to heave,
And noxious airs begin to crawl along,
They creep and wind like unto mist and cloud,
Slowly, and everything upon their way [45]
They disarrange and force to change its state.
It happens, too, that when they've come at last
Into this atmosphere of ours, they taint
And make it like themselves and alien.
Therefore, asudden this devastation strange, [50]
This pestilence, upon the waters falls,

---

7   *Gades*: Modern-day Cádiz, in southwestern Spain.
8   *The elephant-disease*: Probably elephantiasis, or the swelling and hardening of body parts (caused by a range of factors); here, thought to be endemic to Egypt. However, some translators render this as "leprosy."
9   *In Attica the feet are oft attacked*: A reference to gout, which Lucretius says is especially common in central Greece. Attica is the region that contains Athens.
10 *And in Achaean lands the eyes*: The line leaves off that the eyes "are oft attacked." Poor eyesight was common in Western Greece.
11 *'Tis a variable air that causes this*: Illnesses may be caused by different climates and this makes people more susceptible to the diseases of unfamiliar climates.

Or settles on the very crops of grain
Or other meat of men and feed of flocks.
Or it remains a subtle force, suspense
In the atmosphere itself; and when therefrom [55]
We draw our inhalations of mixed air,
Into our body equally its bane
Also we must suck in. In manner like,
Oft comes the pestilence upon the kine,[12]
And sickness, too, upon the sluggish sheep. [60]
Nor aught it matters whether journey we
To regions adverse to ourselves and change
The atmospheric cloak, or whether Nature
Herself import a tainted atmosphere
To us or something strange to our own use [65]
Which can attack us soon as ever it come.

---

12 *Kine*: Cattle.

Letters to Lucilius on Sickness and Death*

SENECA
(Roman, ca. 4 BCE–65 CE)

> Lucius Annaeus Seneca, or Seneca the Younger, was a Roman philosopher and playwright whose philosophical works were especially influential from the Middle Ages through the eighteenth century. Seneca's work was important to the Stoics, who sought happiness (as many philosophies do) by means of wisdom—and in particular, the wisdom to recognize what we can and cannot control. The goal, then, was to use reason (something possessed only by adult humans, according to the Stoics) to overcome passions and fears. In the two letters here, written around 65 CE, Seneca uses the epistolary (letter-writing) form. He writes to his friend, the Roman official Lucilius, though the letters were also written for a broader audience. As you read, consider the Stoic principles Seneca describes related to illness and our inevitable mortality.

---

* Reprinted from Seneca, *Ad Lucilium Epistulae Morales*, trans. Richard M. Gummere (London: Heinemann, 1917), 360–64, 424–27. Internet Archive.

Letter 54. On Asthma and Death

My ill-health had allowed me a long furlough, when suddenly it resumed the attack. "What kind of ill-health?" you say.¹ And you surely have a right to ask; for it is true that no kind is unknown to me. But I have been consigned, so to speak, to one special ailment. I do not know why I should call it by its Greek name; for it is well enough described as "shortness of breath."² Its attack is of very brief duration, like that of a squall at sea; it usually ends within an hour. Who indeed could breathe his last for long? I have passed through all the ills and dangers of the flesh; but nothing seems to me more troublesome than this. And naturally so; for anything else may be called illness; but this is a sort of continued "last gasp." Hence physicians call it "practicing how to die." For some day the breath will succeed in doing what it has so often essayed. Do you think I am writing this letter in a merry spirit, just because I have escaped? It would be absurd to take delight in such supposed restoration to health, as it would be for a defendant to imagine that he had won his case when he had succeeded in postponing his trial. Yet in the midst of my difficult breathing I never ceased to rest secure in cheerful and brave thoughts.³

"What?" I say to myself; "does death so often test me? Let it do so; I myself have for a long time tested death." "When?" you ask. Before I was born. Death is non-existence, and I know already what that means. What was before me will happen again after me. If there is any suffering in this state, there must have been such suffering also in the past,

---

1   The "you" to whom Seneca addresses the letters is, ostensibly, his friend Lucilius, a government official in Sicily during the reign of Nero (54–68 CE). It is not known whether he ever actually sent the letters, or whether they were exclusively written for the purpose of public circulation. Scholars seem to agree that Seneca did intend them to be presented to the public eventually.
2   *It is well enough described as "shortness of breath"*: Asthma is the Greek name Seneca doesn't want to use.
3   One important principle of Stoicism is that a person should endeavor to be "apathetic"—not in our modern sense of not caring—but rather to be free from the excessive influence of the *pathē* (the emotions, and particularly fear and desire). By avoiding being manipulated by passionate responses, the Stoic could achieve contentment (and even joy).

before we entered the light of day. As a matter of fact, however, we felt no discomfort then. And I ask you, would you not say that one was the greatest of fools who believed that a lamp was worse off when it was extinguished than before it was lighted? We mortals also are lighted and extinguished; the period of suffering comes in between, but on either side there is a deep peace. For, unless I am very much mistaken, my dear Lucilius, we go astray in thinking that death only follows, when in reality it has both preceded us and will in turn follow us. Whatever condition existed before our birth, is death. For what does it matter whether you do not begin at all, or whether you leave off, inasmuch as the result of both these states is non-existence?

I have never ceased to encourage myself with cheering counsels of this kind, silently, of course, since I had not the power to speak; then little by little this shortness of breath, already reduced to a sort of panting, came on at greater intervals, and then slowed down and finally stopped. Even by this time, although the gasping has ceased, the breath does not come and go normally; I still feel a sort of hesitation and delay in breathing. Let it be as it pleases, provided there be no sigh from the soul.[4] Accept this assurance from me: I shall never be frightened when the last hour comes; I am already prepared and do not plan a whole day ahead. But do you praise and imitate the man whom it does not irk to die,[5] though he takes pleasure in living. For what virtue is there in going away when you are thrust out? And yet there is virtue even in this: I am indeed thrust out, but it is as if I were going away willingly. For that reason the wise man can never be thrust out, because that would mean removal from a place which he was unwilling to leave; and the wise man does nothing unwillingly. He escapes necessity, because he wills to do what necessity is about to force upon him. Farewell.

---

4 *Let it be as it pleases, provided there be no sigh from the soul*: That is, let his breath hesitate because of asthma, not fear.
5 *The man whom it does not irk to die*: Reserve praise for the person who does not fear death even though they enjoy life.

Letter 61. On Meeting Death Cheerfully

Let us cease to desire that which we have been desiring. I, at least, am doing this: in my old age I have ceased to desire what I desired when a boy. To this single end my days and my nights are passed; this is my task, this the object of my thoughts,—to put an end to my chronic ills. I am endeavoring to live every day as if it were a complete life. I do not indeed snatch it up as if it were my last; I do regard it, however, as if it might even be my last. The present letter is written to you with this in mind,—as if death were about to call me away in the very act of writing. I am ready to depart, and I shall enjoy life just because I am not over anxious as to the future date of my departure.

Before I became old I tried to live well; now that I am old, I shall try to die well; but dying well means dying gladly. See to it that you never do anything unwillingly. That which is bound to be a necessity if you rebel, is not a necessity if you desire it. This is what I mean: he who takes his orders gladly, escapes the bitterest part of slavery,—doing what one does not want to do. The man who does something under orders is not unhappy; he is unhappy who does something against his will. Let us therefore so set our minds in order that we may desire whatever is demanded of us by circumstances, and above all that we may reflect upon our end without sadness. We must make ready for death before we make ready for life. Life is well enough furnished, but we are too greedy with regard to its furnishings; something always seems to us lacking, and will always seem lacking. To have lived long enough depends neither upon our years nor upon our days, but upon our minds. I have lived, my dear friend Lucilius, long enough. I have had my fill; I await death. Farewell.

On the Natural Faculties
(*De naturalibus facultatibus*)*

GALEN

(Greek, ca. 129–200 CE)

Some scholars estimate that nearly ten percent of all Greek literature still surviving was written during the second century CE by Galen of Pergamon, a physician whose medical theories are some of the most influential in Western society. Galenism was a dominant medical system for centuries, and continued to influence medicine into the nineteenth century. Among his many contributions, Galen's commentaries on Hippocrates (see pp. 26–30) seem to have cemented the theory of the four humors, which in turn became a key concept of Galenism. Included is an excerpt framed as a challenge to a major physician and his followers who did not adhere to humoral theories. As you read, consider his argument for the existence of the four humors and their importance for diagnostics and treatment.

---

* Reprinted from Galen, *On the Natural Faculties,* trans. Arthur John Brock (New York: G. P. Putnam's Sons, 1916; Project Gutenberg, 2013), bk. 2, chap. 9, 196–208.

[A Defense of the Four Humors]

Bodies act upon and are acted upon by each other in virtue of the Warm, Cold, Moist and Dry. And if one is speaking of any activity, whether it be exercised by vein, liver, arteries, heart, alimentary canal, or any part, one will be inevitably compelled to acknowledge that this activity depends upon the way in which the four qualities are blended.[1] Thus I should like to ask the Erasistrateans[2] why it is that the stomach contracts upon the food, and why the veins generate blood. There is no use in recognizing the mere fact of contraction, without also knowing the *cause*; if we know this, we shall also be able to rectify the failures of function. "This is no concern of ours," they say; "we do not occupy ourselves with such causes as these; they are outside the sphere of the *practitioner*, and belong to that of the *scientific investigator*." Are you, then, going to oppose those who maintain that the cause of the function of every organ is a natural eucrasia, that the dyscrasia[3] is itself known as a *disease*, and that it is certainly by this that the activity becomes impaired? Or, on the other hand, will you be convinced by the proofs which the ancient writers furnished? Or will you take a midway course between these two, neither perforce accepting these arguments as true nor contradicting them as false, but suddenly becoming skeptics—Pyrrhonists, in fact?[4] But if you do this you will have to shelter yourselves behind the Empiricist

---

1   The theory of the four humors is based around the notion (rooted in ancient Greek philosophy, like that of Empedocles and Plato) that physical matter is composed of the four elements of fire, air, water, and earth, with respective qualities of warmth, coldness, moistness, and dryness. For Galen, the humors represent these qualities in the human body, which exist in a balance.
2   *Erasistrateans*: Followers of Erasistratus, one of the most prominent physicians in Hellenistic Greece. Particularly important for his contributions to anatomy and physiology, Erasistratus was among those who did not ascribe to the humoral theories of Hippocrates that Galen works to cement—as such, Galen takes direct aim at Erasistratus throughout this work.
3   *Eucrasia*: Greek for "good mixture" or "balance" leading to the state of health; *Dyscrasia*: Greek for "bad mixture" or "imbalance" leading to disease.
4   *Pyrrhonists*: Followers of Pyrrho of Elis (ca. 360–270 BCE), founder of the ancient philosophical school of skepticism, which sought wisdom through the suspension of judgment and refraining from statements of certain knowledge.

teaching.[5] For how are you going to be successful in treatment, if you do not understand the real essence of each disease?[6] Why, then, did you not call yourselves Empiricists from the beginning? Why do you confuse us by announcing that you are investigating natural activities with a view to treatment? If the stomach is, in a particular case, unable to exercise its peristaltic and grinding functions, how are we going to bring it back to the normal if we do not know the *cause* of its disability? What I say is that we must cool the over-heated stomach and warm the chilled one; so also we must moisten the one which has become dried up, and conversely; so, too, in combinations of these conditions; if the stomach becomes at the same time warmer and drier than normally, the first principle of treatment is at once to chill and moisten it; and if it become colder and moister, it must be warmed and dried; so also in other cases.[7] But how on earth are the followers of Erasistratus going to act, confessing as they do that they make no sort of investigation into the cause of disease? For the fruit of the inquiry into activities is that by knowing the causes of the dyscrasiae one may bring them back to the normal, since it is of no use for the purposes of treatment merely to know what the activity of each organ is.

Now, it seems to me that Erasistratus is unaware of this fact also, that the actual disease is that condition of the body which, not accidentally, but primarily and of itself, impairs the normal function. How, then, is he going to diagnose or cure diseases if he is entirely ignorant of what they are, and of what kind and number? As regards the stomach, certainly, Erasistratus held that one should at least investigate *how* it digests the food. But why was not investigation also made as to the primary

---

5   *Empiricist*: A person who believes in the philosophy of empiricism, the idea that human knowledge can only be gathered through sensory experience. Galen, for his part, believes that the practice of medicine—and knowledge about diseases—requires both experience and reason.
6   Erasistratus believed that diseases should be treated based on symptoms—that is, no matter the cause of an illness, if it shares symptoms with another condition a similar treatment will work.
7   The idea here is that opposites cure opposites by restoring balance and harmony. This is sometimes referred to as the theory of contraries or the theory of opposites. Compare this to the theory of similars, which holds that "like cures like."

originative cause of this? And, as regards the veins and the blood, he omitted even to ask the question "*how?*"

Yet neither Hippocrates nor any of the other physicians or philosophers whom I mentioned a short while ago thought it right to omit this; they say that when the heat which exists naturally in every animal is well blended and moderately moist it generates blood; for this reason they also say that the blood is a *virtually* warm and moist humor, and similarly also that yellow bile[8] is warm and dry, even though for the most part it appears moist. (For in them the *apparently* dry would seem to differ from the *virtually* dry.) Who does not know that brine and sea-water preserve meat and keep it uncorrupted, whilst all other water—the drinkable kind—readily spoils and rots it? And who does not know that when yellow bile is contained in large quantity in the stomach, we are troubled with an unquenchable thirst, and that when we vomit this up, we at once become much freer from thirst than if we had drunk very large quantities of fluid? Therefore this humor has been very properly termed warm, and also virtually dry. And, similarly, *phlegm* has been called cold and moist; for about this also clear proofs have been given by Hippocrates and the other Ancients.

Prodicus also, when in his book "On the Nature of Man" he gives the name "phlegm" (from the verb πεφλέχθαι) to that element in the humors which has been burned or, as it were, over-roasted, while using a different terminology, still keeps to the fact just as the others do;[9] this man's innovations in nomenclature have also been amply done justice to by Plato. Thus, the white-colored substance which everyone else calls *phlegm*, and which Prodicus calls *blenna* [mucus], is the well-known cold, moist humor which collects mostly in old people and in those who have been chilled in some way, and not even a lunatic could say that this was anything else than cold and moist.

If, then, there is a warm and moist humor, and another which is

---

8   *Yellow bile*: Also known as choler.
9   Here Galen refers to Prodicus of Ceos (ca. 465–395 BCE), a Greek philosopher and contemporary of Plato, who was well known for being overly particular in his definitions of terms; Prodicus used the term Πεφλέχθαι (*pephlekthai*), meaning "to have been burnt," as an etymology for "phlegm," to help define it specifically as a humor that has been overheated.

warm and dry, and yet another which is moist and cold,[10] is there none which is virtually *cold and dry*? Is the fourth combination of temperaments, which exists in all other things, non-existent in the humors alone? No; the *black bile*[11] is such a humor. This, according to intelligent physicians and philosophers, tends to be in excess, as regards seasons, mainly in the fall of the year, and, as regards ages, mainly after the prime of life.[12] And, similarly, also they say that there are cold and dry modes of life, regions, constitutions, and diseases. Nature, they suppose, is not defective in this single combination like the three other combinations, it extends everywhere.

At this point, also, I would gladly have been able to ask Erasistratus whether his "artistic" Nature[13] has not constructed any organ for *clearing away* a humor such as this. For whilst there are two organs for the excretion of urine, and another of considerable size for that of yellow bile, does the humor which is more pernicious than these wander about persistently in the veins mingled with the blood? Yet Hippocrates says, "Dysentery is a fatal condition if it proceeds from black bile"; while that proceeding from yellow bile is by no means deadly, and most people recover from it; this proves how much more pernicious and acrid in its potentialities is black than yellow bile. Has Erasistratus, then, not read the book, "On the Nature of Man," any more than any of the rest of Hippocrates's writings, that he so carelessly passes over the consideration of the humors? Or, does he know it, and yet voluntarily neglect one of the finest studies in medicine? Thus he ought not to have said anything about the *spleen*, nor have stultified himself by holding that an artistic Nature would have prepared so large an organ for no purpose. As a matter of fact, not only Hippocrates and Plato—who are no less

---

10 This refers to blood, yellow bile (or choler), and phlegm, respectively.
11 *Black bile*: Also known as melancholy.
12 In addition to having the combined qualities (of warm/cold/moist/dry) that linked to elements, the humors were also understood to be tied to seasons of the year and stages of human life. A humor would be more likely to exceed its ideal quantity in the season or stage with which it was linked.
13 Elsewhere, Galen tells us that Erasistratus believed that Nature took an active hand in designing, like an artist, and "at the beginning, well and truly shaped and disposed all the parts of the animal" (bk. II, chap. 3).

authorities on Nature than is Erasistratus—say that this viscus also is one of those which cleanse the blood, but there are thousands of the ancient physicians and philosophers as well who are in agreement with them. Now, all of these the high and mighty Erasistratus affected to despise, and he neither contradicted them nor even so much as mentioned their opinion. Hippocrates, indeed, says that the spleen wastes in those people in whom the body is in good condition, and all those physicians also who base themselves on experience agree with this. Again, in those cases in which the spleen is large and is increasing from internal suppuration, it destroys the body and fills it with evil humors; this again is agreed on, not only by Hippocrates, but also by Plato and many others, including the Empiric physicians. And the jaundice which occurs when the spleen is out of order is darker in color, and the cicatrices of ulcers are dark. For, generally speaking, when the spleen is drawing the atrabiliary humor[14] into itself to a less degree than is proper, the blood is unpurified, and the whole body takes on a bad color. And when does it draw this in to a less degree than proper? Obviously, when it [the spleen] is in a bad condition. Thus, just as the kidneys, whose function it is to attract the urine, do this badly when they are out of order, so also the spleen, which has in itself a native power of attracting an atrabiliary quality, if it ever happens to be weak, must necessarily exercise this attraction badly, with the result that the blood becomes thicker and darker.

Now all these points, affording as they do the greatest help in the diagnosis and in the cure of disease were entirely passed over by Erasistratus, and he pretended to despise these great men—he who does not despise ordinary people, but always jealously attacks the most absurd doctrines. Hence, it was clearly because he had nothing to say against the statements made by the ancients regarding the function and utility of the spleen, and also because he could discover nothing new himself, that he ended by saying nothing at all.

---

14 *The atrabiliary humor*: Black bile (melancholy).

A Treatise of the Small-Pox and Measles
(*Kitab al-Judari wa al-Hasbah*)*

RHAZES [ABŪ BAKR MUHAMMAD IBN ZAKARĪYĀ RĀZĪ]
(Iranian, 865–ca. 925 CE)

Born in the second half of the ninth century in Iran, physician and alchemist Abū Bakr Muhammad ibn Zakarīyā Rāzī (later latinized as "Rhazes"), is among the most prolific and influential medieval practitioners and scientists. His work ranges widely, and includes alchemy (the precursor to modern chemistry and pharmacology), surgery, nutrition, medical philosophy and ethics, and the epidemiology, diagnosis, and treatment of diseases. His body of work contains advances in obstetrics, pediatrics, and ophthalmology—among many other contributions. This excerpt from yet another of his critical works is the earliest comprehensive study of smallpox and measles, epidemics which ravaged the world until the introduction of effective vaccines in the twentieth century. As you read, consider his approach to describing smallpox and its treatment.

* Reprinted from Abū Bakr Muhammad ibn Zakarīyā Rāzī, *A Treatise on the Small-Pox and Measles,* trans. William Alexander Greenhill (London: Sydenham Society, 1848), 27–33, 37–40, 44–46, Wellcome Collection.

Chapter I

Of the causes of the Small-Pox; how it comes to pass that hardly any one escapes the disease; and the sum of what Galen says concerning it.

...As to the moderns, although they have certainly made some mention of the treatment of the Small-Pox, (but without much accuracy and distinctness,) yet there is not one of them who has mentioned the cause of the existence of the disease, and how it comes to pass that hardly anyone escapes it, or who has disposed the modes of treatment in their right places. And for this reason we hope that the reward of that man who encouraged us to compose this treatise, and also our own, will be doubled, since we have mentioned whatever is necessary for the treatment of this disease, and have arranged and carefully disposed every thing in its right place, by God's permission.

We will now begin therefore by mentioning the efficient cause of this distemper,[1] and why hardly any one escapes it; and then we will treat of the other things that relate to it, section by section: and we will (with God's assistance,) speak on every one of these points with what we consider to be sufficient copiousness.

I say then that every man, from the time of his birth till he arrives at old age, is continually tending to dryness; and for this reason the blood of children and infants is much moister than the blood of young men, and still more so than that of old men.[2] And besides this it is much hotter; as Galen testifies in his Commentary on the "Aphorisms," in which he says that "the heat of children is greater in quantity than the heat of young men, and the heat of young men is more intense in quality." And this also is evident from the force with which the natural processes,

---

1 *The efficient cause of this distemper*: According to the Greek philosopher Aristotle, the "efficient cause" is the source of a thing or of a change to it (such as a parent to a child). So here, Rhazes is seeking the etiology, or origin, of smallpox.
2 Humoral theory holds that the four humors are each composed of a combination of qualities (moist or dry and cold or hot). These would occur in a particular balance in each individual, and that balance could shift over the seasons and stages of life. Here Rhazes notes that older people tend towards excesses of melancholy (or black bile), which is dry and cold.

such as digestion and growth of body, are carried on in children. For this reason the blood of infants and children may be compared to must,[3] in which the coction[4] leading to perfect ripeness has not yet begun, nor the movement towards fermentation taken place; the blood of young men may be compared to must, which has already fermented and made a hissing noise, and has thrown out abundant vapors and its superfluous parts, like wine which is now still and quiet and arrived at its full strength; and as to the blood of old men, it may be compared to wine which has now lost its strength and is beginning to grow vapid and sour.

Now the Small-Pox arises when the blood putrefies and ferments, so that the superfluous vapors are thrown out of it, and it is changed from the blood of infants, which is like must, into the blood of young men, which is like wine perfectly ripened: and the Small-Pox itself may be compared to the fermentation and the hissing noise which take place in must at that time. And this is the reason why children, especially males,[5] rarely escape being seized with this disease, because is it impossible to prevent the blood's changing from this state into its second state, just as it is impossible to prevent must (whose nature is to make a hissing noise and to ferment,) from changing into the state which happens to it after its making a hissing noise and its fermentation. And the temperament of an infant or child is seldom such that it is possible for its blood to be changed from the first state into the second by little and little, and orderly, and slowly, so that this fermentation and hissing noise should not show itself in the blood: for a temperament, to change thus gradually, should be cold and dry; whereas that of children is just the contrary, as is also their diet, seeing that the food of infants consists of milk; and as for children, although their food does not consist of milk, yet it is nearer to it than is that of other ages; there is also a greater mixture in their food, and more movement after it; for which reason it is seldom that a child escapes this disease. Then afterwards alterations take place

---

3   *Must*: Freshly crushed fruit that is fermented and eventually strained for the production of wine.
4   *Coction*: Heating or boiling.
5   *Especially males*: Humoral theory held that male bodies were naturally hotter and more dry, whereas female bodies were naturally colder and more moist.

in their condition according to their temperaments, regimen, and natural disposition, the air that surrounds them, and the state of the vascular system both as to quantity and quality, for in some individuals the blood flows quickly, in others slowly, in some it is abundant, in others deficient, in some it is very bad in quality, in others less deteriorated.

As to young men, whereas their blood is already passed into the second state, its maturation is established, and the superfluous particles of moisture which necessarily cause putrefaction are now exhaled; hence it follows that this disease only happens to a few individuals among them, that is, to those whose vascular system abounds with too much moisture, or is corrupt in quality with a violent inflammation; or who in their childhood have had the Chicken-Pox,[6] whereby the transition of the blood from the first into the second state has not been perfected. It takes place also in those who have a slight heat, or whose moisture is not copious; and to those who had Chicken-Pox in their childhood, and are of a dry, lean habit of body, with slight and gentle heat; and who when they become young men, used a diet to strengthen and fatten their body, or a diet which corrupted their blood.

And as for old men, the Small-Pox seldom happens to them, except in pestilential, putrid, and malignant constitutions of the air, in which this disease is chiefly prevalent.[7] For a putrid air, which has an undue proportion of heat and moisture, and also an inflamed air, promotes the eruption of this disease, by converting the spirit and the two ventricles of the heart to its own temperament, and then by means of the heart converting the whole of the blood in the arteries into a state of corruption like itself.

---

6   The translator, Greenhill, tells us this means literally a "light (or mild) Small-Pox" in the Greek translation.
7   This is a reference to the theory of miasma, which held that "bad air," such as that emanating from rotting matter, spread disease.

Chapter II

A specification of those habits of body which are most disposed to the Small-Pox; and of the seasons in which these habits of body mostly abound.

The bodies most disposed to the Small-Pox are in general such as are moist, pale, and fleshy; the well-colored also, and ruddy, as likewise the swarthy when they are loaded with flesh; those who are frequently attacked by acute and continued fevers, bleeding at the nose, inflammation of the eyes, and white and red pustules, and vesicles; those that are very fond of sweet things, especially, dates, honey, figs, and grapes, and all those kinds of sweets in which there is a thick and dense substance, as thick gruel, and honey-cakes, or a great quantity of wine and milk.

Bodies that are lean, bilious, hot, and dry, are more disposed to the Measles than to the Small-Pox; and if they are seized with the Small-Pox, the pustules are necessarily either few in number, distinct, and favorable, or, on the contrary, very bad, numerous, sterile, and dry, with putrefaction, and no maturation.

Lastly, those bodies that are lean and dry, and of a cold temperament are neither disposed to the Small-Pox nor to the Measles; and if they are seized with the Small-Pox, the pustules are few, favorable, moderate, mild, without danger, and with a moderate light fever from first to last, because such constitutions extinguish the disease.

I am now to mention the seasons of the year in which the Small-Pox is most prevalent; which are, the latter end of the autumn, and the beginning of the spring; and when in the summer there are great and frequent rains with continued south winds, and when the winter is warm, and the winds southerly.

When the summer is excessively hot and dry, and the autumn is also hot and dry, and the rains come on very late, then the Measles quickly seize those who are disposed to them; that is, those who are of a hot, lean, and bilious habit of body.

But all these things admit of great differences by reason of the diversity of countries and dwellings, and occult dispositions in the air, which necessarily cause these diseases, and predispose bodies to them; so that they happen in other seasons besides these. And there it is necessary to use great diligence in the preservation from them, as soon as you see them begin to prevail among the people; as I shall mention in the sequel.

Chapter V

On the preservation from the Small-Pox before the appearance of the disease, and the way to hinder the multiplying of the pustules after their appearance.

It is necessary that blood should be taken from children, youths, and young men who have never had the Small-Pox, or have had only the Chicken-Pox, (especially if the state of the air, and the season, and the temperament of the individuals be such as we have mentioned above,) before they are seized with a fever, and the symptoms of the Small-Pox appear in them. A vein may be opened in those who have reached the age of fourteen years; and cupping-glasses must be applied to those who are younger; and their bed-rooms must be kept cool.[8]

Let their food be such as extinguishes heat; soup of yellow lentils, broth seasoned with the juice of unripe grapes, acid minced meat, kid's-foot jelly, the strained liquor of *sicbáj*,[9] veal broth, broth made of woodcocks, hens, and pheasants, and the flesh of these birds minced and dressed with the juice of unripe grapes. Their drink should be water cooled with snow, or pure spring water cold, with which their dwellings may also be sprinkled. Let them frequently eat acid pomegranates, and suck the inspissated juices[10] of acid and styptic fruits, as of pomegranates, warted-leaved rhubarb, acid juice of citrons, juice of unripe grapes, Syrian white mulberries, and the like. Where the temperament is hot,

---

8   Bloodletting was a common treatment, thought to help remove excess humors from the body. Precise instructions regarding the practice included restrictions based on age, pregnancy, strength and weakness, and seasonal changes.

9   *Sicbaj*: According to the translator, this consisted of different kinds of minced flesh-meat, dressed with vinegar and honey, or with acid syrup, to which were sometimes added raisins, a few figs, and chiches (chick-peas).

10 *Inspissated*: Thickened or congealed.

and there is much inflammation, the patient may take in the morning barley water carefully prepared, to which is added a fourth part of acid pomegranate juice. But if the heat be less, barley gruel and sugar may be given in the morning, and vinegar, lentils, and especially juice of unripe grapes, may be added to the food; for by means of these you will be able to thicken and cool the blood, so as to prevent the eruption breaking out. This regimen is of great service in all times of pestilence, for it diminishes the malignity of pestilential ulcers, and boils, and prevents pleurisies, quinsies,[11] and in general all distempers arising from yellow bile and from blood.

In the middle of the day let the patient wash himself in cold water, and go into it, and swim about in it. He should abstain from new milk, wine, dates, honey, and in general from sweet things; and dishes made by a mixture of flesh, onions, oil, butter, and cheese; from lamb, beef, locusts, young birds, high-seasoned things, and hot seeds. When the season is pestilential and malignant, or the temperament is hot and moist and liable to putrefaction, or hot and dry and liable to inflammation, together with this regimen the patient must take remedies which we are about to describe. To those who are of a hot, dry, inflammable temperament give those garden herbs which are cooling, moist, and extinguish heat, such as purslain, Jew's mallow, strawberry blite, and also gourds, serpent cucumbers, cucumbers, and water melons.

As to melons, especially sweet ones, they are entirely forbidden; and if the patient happen to take any, he should drink immediately after it the inspissated juices of some of the acid fruits. He may be allowed soft fish, and butter-milk.

With respect to those who are fat, fleshy, and of a white and red complexion, you may be content to let them eat such food as we first mentioned, consisting of any cooling and drying things. They should be restricted from labor, bathing, venery, walking, riding, exposure to sun and dust, drinking of stagnant waters, and eating fruits and vegetables that are blasted or moldy. Let their bowels be kept open, when there is occasion for it, with the juice of Damask plums and sugar, and whey

---

11   *Pleurisy*: An inflammation of the tissue around the lungs; *Quinsy*: A peritonsillar abscess.

and sugar. And let them abstain from figs and grapes; from the former, because they generate pustules, and drive the superfluous parts to the surface of the skin; and from the latter, because they fill the blood with flatulent spirits, and render it liable to make a hissing noice, and to undergo fermentation. If the air be very malignant, putrid, and pestilential, their faces may be constantly bathed with sanders water and camphor, which (with God's permission,) will have a good effect.

As to sucking infants, if they are above five months old, and fat, fair, and ruddy, let them be cupped; and let the nurse be managed with regard to diet in the manner we have mentioned. And let those infants that are fed on bread have those things which we have mentioned in a proper quantity....

But when the fever arises which is accompanied by symptoms of the Small-Pox, this regimen is not to be used, except after much observation, inquiry, and caution. For a mistake here is very dangerous; and for this reason, because that blood, when it ferments, is inflated and increased, and Nature, according to the temperament of the patient, is endeavoring to expel all its superfluous parts to the surface or to the members of the body; if, then, the cooling and thickening which you intend does not bring back the blood to a cooler and thicker state than it was in before its ebullition, the ebullition will break out a second or third time; and thus it will happen that you will be acting against Nature, and disturbing her in her work. Nor is it possible for the ebullition, if it be vehement, to be checked but by remedies in which there is great danger, and which do in a manner greatly congeal and coagulate the blood, (such as opium, hemlock, a great quantity the expressed juice of lettuce, black nightshade, and the like) and by the constant and excessive use of the regimen which we have just mentioned. And the congelation of the blood and the extinction of the natural heat at the same time, from the excessive use of these remedies, is not safe. Besides, even if you do employ them to excess, you will not be able to extinguish the ebullition and to restrain the violence of the unnatural heat; for by this excess you at the same time depress the power which the natural heat has of resisting what is hostile to itself; and you extinguish this and the unnatural heat together. And this I here mention to you (a matter which some physicians pass over from ignorance, and some from avarice, that they alone may receive profit from it) in order that *you* may not offend against nature, as do they; by permission of the Almighty and glorious God.

When you perceive symptoms of the Small-Pox, and you see a distention of the body, frequent stretching, pain in the back, redness of the complexion and of the eyes, a very violent headache, a strong and full pulse, a shortness of breath, a red and turbid urine, and the body hot to the touch, like that of a man who has been in a bath; and when also the body is fleshy, and the patient's diet has been such as produces plenty of blood: then take from him a large quantity of blood, even until fainting comes on. It is best to take it from the basilic vein,[12] or from some of its branches; if this cannot be found, then from the inner vein; and if this cannot be found, then from the cephalic. But when the basilic and its branches cannot be found, it is better to take the blood from the popliteal vein, or the saphena,[13] because these draw the blood from the greater veins in the abdomen more than the cephalic does. When these symptoms do not run very high, although they are distinctly manifest, then take away less blood; and when they have but slight force, then draw but little blood; and afterwards proceed in the cure with extinguents, as I have already mentioned. When you find that by the use of extinguents the feverish heat is moderated, and the pulse and breathing are returned to their natural stated, you should still continue to employ these remedies,—for by their means you will entirely drive away the ebullition of the Small-Pox.

In order more effectually to perform this extinction, let the patient drink water made cold in snow to the highest degree, several times and at short intervals, so that he may be oppressed by it, and feel the coldness of it in his bowels. If, after this, he should continue to be feverish, and the heat should return, then let him drink it a second time, to the quantity of two or three pints or more, and within the space of half an hour: and if the heat should still return, and the stomach be full of water, make him vomit it up, and then give him some more. If the water finds a passage, either by sweat or by the urine, then you may be sure that the patient is in a fair way of being restored to health; but if you do not see

---

12 *Basilic vein*: A large, superficial vein that runs along the inner arm.
13 *The popliteal vein, or the saphena*: Two veins on the back of the leg.

that the water has found a passage, or you find that the heat is increased, and returns as it was at first, or even is more violent, then omit giving the cold water in large quantities at several times, and have recourse to the other extinguents which I have described. And if you see them relieve the patient in the way I have mentioned, then persist in the use of them; if, however, you see that there arises any anxiety and inquietude after taking them, or that the anxiety and inquietude is altogether vehement and immoderate, then you may be sure that it is impossible to prevent the eruption of the Small-Pox or Measles.

Causes and Cures
(*Causae et curae*)*

HILDEGARD VON BINGEN
(German, 1098–1179)

The Abbess Hildegard von Bingen is perhaps most renowned as a twelfth-century mystic. By her own account, she began having religious visions at the age of five and was sent to live at a Benedictine monastery around the age of eight. There, she was enclosed with the anchoress Jutta[1] and trained as a nun, eventually becoming head of the convent. She continued to have religious visions and began writing widely, producing works of music, an early example of a morality play, and texts exploring science and medicine. *Causes and Cures* (*Causae et curae*) is a text that considers the human body and its relationship to the natural world as well as a range of illnesses and ailments for which she offers remedies. This new translation from the original Latin includes her work on migraine headaches, a condition that many modern scholars believe she may herself have experienced and that may have accompanied some of her visions. As you read, consider her description of this painful condition and its treatment.

---

1   Anchorites were permanently enclosed in cells attached to churches to focus on their faith. Upon enclosure, the priest recited the office of the dead to symbolize the earthly death of the anchorite. In many cases, the walls were bricked up. The cells contained small windows that allowed the anchorites to witness mass and offer spiritual guidance to members of the community (and so that servants could deliver food and carry away waste).

---

* Translated from Hildegard von Bingen (Hildegardis), *Causae et curae*, ed. Paul Kaiser (Leipzig, Germany: In aedibus B.G. Teubneri, 1903), 90–91, 166–67 (my own translation), Google Books.

Book II: Concerning Migraines

Migraines arise from melancholy and from all the bad humors which are in a person,[2] and half of a person's head is seized at a time, rather than every part at once: so it is now in the right part of the head, now in the left. Evidently, when the humors are overabundant, the migraine seizes the right part, however, when it is melancholy that has become excessive, it's the left part. Migraine has such great strength by itself, that if it were to seize the whole head of a person simultaneously, the person could not endure it. And it is very difficult to drive it out, because it is difficult to calm melancholy and the bad humors at the same time.

Book III: Concerning Migraines

Let whoever may be suffering a migraine take aloe and twice as much myrrh, and reduce this into a fine powder, and then let them take fine wheat flour and add oil of poppy to these and thus make a dough, like a leavened dough, and with this let them cover the entire head all the way to the ears and all the way to the neck. Place a felt cap over the head, and thus over three days—night and day—leave it on the head. For the heat of aloe and dryness of myrrh, once tempered with the sweetness of wheat flour and the coldness of poppy oil, calms this pain of the head. And this ferment presently returns fatness to the brain.

---

2   *From melancholy and from all the bad humors which are in a person*: Melancholy (or black bile) is one of the four humors, along with choler (yellow bile), blood, and phlegm. According to the humoral theory, these exist in an individual's body in a particular balance, and when those humors fall out of balance or are corrupted, sickness ensues.

The Salernitan Regimen of Health
(*Regimen sanitatis Salernitanum*)*

UNKNOWN

(Italian, ca. twelfth century)

This didactic (educational) poem, originally in Latin, provided domestic medical advice of the kind that could be followed at home without a doctor. The twelfth-century poem builds on principles upheld by the renowned medical school of Salerno in Italy, Europe's first medical school. The work was incredibly popular. At least one-hundred different manuscript copies (literally meaning "written by hand") have been found. After the printing press arrived in Europe in the mid-fifteenth century, around three hundred editions were printed across multiple languages. Some scholars have argued that the poem's influence, extending beyond the realm of practical medicine, can be seen in several of William Shakespeare's plays as well.[1] The poem was originally organized into short pieces of advice called aphorisms. The excerpts here include original translations of these aphorisms as numbered prose sections, for somewhat easier reading. As you read the *Regimen*'s advice, consider the principles of healthy behavior and nutrition, anatomy and physiology, and bloodletting practices, which are all founded on the Galenic (or humoral) tradition.

1 Robert L. Reid, "Humoral Psychology in Shakespeare's *Henriad*," *Comparative Drama* 30, no. 4 (1996/97): 471–502, JSTOR.

---

* Translated from *Regimen sanitatis Salernitanum: A Poem on the Preservation of Health in Rhyming Latin* Verse, ed. Sir Alexander Croke (Oxford: D. A. Talboys, 1830; Biodiversity Library, 2008), 103–48 (my own translation).

[On the Preservation of Health]

The whole school of Salerno wrote to the King of England:[2]

1. If you wish to remain unimpaired, if you wish to remain healthy, take away heavy worries; think it profane to be angry; refrain from undiluted wine, eat less; note it is not vain to rise after dinner; flee from midday naps; do not repress piss, nor clench the anus. If you keep these rules well, you may live a long time.

2. If you should lack doctors, let these three become doctors to you: a happy mind, rest, and moderate diet.

3. Rising in the light of morning, you should wash your hands in ice cold water. You should walk back and forth a little bit, and stretch the limbs a little bit, comb hair, brush teeth. These comfort the brain, and the other members of your body. Having been washed, keep warm; having been nourished, stand or stroll, cool down a little.

4. Let the midday nap be brief or nonexistent for you. Fever, sluggishness, headache, and also catarrh:[3] these arise out of the midday nap.

5. Four things come out of wind retained in the belly: spasm, dropsy, colic, and vertigo.

6. The greatest punishment for the stomach is made out of a great dinner. If you would be light by night, let your dinner be small.

7. You should never eat unless you know your stomach has been purged prior and voided of the food you took before. You shall be able to know for certain from your desire: these are your signs, by a thin diet in your mouth.

8. Peach, apple, pear, milk, cheese, and salted meat, as well as meats of deer, hare, goat, cow: these melancholic foods are the enemy of the sick.

9. Fresh eggs, red wine, rich soups and clear broths are strengthening of nature.

10. Wheat nourishes and fattens, as does milk, new cheese, testicles,

---

2   Which King of England—if any—this refers to is unclear: one theory is that it was addressed to a prince (the son of William the Conqueror) who stopped in Salerno for treatment. However, that son never became king.

3   *Catarrh*: Mucus buildup in an airway, usually the sinuses or throat.

pork, brains, marrow, sweet wine, pleasant-tasting foods, suckable eggs, ripe figs, and young grapes....

12. Alliums, nuts, rue, pear, radish, and theriac:[4] these are antidotes against deadly poison

13. Let the air be pure, habitable, and bright; let it neither be contaminated nor smelling with the foulness of the sewers.

14. If drinking late should do harm to you, drink wine again at an early hour, and it will be medicine. Better wines beget better humors: if it has been darkened, a lazy body returns to you. Let wine be clear, aged, fine, mature, and well-diluted, taken in moderation.

15. Beer should not be sour, but well clear, cooked from strong grain, plenty and aged. Of which, should it be drunk, the stomach is not thence weighed down.

16. You are ordered to take only a small amount of food in the season of spring; but also, the heat of summer does harm to immoderate banquets. You should beware the fruit of Autumn, lest they be grief for you. Take how much of the meal you wish in the season of Winter....

20. If you wish to be healthy, wash hands often. A washing after the table brings together two benefits for you: it cleanses the palms and sharpens the eyes....

25. The drinking of water while eating becomes greatly harmful: it cools the stomach, the food is poised to be undigested....

31. Goat milk is healthy for those with consumption,[5] after that camel's milk, and more nutritious of all is ass milk; more nutritious milk is from cows and sheep. If the head is feverish and hurts, it is not very healthy....

35. Cheese is cold, constipating, coarse and likewise harsh. Cheese and bread is good food for those in good health; if they are not healthy, then do not join the cheese with bread....

51. You should place the seasoning vessel on the table for meals. Salt shuns poison and gives taste to non-delicious foods, for food tastes bad

---

4   *Theriac*: An expensive medicine, made from complex blends of ingredients, often including snake flesh and opium, and thought to act both as an antidote to poisons and as a panacea.
5   *Consumption*: A wasting disease, most often associated with tuberculosis.

except that which is given salt. Very salty food inflames the vision, diminishing sperm and generating scabies, itching, and stiffness.

52. These three tastes are flourishing in heat: the salty, the bitter, the sharp. The astringent becomes cold, just as the styptic, and the tart; oily, tasteless, and sweet foods give moderation....

54. I command for everyone to preserve a customary diet: I approve it to be thus unless change is necessary; it is Hippocrates' testimony that evil diseases are the logical conclusions. A steadfast goal of medicine is a reliable diet, for which, if you lack care, you foolishly guide and cure badly....

60. Doctors do not seem to agree concerning onions: Galen[6] says they are not good for cholerics, but he teaches that they are certainly very healthy for phlegmatics, particularly for the stomach, and to produce a beautiful complexion. By often rubbing ground onions on a place denuded of hairs, you will be able to repair the beauty of the head....

63. The nettle gives sleep to the sick, likewise removes vomiting, it curbs longstanding cough, and relieves colic, banishes cold of the lungs and tumors of the belly, and aids all maladies of the joints....

72. Leeks, through frequent eating, render young women fertile. By means of this, you will be able to withhold a dripping stream of blood....[7]

75. Fear, prolonged hunger, vomiting, a blow, accidents, drunkenness, and cold cause ringing in the ear.

76. The bath, wines, Venus, wind, pepper, alliums, smoke, leeks with onions, lentils, crying, beans, mustard, the sun, sexual intercourse, fire, labor, a blow, sharp things, and dust: these damage the eyes. But staying awake at night hurts them more....

81. Man is composed out of 219 bones, 32 teeth, and 365 veins.

82. Four humors constitute the human body: blood, choler (yellow bile), phlegm, melancholy (black bile). Earth corresponds with melancholy; water to phlegm; air to blood; fire to choler.[8]

---

6 *Galen*: The physician Galen of Pergamon (129–ca. 210 CE), one of the most important and prolific of medical figures of the ancient world. His works relied heavily on those of Hippocrates (see pp. 26–30), and his views on medicine and anatomy, which included the theory of the four humors, would dominate Western medicine for over a millennium.
7 Many translations render this as "nosebleed."
8 The foundation of humoral theory is the notion that the body is composed of a

83. Those who are sanguine[9] are fat and merry by nature; they always desire to hear rumors repeated, Venus and Bacchus delight them; dishes of food, having laughed, and speaking pleasant words make this person cheerful. They are skillful and more apt in all studies. Rage does not move them groundlessly. They are abundant in giving, loving, cheerful, laughing, ruddy in complexion, singing, fleshy, audacious enough, and kind.

84. And it is the humor of choler which is capable of violent action. This type of person longs to outdo all others; this type learns lightly, eats much, and, having been stimulated, grows. From there he is magnanimous, gives abundantly, seeking the highest status; hairy, deceitful, easily enraged, wasteful, audacious, astute, slender, dry of nature, and yellow in complexion.

85. Phlegm bestows moderate strength, and the phlegmatic is broad and short. Phlegm makes fat and renders blood mediocre. The phlegmatic is idleness, not study, but surrenders bodies to sleep; dull in feeling, slow of motion, sluggish, and drowsy. This drowsy, sluggish person, great in quantity of spit, is dull in feeling, fat, and in appearance, pale in complexion.

86. The sad substance of black melancholy remains, which renders people depraved, very sad, and uncommunicative. They are vigilant in studies, and the mind is not devoted to sleep: they deliver on what they have proposed to do, and consider that nothing is prudent for themselves. They are envious and sad, wanton, and skillful misers, not lacking in guile, timid, and sallow in complexion.

87. These are the humors which bestow a complexion on each person: from phlegm a white complexion is produced in all things, from blood is produced a ruddy complexion, and a ruddy one from choler. If blood should offend by overflowing, the face blushes, the eyes are

---

particular balance of each of the four humors, which in turn each have qualities (either hot or cold, and either moist or dry). This aligns them with the four elements: melancholy is cold and dry, phlegm is cold and moist, blood is warm and moist, and choler is hot and dry.

9   The humors were also associated with physical characteristics, and for many theorists, with temperament. The "sanguine" body type and temperament is that in which blood is the dominant humor.

prominent, the cheeks are swollen, and the body is excessively weighed down. And the pulse is fast, full, and soft, extraordinary pain is produced, especially in the forehead, and there is constipation of the belly, and there is a dry tongue and thirst, and the dreams are full of redness, sweetness of the spit is present, and all bitter things are sweet.

88. Those younger than seventeen year hardly seek phlebotomy.[10] The more productive spirit departs through phlebotomy: the spirits are soon multiplied from drinking wine, and any humoral damage is slowly repaired by means of food. Phlebotomy clarifies the eye, makes the mind and brain whole, causes the marrow to be warm, will purge the internal organs, tames the stomach and abdomen, gives pure feeling, gives sleep, abolishes boredom, and produces and increases the hearing, voice, and strength.

89. Three months are good for phlebotomy: May, September, April; and these are lunar months, and are just like Hydra days.[11] On the first day of the first (May), and the last day of the latter (September and April), neither draw blood nor consume goose-meat. In the elderly or young, if the veins are full with blood, an incision of the vein contributes well in all months. These are the three months—May, September, April, in which you should draw blood in order to live a long time.

90. A cold nature, cold regions, extraordinary pain, after bathing or sexual intercourse, extreme youth and very old age, extended illness, overindulgence of drink and food; if the feeling of the stomach is frail or thin, and it is squeamish, it is not for you to be phlebotomized.

91. What should you do when you want to undergo phlebotomy—either when you are letting blood or when you will do so? Ointment, drinking, bathing, bandage or movement: all ought to be borne in mind for you.

92. Phlebotomy gladdens the sorrowful, pacifies the irate, and makes lovesick people not lose their minds.

93. Make the incision moderately large, in order that the more productive vapor and the freer blood may exit quickly.

---

10 *Phlebotomy*: The practice of bloodletting, one of the purgative methods of relieving an imbalance in the humors.
11 *Hydra days*: Days connected to the astronomical constellation Hydra.

94. After blood has been drawn, be vigilant for six hours, lest the vapor of sleep strike your sensible body. Lest you should damage your nerves, the incision should not be deep for you. After blood has been purged, you should not enjoy food immediately.

95. When you have had blood drawn, solemnly avoid all milk; a person having been phlebotomized avoids drinking. Avoid the cold, which is enemy of bloodletting, cloudy air will be forbidden. When blood has been drawn, the spirit rejoices in light breeze. Rest is suitable for all, but movement is very harmful.

96. Draw blood at the beginning of acute and very acute illnesses. Take a great deal of blood from those of middle age, but take from each child and elderly person very little. In the Spring take double, in the remaining seasons take the standard amount.

97. In Summer and Spring, draw blood from the right side; in Fall and Winter, from the left. These four members—the head, heart, feet, and liver—need clearing. In Spring purge the heart, do the liver in summer, and the remaining follow the order of the seasons.

98. Opening the salvatella vein[12] gives you the most small gifts: it purges the liver, spleen, chest, diaphragm, and voice, and takes away pain of the heart.

99. If your headache comes from drinking, you should drink spring water; acute fever is actually caused from excessive drinking. If the crown and front of the head is oppressed by burning pain, kind of rub the temples and forehead at the same time, and wash likewise with warm, cooked black nightshade.

100. The season of summer dries fasting bodies. Use emetics in any month, it also purges noxious humors, and washes the whole circuit of the stomach. Spring, Autumn, Winter, and Summer govern the year. The season of Spring the air is warm and humid, and there may be no better time for bloodletting. At that time, the use for man of Venus should be moderate, and likewise movement of the body, loosening of the belly,[13] sweat, and baths. The body should be purged at that time with medicines. Summer, by custom, warms and dries; and red choler

---

12 *Salvatella vein*: A narrow vein on the back of the little finger.
13 *Loosening of the belly*: The use of laxatives.

should be recognized as ruling chiefly at that time. Humid, cold dishes ought to be given, Venus should be beyond consideration, baths are not beneficial, bloodletting should be rare, rest is useful, and drinking should be done with moderation.

On Wounds and Fractures*

GUY DE CHAULIAC
(French, 1300–1368)

By the time the French physician and surgeon Guy de Chauliac composed his seven volume *Chirurgia magna* (Great Surgery) in 1363, surgery was a well-established practice around the world. De Chauliac himself was trained in several of the best medical schools in Europe and acted as personal physician to three popes. The work, based on Galenic principles and Islamic medicine (including that of Rhazes), established him as the preeminent surgeon of fourteenth century Europe, and it would be used as a surgical textbook for centuries to follow. This excerpt comes from a shortened but often quoted 1923 translation of *Chirurgia magna* published under the title *On Wounds and Fractures*. As you read, consider what characteristics and ethical principles de Chauliac requires of surgeons.

---

* Reprinted from Guy de Chauliac, *On Wounds and Fractures*, trans. W. A. Brennan (Chicago: W. A. Brennan, 1923), xiii. Google Books.

What the Surgeon Ought to Be

The conditions necessary for the surgeon are four: first, he should be learned; second, he should be expert; third, he must be ingenious, and fourth, he should be able to adapt himself. It is required for the first that the surgeon know not only the principles of surgery, but also those of medicine in theory and practice; for the second, he should have seen others operate; for the third, that he should be ingenious, of good judgment and memory to recognize conditions, and for the fourth, that he be adaptable and able to accommodate himself to the circumstances. Let the surgeon be bold in all sure things, and fearful in dangerous things; let him avoid all faulty treatments and practices. He ought to be gracious to the sick, considerate to his associates, cautious in his prognostications. Let him be modest, dignified, gentle, pitiful, and merciful; not covetous or an extortionist of money; but rather let his reward be according to his work, to the means of the patient, to the quality of the issue, and to his own dignity.

The Book of Margery Kempe*

MARGERY KEMPE
(English, ca. 1373–1438)

Little was known of Christian mystic Margery Kempe's work until the full-length manuscript of her book was found in 1934 in the cupboard of an English manor house. Identified by American scholar Hope Emily Allen, Kempe's rediscovered manuscript has been called the first work of autobiography in English. It details the life of a relatively middle-class woman, recounted in her own words and written down by a scribe around 1430. Kempe's story takes a surprising turn when an extended illness leads to a divine encounter with Jesus Christ after the birth of her first child. After this, she became a mystic and pilgrim. While female mystics were often nuns, anyone with the means to travel could embark on pilgrimages to holy sites, and the practice was common. Included here, in an original translation from the Middle English, are two excerpts detailing some of the tribulations Kempe faced. As you read, consider the account of her bodily and mental health.

Book 1, Chapter 1

A short treatise about a creature[1] who lived in great ostentatious wealth and pride towards the world, who then was drawn to our Lord by great poverty, sickness, shame and great rebuking from many diverse countries and places. Of her many tribulations some shall be shown below—not in the order in which it all happened, but as the creature could remember them when the story was written (because it was twenty years and more from the time this creature had forsaken the world and busily joined with our Lord before this book was written). Despite this, this creature had great advice in writing down her tribulations and her feelings. And a white friar offered to write if she wanted, but she was warned in her spirit that she should not write so soon. And many years after she was bid in her spirit to write.

And even then it was written first by a man who could neither write well in English nor German. So it was unable to be read except by special grace, for there was so much verbal abuse and slander of this creature that few men would believe her. And so, at last, the priest was strongly moved to write this treatise; and he could not effectively read it for four years altogether. And then because of the requests of this creature, and compelling of his own conscience, he tried again to read it and it was much easier than it was previously. And so he began to write in the year of our Lord 1436, on the next day after Mary Magdalen, according to the information provided by this creature.

When this creature was twenty years of age or somewhat more, she was married to a worshipful Burgess and was with child in short time, as nature would have it. And after she had conceived, she was belabored with great attacks of feverish illness until the child was born. And then, due to the difficulty she had in childbirth and the previous sickness, she despaired of her life, supposing that she might not live. And then she sent for her confessor, for she had a thing on her conscience which she had never told anyone before that time in all her life; for she was always hindered by her enemy the devil, who was constantly saying to

---

1 *A short treatise about a creature*: Uses the third-person, including the term "creature," to refer to herself throughout the work.

her while she was in good health that she needed no confession, but could do penance by herself alone and all would be forgiven, for God is merciful enough. And therefore this creature often did great penance, by fasting on bread and water, and by other deeds of alms with devout prayers—but she would not share her sins in confession. And any time she was sick or diseased the devil said in her mind that she should be damned, for she was not shriven of that default.

Because of that, after that her child was born, she did not trust her life, and sent for her confessor (as I said before), fully desiring to be shriven of all her lifetime as near as she could. And when she came to the point of saying that thing which she had so long concealed, her confessor was a little too hasty and began to chastise her harshly before then she had fully explained her intention. And so she would say no more, no matter what he did. And at once, because of the fear she had of damnation on the one hand and his sharp rebukes on the other hand, this creature went out of her mind and was extraordinarily troubled and burdened with spirits for half a year, eight weeks, and a few days.

And throughout this time she saw (as she thought) devils open their mouths, all lit up with burning flames of fire, as though they would swallow her up: sometimes rearing up at her, sometimes threatening her, sometimes pulling her and tugging at her, both night and day during the that whole time. And also the devils screamed at her with great threats, and commanded her to forsake her Christendom, her faith, and deny her God, his mother and all the saints in heaven, her good works and all good virtues, her father, her mother, and all her friends. And so she did.

She slandered her husband, her friends, and her own self, she spoke many a rebuking word and many a malicious word. She recognized neither virtue nor goodness; she desired all wickedness, and whatever the spirits tempted her to say and do, so she said and did. She would have killed herself many times in her agitation, and would have been damned with them in hell. And, in evidence of this, she bit her own hand so violently that it was seen all her life after. And also she tore apart the skin on her body right against her heart with her nails, fearsomely, for she had no other instruments. And she would have done worse except she was bound and firmly kept both day and night so that she might not do what she wanted.

And when she had long been burdened by these and many temptations, so that men thought she should never escape from them nor live, then one time as she lay alone and her keepers were away from her, our Merciful Lord Christ Jesus (ever to be trusted, and worshiped be his name, never forsaking his servant in time of need), appeared to this creature who had forsaken him. He appeared in the likeness of a man most pleasant, most beautiful, and most amiable that ever might be seen with a human's eye, wearing a mantel of purple silk, sitting up on her bed's side looking upon her with such a blessed presence that she was strengthened in all her spirits. He said to her these words: "Daughter, why have you forsaken me, though I never forsook you?"

And as soon as He had said these words, she saw—truly—how the air opened as bright as any lightning. He rose up into the air, not very hastily and quickly, but beautifully and slowly, so that she might well behold him in the air until it was closed again. And right away the creature was stabilized in her wits and in her reason as well as ever she had been before.

And she begged her husband as so soon as he came to her that she might have the keys to the pantry so she could have her meat and drink as she had done before. Her maidens and her keepers counseled him he should deliver her no keys, for they said she would just give away all the goods there, for she didn't know what she was saying (as they supposed). Nevertheless her husband, ever having tenderness and compassion for her, commanded they should deliver to her the keys, and she took her meat and drink as her bodily strength would allow. Then she recognized her friends and her servants and all others that came to her to see how our Lord Jesus Christ had worked his grace in her—so blessed may he be whoever is near in tribulation. Even when men think He is far from them, He is very near through his grace. Afterward, this creature did all the other duties that belonged to her wisely and sadly enough, although she did not know the true spiritual ecstasy of our Lord.

Book 1, Chapter 56

Afterward, God punished her with many great and diverse sicknesses; she had the flux[2] a long time—until she was anointed, expecting to die. She was so feeble that she could not hold a spoon in her hand. Then our Lord Jesus Christ spoke to her in her soul and said that she would not die yet, then she recovered again for a little while. Soon after she had such a great sickness in her head, and afterwards in her back, that she worried she would lose her mind from it. After she recovered from all these sicknesses, in just a short time another sickness followed that was set in her right side and lasted for all but eight weeks (occurring at different times) over eight years. Sometimes she had it once in a week lasting sometimes thirty hours, sometimes twenty, sometimes ten, sometimes eight, sometimes four, sometimes two. It was so hard and sharp that she had to clear out everything in her stomach, as bitter as if it had been gall, neither eating nor drinking while the sickness endured but constantly groaning until it was gone.

Then she would say to our Lord, "Oh, blissful Lord, why would you become a man and suffer so much pain for my sins and for all men's sins so that we shall be saved, and yet we are so unkind to you, Lord. And I, most unworthy, cannot suffer this little pain? Oh Lord, for your great pain have mercy on my little pain—for the great pain you suffered give me not as much as I deserve, because I cannot bear as much as I deserve. And if you decide, Lord, that I must bear it, send me patience; otherwise, I may not suffer it. Oh, blissful Lord, I would rather suffer through all the malicious words that men might say about me and that all clerks would preach against me for your love, (as long as it hindered no one's soul), than suffer through this pain that I have. To suffer malicious words for your love hurts me not at all. And the world may take nothing from me but worship and worldly goods, and I set no stock by the worship of the world. And all manner of worldly goods and honor, and all manner of loves on earth, I pray the Lord forbid me from having—namely all those loves and goods of any earthly thing which could

---

2   *The flux*: An early term for dysentery (a type of gastroenteritis) that literally means "flowing."

decrease my love against you or lessen my spiritual reward in heaven. And all manner of loves and goods which you know in your godhead would increase my love for you, I pray that you grant me those, for your mercy to your everlasting worship."

Sometimes even in spite of that, the said creature had great bodily sickness; yet the passion of our merciful Lord Christ Jesus worked in her soul so that for the time she did not feel her own sickness, but wept and sobbed in remembrance of our Lord's passion (as though she saw him with her bodily eyes, suffering pain and passion right in front of her). After eight years had passed, her sickness departed, so that it came back not week by week as it did before. But then her cries and her weeping increased so much that the priests dared not administer the sacrament to her openly in the church but only privately in the prior's chapel at Lynn, far from people's earshot. And in that chapel she had such high contemplation and so much intimate talk with our Lord because she was pushed out of church for His love, that she cried when she was given the sacrament—as if her body and her soul should have split apart—so much so that two men held her in their arms until her crying stopped, for she could not bear the abundance of love that she felt in the precious sacrament (which she steadfastly believed was truly God and man in the form of bread). Then our blissful Lord said in her mind, "Daughter I will not have my grace hidden that I give you; for the more intent that people are to hinder it and prevent it, the more I shall spread it abroad and make it known to all the world."

Syphilis: or, the French Disease
(*Syphilis sive morbus gallicus*)*

GIROLAMO FRACASTORO
(Italian, ca. 1476–1553)

In the late fifteenth century, a sexually transmitted infection caused by the bacterium *Treponema pallidum* began its rampage across Europe. Everywhere it spread, it was promptly blamed on another nation. Often called the "French Disease" or "French Pox," it was also labeled the "Italian," "Spanish," "Polish," and "Christian" disease, depending on one's location and politics. Italian poet and doctor of medicine and natural philosophy Girolamo Fracastoro gave the disease its common modern name "syphilis" in his three-book didactic (educational) poem in 1530. The poem describes the disease and its contemporary treatments and offers a poetic and mythological imagining of the disease's origins as a punishment heaped upon a shepherd. As you read the excerpts, consider Fracastoro's discussion of the nature of the disease—which includes an important idea similar to our modern germ theory—and the tale of the Shepherd Syphilus.

---

* Reprinted from *Hieronymus Fracastor's Syphilis: From the Original Latin*, trans. Solomon Claiborne Martin (St. Louis: The Philmar Company, 1911), 18–23, 53–57, Google Books.

[On the Nature of Syphilis]

A subtle poison at once spreads itself in the ether and disseminates its pernicious effluvia throughout the immensity of space.

What was the origin of this poison? Are we to believe that the sun's rays, associated with the malign influence of the stars, raised from the bosom of the earth and of the waters unhealthful vapors which spread in the air contagious miasms,[1] the germs of a disease[2] as yet unknown? Or, on the other hand, were these miasms engendered in the upper regions of the atmosphere, from which as a consequence, they descended among us? It cannot be told, how many mysteries of the sky unfold to our eyes, how difficult it is to go back to the origin of causes, which at times are separated from their effects by long series of years, and at others are mingled with events in an inextricable confusion.

Add to this that Nature may vary at its will the influence of epidemic miasms. Thus, at times, the infected air pours its poisons only on vegetation, killing the flowers and the tender buds, tainting the wheat with an unclean rust, destroying all hopes of crops, changing seeds as deep as the very bosom of earth. At other times it is the animals only that are struck, and that, either all at once, or only a few among all. I remember, for instance, in a year that was remarkable not only for an unusual and suspicious fertility of the soil, but also by an excessive frequency of Southern winds and of autumnal rains, that all goats—and only goats— were affected by disease. They came out of the sheds full of vigor and health; then, at the same moment that they were cheerfully browsing the grass of the meadows, they were attacked with a suffocating cough, a certain prelude of death. They were then seen to turn convulsively on themselves and fall exhausted, among their companions, and soon give

---

1 *Contagious miasms*: Miasma, or "bad air," was thought to cause disease, especially in places where it gathered densely.
2 The germ theory of disease (our current leading theory of disease, which holds that disease is caused by microorganisms infecting hosts) would not become dominant over humoral theory until well into the nineteenth century, but versions of the idea occurred periodically from ancient periods onward. Fracastoro offers one such version in his works, and scholars believe that his work was influenced by that of Lucretius (see pp. 31–36).

up their last breath. Then, a surprising thing; in the spring and in the summer which followed, it became the turn of the various cattle, whom a malignant fever decimated to the point of almost completely destroying them. As a matter of fact, celestial influences are varied in an infinite degree like the events derived from them, and to each one of them is intimately bound a certain order of phenomena.[3]

And on the other hand, what diversity in the morbid germs, what oddity in their effects! You shall judge of them.

The miasms contained in the atmosphere are found in direct contact with the eyes; well, it is not only the eyes that they affect, it is the lung that they will reach in the depths of the chest! In the same manner also we occasionally see the tender grape preserve itself intact next to hardier fruits which die away; and when, in its turn, it dies, either by impoverishment of the seed, or by a swelling or a shrinking of its pores, it is never so except under the influence of causes that are proper to it.

Let us now study the symptoms of this scourge which a celestial influx has caused and reproduced after centuries that it was forgotten. This disease does not affect the dumb inhabitants of the wave, nor the wild beasts of the forests, nor the birds of the sky, nor horses nor cattle. It only has to do with man; man alone is its prey.

In the human body, it is the blood that it attacks at first, and, feeding on naught but fat and viscid humors, it is on the fat and corrupted parts of this fluid that it preferably attaches itself.

Here especially, O muse, I claim thy help to limn the picture of this execrable pestilence. Deign also to inspire me, Apollo, god of the day, god of poetry,[4] and make matters such that my work may, thanks to thee, remain through coming centuries. A day, in fact, may perhaps come when our great grand nephews will take the pleasure of consulting the description of a forgotten disease. Forgotten, yes, for no one doubts at a given time this disease will return into the clouds of nothingness. And

---

3 Astrology was thought to have a profound influence on health; astrological medicine associated each of the planets, the sun and moon, and the astrological signs with various diseases and parts of human anatomy in a practice called *melothesia*.
4 *Apollo, god of the day, god of poetry*: This Greek god is also associated with medicine, sickness, and health, and is the father of Asclepius, the god of medicine.

no one doubts also but that, after another series of centuries, it will return to the light, to afflict anew the world and once more spread terror among the peoples of another age.

One of the most surprising of facts is that, after having contracted the germ of the contagion, the victim attacked by the scourge does not often present any lesion that is well marked before the moon has four times accomplished its travels. The disease, in fact, does not show itself at once by accusing symptoms directly that it has penetrated the organism. For a certain time it broods in silence, as if it were gathering its forces for a more terrible explosion. During this period, at all events, a strange languor seizes the patient and depresses his whole being; his mind seems heavy, his limbs are soft, and weakening, fail for work; the eye loses its flash and the face is depressed in its expression and has become pale.

It is on the organs of generation[5] that the virus first is transported, to irradiate from there to the neighboring parts and on the regions of the groin.

Soon after, more well defined symptoms show themselves. When the light of day disappears to give place to the shades of night, at the time when the inner heat of living bodies leaves the peripheral parts to concentrate upon the viscera, atrocious pains suddenly burst forth in the limbs charged with vitiated humors and torture the articulations, the arms, the shoulders, the calves. It is because at that moment, vigilant Nature, an enemy of all impurity, is at work to react against the putrid ferments which the disease has introduced into the veins and with which it has penetrated all the humors,[6] all the nourishing juices of the organisms. She strains to drive them away; she energetically fights against them. But they resist; thick, viscid, not displacing themselves except slowly, they fix themselves on the muscles, they attach themselves to the exsanguined framework of the tissues, and give rise to horrible sufferings wherever they adhere.

---

5   *Organs of generation*: Reproductive organs.
6   The four humors (blood, phlegm, black bile or melancholy, and yellow bile or choler) were thought to be critical to health, and required careful balance in the body; if they putrefied, overflowed, or diminished in excess, a person would become sick.

The most subtle of these morbid humors, those which are the most easily evacuated, take refuge either in the skin or in the extremities of the limbs. They then produce hideous eruptions on those points and these exanthems[7] soon spread over the whole body and cover the face with a repulsive mask.

Unknown up to our days, these eruptions consist of pustules and conical pimples, which, gorged with corrupted liquids, are not slow in opening to allow the escape of a mucous and virulent sanious liquid.[8] Even, sometimes, the pimples that are similar develop in the depths of organs and noiselessly corrode the tissues. It is thus that horrible ulcers are seen covering the limbs, denuding the bones, eating the lips and penetrating the throat, from which there only issues a weak and plaintive voice.

At other times, again, there exhales from the skin thick humors which dry into fearsome crusts on the surface of the integument. Like these are seen the viscid juices which come from the cherry tree or the almond tree condensing in a gummy callus on the bark of these trees.

Ah! how many patients, sorrowful victims of this plague have contemplated with horror their faces and their bodies covered with the hideous taints, deploring their youth destroyed in its bloom, and have cursed the gods and threatened the sky! Unfortunates! Night which pours sweet repose upon all nature, has no more charms for them, for sleep has fled from their eyes. For them, in the same manner, aurora comes without attractions, for day like night recalls their pains. The pleasures of the table, joyous feasts, the intoxicating gifts of Bacchus, the festivities of the city, the delights of the country, nothing smiles for them any more. Vainly do they search for a respite to their sufferings on green banks made pleasant by the purling of streams, in the shade of valleys, and in the solitude of mountains. Desperate, lost, they return addressing ardent prayers to the gods, burning expiatory incense in the temples, loading altars with rich gifts. Useless trouble! The gods remain deaf to their voices and disdain their sacrifices.

---

7 *Exanthems*: Rashes, usually extensive.
8 *Sanious liquid*: A thin, greenish discharge composed of serum and pus.

[The Mythical Origin of Syphilis]

But a time came, alas! in which corruption and impiety slipped in among us, in which the sacred altars of our fathers were devoted to contempt. The punishment of such a crime did not take time to come, for from that period dates for us a series of misfortunes which I would be unable to recite. It was, at first, that famous island[9] to which Atlas had given his name, that queen of the seas, Atlantic, that a fearful cataclysm shook to its very foundations, and which threw itself in the bosom of those waves which were formerly subject to its empire. Then the anger of heaven turned itself against our flocks, and we saw disappear to the last young of this giant animal of which nothing has survived among us but a memory. As a result, we have nothing to offer to our gods but the blood of foreign victims, born under a sky which is not ours. Later on yet, the anger of the gods and the vengeance of Apollo unchained upon us the terrible scourge of which thou hast seen the ravages. This disease has spread itself in all our cities, and very few among us escape its cruel attacks. It is for the purpose of conjuring him and to propitiate him that our fathers established these expiatory sacrifices, of whose origin it remains for me to tell thee.

According to an ancient tradition, even here, on the banks of this river, a shepherd of the name of Syphilus watched innumerable flocks of King Alcithous. It was the period of the Solstice, and Sirius[10] threw the fire of his rays on these fields. A torrid heat burned the earth; the forests had no shade, the breeze was no longer cool. Syphilus saw his animals dying; seized with indignation, exasperated by his own sufferings, he threw to Sirius a threatening look and thus addressed the god:[11] "What! we honor thee as the father and the creator of all things, we erect to thee altars, we offer to thee our incense, we sacrifice to thee victims

---

9 *That famous island*: Atlantis, first mentioned in philosophical dialogues of Plato (ca. 428–ca. 347 BCE), was legendarily described as an advanced and powerful island society that sank into the sea.
10 *Sirius*: The Dog-star—and god—Sirius, the brightest star in the constellation Canis Major, was thought to cause summertime droughts and heatwaves (and gave us the phrase "the dog days of summer").
11 Other translations render the god here as Apollo, god of the sun.

without number, and this is our reward, this is the care that thou takest of the flocks of my King! Ah! it is jealousy without doubt that is devouring thee! Thou who hast in the heavens, it is said but one bull, but one ram, with a hectic dog to watch this great drove, thou hast not borne in view without envy our thousands of cattle, our thousands of sheep with the white fleece. Fool that I am. It is not to thee, it is to Alcithous that I should render divine honors. If that great King commands so many peoples, if so many seas obey his laws, it is because, most assuredly, his power is greater than thine and that of all the other gods. He, at least, will know how to guard our flocks, to give them cool shelter, and to furnish them with green shades."

He had spoken, and without waiting he erected an altar on the neighboring mountain; he then rendered divine honors to Alcithous. Shepherds and plowmen soon follow this impious example; and incense no longer smokes, the blood of victims is no longer poured out in honor of the new god.

Alcithous received these homages with intoxication. From the top of his throne, in the midst of his assembled peoples, he proclaimed himself the sovereign of the world; he decreed that in future, to him alone were divine honors to be rendered. "Let the gods," said he, "divide the heavens among them; they have nothing to look after among the things here below!"

But Sirius,[12] whom nothing escapes, Sirius who with one look embraces the universe, could not see without indignation such sacrileges. In his anger, he charges his rays with pestilential poisons and virulent miasms, which simultaneously infect the air, the earth and the waters. At once upon this criminal earth there arises an unknown plague. Syphilus is the first attacked by it, on account of having been the first to profane the sacred altars. A hideous leprosy covers his body; fearful pains torture his limbs and banish sleep from his eyes. Then, this terrible disease—known since then among us by the name of Syphilis—does not take long to spread in our entire nation, not even sparing our King himself.

---

12 Again, other translations render this as Apollo—a logical choice, given his association with both the Sun and sickness—either way, the suggestion here is that Syphilus is offending the Sun itself, and reaps the consequences.

Our fathers then, in their alarm, ran to ask the nymph America, who gives the sacred oracles in the woods of Carthese. They ask her the cause of the disease which is afflicting them; they implore of her a remedy for their sufferings.

"Impious mortals," answers the nymph, "you have had the presumption to equal yourselves to the gods, and today you suffer the punishment of your crime. Go, go without loss of time, to implore your pardon of the god whom you have offended; re-erect those altars and offer to him those sacrifices which are his due. Perhaps you may, in this manner, appease his anger. But do not hope to see the end of the scourge that is afflicting you. This disease shall be eternal, and whosoever shall be born on this earth will suffer from its attacks; Apollo has sworn it by the Styx and by immutable Destiny. Here at all events, is how you may obtain relief to your sufferings. Choose in your flocks a white heifer and a black one; sacrifice the first to Juno and the second to Cybele.[13] Juno will scatter in the air propitious germs which, received and fecundated in the bosom of Cybele, produce a tree with green branches. That tree is your savior."[14]

Thus spoke the nymph, whose voice shook the cave and the neighboring wood. A chill of terror occurred at this sinister prophecy. Nevertheless, the commands of the nymph were obeyed; the altars were re-erected; two heifers were sacrificed, the white one and the other black, in honor of Juno and of Cybele.

Then suddenly, O unheard prodigy and true prodigy (I attest for it the gods and the names of our fathers), an unknown tree arises from the bosom of the earth, spreads its branches and develops its luxuriant crown of foliage. It is from the fruitful trunk of this tree that the neighboring forest was born.

Our high priest at once prescribes new sacrifices in honor of Apollo.

---

13 Juno is the queen of the gods in the Roman pantheon; Cybele is a mother goddess imported to Greece from Anatolia (now in modern-day Turkey).

14 *That tree is your savior*: Juno provides seeds from the Guaiacum tree, which is native to the subtropics and tropics of America and was first brought back to Europe from the Caribbean by Spanish colonizers in the sixteenth century. It was widely believed to be a medical remedy for syphilis. Substances derived from the tree are still used in food and medicine (notably the expectorant guaifenesin).

He insists upon an expiatory victim, and fate chooses Syphilus to pay with his life for the crime of the nation.

The sacrifice is being prepared. Already the ribbons and the sacred cakes are deposited on the altar; already the iron threatens the breast of the victim, when all at once Juno and Sirius, whose anger has been appeased, substitute for the shepherd Syphilus a young bull who receives the fatal blow and alone pays with the price of his blood the outrage done to the gods.

The Castle of Health*

SIR THOMAS ELYOT
(English, ca. 1490–1546)

Diplomat and author Sir Thomas Elyot was a skilled researcher, careful reader, and keen thinker, not a physician. However, when Elyot's *Castle* was initially published around 1539, it was the first comprehensive guide to health published in English for regular people to use in their homes—a genre called a "regimen" (see also pp. 59–66). The title plays on a common metaphor in which the human body is described in architectural terms, as a house, castle, or fortress. It was an incredibly popular work, and many others like it soon followed. Physicians, however, were not thrilled by the prospect of medical knowledge being published in the common language for just anyone to access. European medical texts were traditionally published in Latin, a language that relatively few could read and write. In the excerpt, which is drawn from the Proem (or Preface) added to later editions of the work, consider Elyot's defense of his choice to write the work and make it available to all who could read English.

---

* Reprinted from Sir Thomas Elyot, preface to *The castell of health, corrected, and in some places augmented by the first author thereof, Sir Thomas Elyot Knight* (London, 1595; Early English Books Online Text Creation Partnership, 2011).

The Proem

...And although I have never been at Montpelier, Padua, nor Salerno,[1] yet have I found some thing in Physic,[2] whereby I have taken no little profit concerning mine own health. Moreover I wot not[3] why physicians should be angry with me, since I wrote and did set forth the *Castle of Health* for their commodity, that the uncertain tokens of urines, and other excrements[4] should not deceive them, but that by the true information of the sick man, by me instructed, they might be the more sure to prepare medicines convenient for the diseases.

Also to the intent that men observing a good order in diet, and preventing the great causes of sickness, they should of those maladies the sooner be cured. But if physicians be angry, that I have written Physic in English, let them remember that the Greeks wrote in Greek, the Romans in Latin, Avicenna[5] and the other in Arabic, which were their own proper and maternal tongues. And if they had been as much attached with envy and covetousness, as some now seem to be, they would have devised some particular language with a strange cipher or form of letters, wherein they would have written their science, which language or letters no man should have known, that had not professed and practiced Physic: but those although they were Paynims and Jews,[6]

---

1 *Montpelier, Padua, nor Salerne*: Three of the most prominent centers for medical study and education; Salerno, for instance, develops the principles that underlie the *Regimen sanitatis salernitanum*.
2 *Physic*: Meaning medicine; this is where we get the term "physician" (one who practices "physic").
3 *I wot not*: I don't understand.
4 *Uncertain tokens of urines, and other excrements*: Exactly how it sounds: much of medical diagnosis happened by careful examination of human waste. We still do this today but in more sanitary conditions.
5 *Avicenna*: Ibn Sina (known in Europe as Avicenna) is one of western medicine's most important figures; born in Iran in 980 CE, he was also a prominent Muslim poet and philosopher (though scholars disagree about what branch of Islam he adhered to).
6 *Paynims and Jews*: Paynim is an archaic term for heathens or pagans that was most frequently applied to Muslims. The terminology here is not without prejudice: Muslims and Jews were widely discriminated against. However, Elyot's main point is that Christians are being outperformed in the act of charity by non-Christian

yet in this part of charity they far surmounted us Christians, they that would not have so necessary a knowledge as Physic is, to be hid from them which would be studious about it.

Finally God is my Judge, I write neither for glory, reward, nor promotion, only I desire men to deem well mine intent, since I dare assure them, that all that I have written in this book, I have gathered of most principal writers in Physic. Which being thoroughly studied, and remembered, shall be profitable (I doubt not) unto the reader, and nothing noxious to honest physicians, that do measure their study, with moderate living and Christian charity.

cultures who make essential knowledge accessible to all.

The Herbal, or General History of Plants*

JOHN GERARD
(English, 1564–1637)

It's no secret that plants have, in addition to their nutritional properties, medicinal properties as well. By the sixteenth century, European colonial expansion into parts of Africa, the Americas, and Asia resulted in major advancements and increased interest in the study of botany. Out of this, a genre of writing called the "Herbal" took shape that cataloged plants and their uses in print. In his 1597 edition of his *Herbal*, English botanist John Gerard modifies a translation of the work of Rembert Dodoens, a prominent Flemish botanist, and adds new details, including descriptions of a range of plants from the Americas and additional illustrations. Gerard's *Herbal* became among the most prominent and influential work of its kind, listing detailed information about known varieties of plants, their appearance and growing seasons, and the dietary and medicinal properties they offered. Included here is an excerpt on the willow tree, now known to produce salicin, from which salicylic acid and aspirin are derived.

---

* Reprinted from John Gerard, *The Herball or Generall Historie of Plantes* (London: John Norton, 1597), chap. 51, 1202, 1205–6. Internet Archive.

Of the Willow Tree

The kinds: There are diverse sorts of Willows contained under sundry titles: the Oziar, the Sallow, the Rose Willow, the common Withy, and the Dwarf Willow, or Withy [See Illustration 1]....

The place: These Willows grow in diverse places of England; the Rose Willow grows plentifully in Cambridgeshire, by the river, and ditches there in Cambridgetowne they grow abundantly about the places called Paradise, and Hellmouth, in the way from Cambridge to Grantchester. I found the dwarf Willows growing near to a bog or marsh ground, at the further end of Hampstead heath upon the declining of the hill, in the ditch that encloses a small cottage there, not half a furlong from the said house or cottage.

The time: The Willows do flower at the beginning of the Spring....

The temperature: The leaves, flowers, seed, and bark of the Willows, are cold and dry in the second degree, and astringent.

The virtues: The leaves and bark of Withy or Willows do stay the spitting of blood, and all other flux of blood whatsoever, in man or woman, if the said leaves and bark be boiled in wine and drunk.

The green boughs with the leaves may very well be brought into chambers, and set about the beds of those that be sick of agues:[1] for they do mightily cool the heat of the air, which thing is a wonderful refreshing to the sick patients.

The barks have like virtues: Dioscorides[2] writes, that these being burnt to ashes, and steeped in vinegar, take away corns and other like risings in the feet and toes: diverse [people] says Galen, do slit the bark whiles the Withy is in flowering, and gather a certain juice, with which they use to take away things that hinder the sight, and this is when they are constrained to use a cleansing medicine, of thin and subtle parts.

---

1 *Agues*: Sickness marked by fevers and chills; often associated with malaria.
2 *Dioscorides*: Pedanius Dioscorides (ca. 40–ca. 90 CE) was a Greek pharmacologist and physician; his multivolume *De materia medica* cataloged around 600 different plants, including their medical and dietetic uses, and one thousand simple medicines, and was in constant circulation as a medical guide for over 1,500 years.

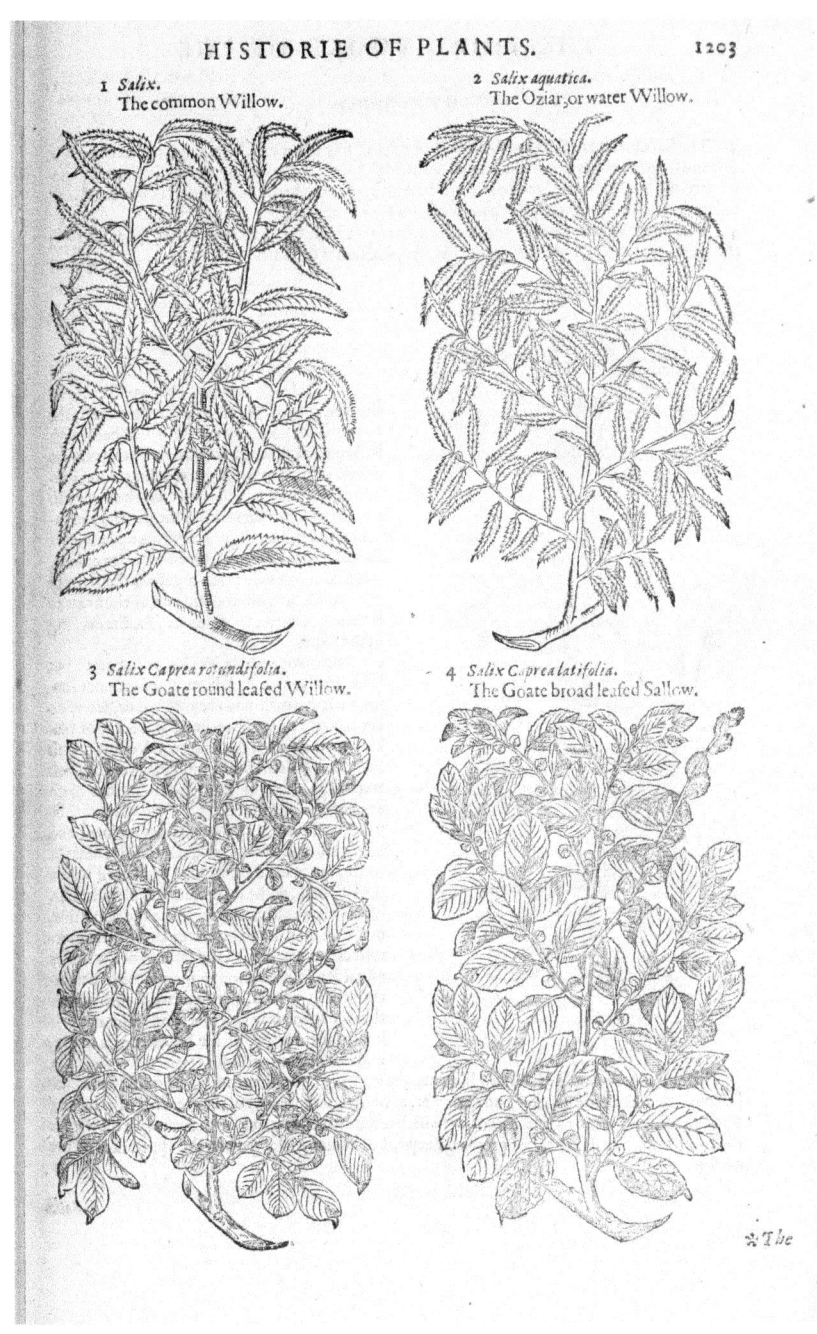

Illustration 1. Drawings of different willow varieties. Reprinted from John Gerard, *The Herball or Generall Historie of Plantes* (London: John Norton, 1597), 1203, Internet Archive.

Seven Defenses
(*Sieben Defensiones*)*

PARACELSUS
(Swiss, ca. 1493–1541)

The Swiss scholar known as Paracelsus[1] stands as one of the most prominent challengers to the longstanding medical thinking of Galenic medicine. Paracelsus proposed a new system of medicine and the treatment of diseases that would shape the fields of chemistry, pharmacology, and toxicology in profound ways, including the development of complex chemical compounds as medicine. This system, known as Paracelsianism, was grounded in alchemy, which was a precursor of modern pharmacology and chemistry, and continued to challenge Galenism after Paracelsus's death. The excerpt is translated from the original German text, which was published during the sixteenth century. As you read, consider Paracelsus's response to the critics of his method, which includes a principle that is still important today: that the size of the dosage determines whether or not something is dangerous.

---

1 Paracelsus was born Philippus Aureolus Theophrastus Bombastus von Hohenheim. According to medical historian Walter Pagel, the name Paracelsus might signal a belief that he was better than the great Roman physician named Celsus (ca. 25 BCE–ca. 50 CE), or it may be a latinizing of Hohenheim, the name of his family's estate. Walter Pagel, *Paracelsus: Introduction to Philosophical Medicine in the Era of the Renaissance* (Basel: S. Karger, 1982), 5ff.

---

* Translation from Theophrast von Hohenheim (Paracelsus), *Sieben Defensiones* [...], ed. Karl Sudhoff (Leipzig: Verlag von Johann Ambrosius Barth, 1915), 23–27 (my own translation), HathiTrust.

The Third Defense: About Writing These New Receipts

But over and above what is reported, is that clamor still greater among the ignorant, alleged, and invented doctors, those who say that my receipts that I write are a poison, a corrosive and an extraction of all the wickedness and toxicity of Nature.[2] To such allegations and outcries, my first question might be—should they be capable of answering or knowing—what might be poison or not poison? Or maybe if, in poison, there might be no Mysterium[3] of Nature? Because in this same point they are ignorant and unknowing of Natural forces. Because what is there that God has created, that is not blessed with a large-scale gift to the good of humanity? Why, therefore, should poison be discarded and scorned, if really not the poison, but rather Nature is sought? I will give you an example, to understand my intention. Look at the toad, how so very a poisonous and offputting an animal it is; look also indeed at the great Mysterium that is in it, regarding the Pestilence. If the Mysterium should be scorned because of the poisonous and off-putting nature of the toad, how much bigger a mockery that would be! Who is it who has composed the recipe of Nature? Has God not done it? Why would I scorn His composition, whether or not what he composes seems inadequate to me? It is He in whose hand all wisdom stands, and He knows where He should place every Mysterium. Why, then, should I be astonished or let myself be afraid—because one portion is poison should I despise the other portion? Each thing should be used for that which it is prescribed, and we should not bear any further shyness about it. For God Himself is the Physician and the Remedy. And every physician should persuade himself of the power of God, which Christ gives us to understand, saying, "If you will drink poison, it will not harm you."[4] So now the poison does not prevail, but rather goes into the body without

---

2   Paracelsus is responding to criticisms of his medicines (the recipes for which were called "receipts"), which used mercury, sulfur, and salt (specifically metallic salts like potassium nitrate—also known as saltpeter). This was in stark contrast to the more common practice of using herbal compounds or "simples" (single-ingredient medicines) for therapeutic purposes.
3   *Mysterium*: The essence or origin of something else.
4   Cf. Mark 16:18, in the Bible.

harm just as we need it after the prescribed manner of Nature; why then should the poison be scorned? Whoever scorns poison, doesn't know what is in poison. For the Arcanum[5] in the poison is so blessed, that the poison neither takes from it nor harms it. But I would not have proffered to you this paragraph because it is sufficient to defend myself, but rather because it is necessary to communicate to you a larger report, so I may give a sufficient account of poison.

How is it that you see in me everything you are full of, and chastise me for a lentil, when melons lie in you? You chastise me for my receipts: look at your own, look how they are! Namely, first, with your purging: where is a purgative in all your books which is not a poison?[6] Or which does not serve Death? Or which may be used without vexation where the dose in its right weight is not considered? Now mark the point of what this is: it is neither too much nor too little. Whoever hits the middle receives no poison. And if I nevertheless did use poison, which you can't prove, but suppose I did use it and gave its proper dose—am I likewise punishable, or not? I want to let everyone see this. You know that theriac[7] is made from the Tyro snake—why do you not scold your theriac, because the poison of this snake is in it? But because you see that it is useful and not harmful, you are silent. If, therefore, my remedy is found to be no less then theriac, why should it pay for the fact that it is new? Why shouldn't it be just as good as an old remedy? If you would properly reveal every poison, what is there that is not a poison? All things are poison, and nothing is without poison: the dose alone makes a thing not poison. As an example, every dish and every drink, if it is ingested over its dose, then it becomes poison; the outcome proves it. I also concede that poison is poison: but that it might for that reason be discarded? That may not be. Now since there is nothing that is not

---

5 *Arcanum*: Element that acts as a remedy.
6 Purgation was a key part of the treatment of sickness in humoral medicine, which held that an imbalance of the four humors in the body led to illness. Purging (by the use of an emetic to induce vomiting, for example) was understood to help restore that balance.
7 *Theriac*: A compound thought to act as an antidote to poison (and sometimes as a panacea); complex in composition, it often contained opium and viper flesh, from which it got its name: θηριακός means "pertaining to venomous beasts."

poison, why do you correct? Only so that the poison does no damage: if I also correct to such an extent, why then do you punish me? You know the *Argentum vivum*[8] is nothing but solely poison, and daily experience proves the same. Now you have this as a custom: you smear the sick with it, much more than a cobbler smears grease on leather; you fumigate with its cinnabar,[9] you wash with its sublimate,[10] and you do not want anyone to say that it is poison. Yet it is poison, and you force such poison into people, saying it is healthy and good, it is corrected with white lead as if it is no poison. Carry to Nuremberg for inspection what I and you write as Receipts, and see that same day who uses poison or not. For you do not know the correction of mercury, nor its dose, but you smear as much as will go on.

One thing I must make you think about: whether your Receipts, which you say are without poison, can cure epilepsy or not, or the gout or apoplexy. Or whether you, through your rose sugar cure St. Vitus's Dance[11] or lunacy, or other similar diseases? Certainly you have not done that with those, nor will you yet do it with them. It must be another thing—why would you hold it against me that I take what I must and should take, for what it is prescribed? I will let Him be responsible for that, Who has composed it thus in the creation of heaven and earth. In addition, since the art is given to us to separate two detestable things from one another, why should poison be said to exist in the first place? Look at my Receipts—is it not my first article, that the good be separated from the bad? Is this separation not my correction? Should

---

8   *Argentum vivum*: Quicksilver, or mercury, a toxic chemical element commonly used in alchemy, and which has been used in many medical contexts. Paracelsus was an early advocate for mercury as a treatment for syphilis—this earned him criticism from many, but mercury would become a dominant therapeutic (despite its danger) through the twentieth century.
9   *Cinnabar*: The bright red solid form of mercury sulfide.
10 Sublimed mercury has been heated with salt niter in a subliming pot called an aludel, and thus transformed into mercury bichloride (or corrosive sublimate), a highly toxic crystalline powder once used in preservation, photography, and as medicine (including for the treatment of syphilis).
11 *St. Vitus's Dance*: The neurological disorder Sydenham's chorea, characterized by uncontrollable movements in certain parts of the body, mainly the hands, legs, and facial muscles.

I not read and use such corrected *Arcanum*, since I can find no malice in the same, and you find even less? You criticize me for the *Vitriolum*,[12] in which there is great secrecy and more benefit than in all the tins of an Apothecary. That it is poison you cannot say. If you say it is corrosive, tell me: in what form? You must take it to that point, otherwise it is not corrosive. Can it be taken to the point of being corrosive? So then it can also be prepared as a sweetness, since they are both side by side. As the preparation is, so too it is with vitriol. And each Simplex is like the same as itself, it is brought through art in many ways into all shapes and forms just as food which stands on the table: if a human eats it, it becomes human flesh; through a dog, dog flesh, through a cat, cat flesh. It is the same with medicine, which becomes what you make of it. If it is possible to make bad from good, so it is also possible to make good from bad. No one should punish a thing who doesn't know its transmutation and who doesn't know what separation does to it. As an example take arsenic, which is one of the highest poisons, and of which a single dram[13] can kill any horse: burn it with saltpeter, and it is no longer a poison—savoring ten pounds is harmless.[14] So see what the distinction is and what the preparation does.

But one who wants to punish should first learn, so that if he punishes, he is not himself chastised. I can perceive your folly and simple-mindedness, that you don't know what you're talking about, and that you must indulge your useless mouths. I write new Receipts, because the old ones do not work. There are new diseases available that desire new Receipts. But watch for this in all my Receipts: I uniformly take what I want, provided that I take just that in which is the *Arcanum* against the disease against which I combat. And note further what I do to it: I separate that which is not *Arcanum* from that which is *Arcanum*, and

---

12 *Vitriolum*: Iron, copper, or zinc sulfate, used in alchemy and medicine.
13 *Dram*: A weight measurement of 60 grains or 1/8 ounce in the Apothecaries' System used for pharmaceutical purposes.
14 A solution of 1% potassium arsenite would come to be named Fowler's Solution, after Thomas Fowler (1736–1801), and would be used as a medicinal tonic for a range of conditions, including syphilis, chorea, and tuberculosis, despite arsenic being carcinogenic. However, simply burning arsenic and saltpeter (potassium nitrate) would not allow for much savoring: the combination explodes when ignited.

give the *Arcanum* its right dose. Now I know I surely have defended my Receipts, and you scold me for them out of your jealous hearts and present your incompetent Receipts instead. If you were of upright conscience, you would stop; but those whose heart is full, you run your mouths in excess. I set here in this work five Defenses, which if you read through them, so you will find the reasons why I make these Receipts from the same simples which you allege to be poison. Why should I pay when I establish the foundation which you don't know to see. If you were skilled in the things in which a doctor should be skilled, you would think differently. But you should realize that whatever appears for the good of the people is not a poison: the only poison is that which brings harm to people—what is not functional for people, but rather is harmful for them. This your humble Receipts can attest, since no art is considered, but just pounding, mixing, and pouring. I have hereby defended and protected myself: my Receipts are administered and applied following the order of Nature, and you yourselves don't know what you're talking about, but rather run your mouths like raging fools, recklessly and without understanding.

The Compendium of Materia Medica (*Bencao Gangmu*)*

LI SHIZHEN
(Chinese, 1518–1593)

Compiled in the late sixteenth century, the *The Compendium of Materia Medica* (*Bencao Gangmu*)[1] collects centuries of knowledge of traditional Chinese medicine. It quickly became the most important work of its kind because of its careful synthesis and revision of prior works. Its author, physician Li Shizhen, spent three decades researching and composing the manuscript, which contains more than eight hundred citations to other works in addition to Li's contributions. The work offers an encyclopedic discussion of 1,892 substances relevant to contemporary medical treatments, along with detailed illustrations and directions for mixing prescriptions. The selection and accompanying illustration concerns various kinds of leafy plants [See Illustration 2]. As you read, consider the illustrations and descriptions of the qualities and uses of each plant described.

1 *Materia medica*: Knowledge of the therapeutic properties of medicinal substances.

* Reprinted from Li Shizhen, *Bencao gamu* (Nanjing, 1596), Wellcome Collection.

[Flora]

The leaves of the trifoliate orange are similar to those of the tangerine. It has thorny branches and bears white blossom. The fruits, which are rather small, resemble citrus aurantium. The leaves are pungent in sapor[2] and warm in thermostatic character.[3] They can harmonize the center and regulate Qi,[4] and are used to treat purulent and bloody diarrhea, painful straining at stool (*liji houzhong*), etc.

The spine date plant resembles the common date. The bark is thin and soft and the wood is red. The fruits are purplish red, rounded and sharp-tasting. The stones are used in medicine: they are sweet in sapor and neutral in thermostatic character. They have the medicinal properties of replenishing and nourishing the heart and liver, calming the mind and arresting sweating, and can be used to treat debilitation-type distress (*xufan*) and insomnia, physical debility and excess sweating, etc.

The dogwood bears red fruits, which resemble spine jujube. They are acid in sapor, neutral in thermostatic character, and have the medicinal properties of replenishing essence/semen (jing) and marrow, and warming the small of the back and the knees. They can be used to treat physical debility and excess sweating, frequent micturition[5] and urinary incontinence, impotence and involuntary ejaculation, etc.

The cape jasmine (also known as *yuetao*, Canton peach) is round and thin-skinned. Those with seven to nine sides are preferred for medicine. They are gathered after frost. They are bitter in sapor and cold in thermostatic character, and have the medicinal properties of clearing

---

2   *Sapor*: Taste; according to traditional Chinese medicine, there are five primary tastes (sour, bitter, sweet, spicy, and salty) as well as bland, astringent, and aromatic. The taste is assessed along with the temperature and direction of action to help understand a substance's potential functions.
3   *Thermostatic character*: Temperature; the five main temperatures are hot, warm, neutral, cool, and cold. This relates not to the serving temperature of the food, but rather its effect on the body.
4   Traditional Chinese medicine understands health as the product of the proper circulation of *qi* (vital energy) and *xuè* (blood), and the balance of *yin* and *yang* (the opposing qualities of *qi*). In a body where these are in disharmony, illness and pain result, requiring their careful regulation.
5   *Micturition*: Urination.

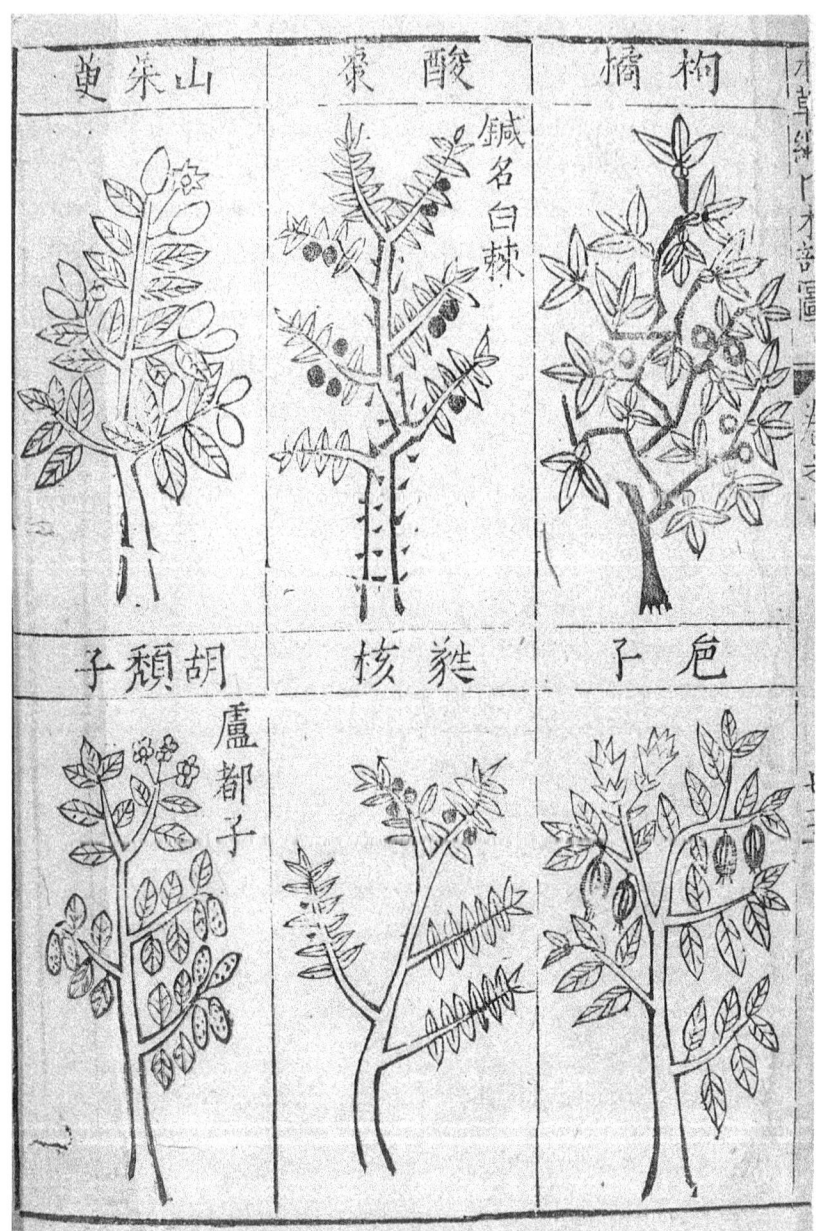

Illustration 2. Medicinally valuable flora. From top right: *Gouju* (trifoliate orange); *suanzao* (spine date); and *shanzhuyu* (dogwood). From bottom left: *zhizi* (cape jasmine, Gardenia jasminoides Ellis); *ruihe* (Prinsepia uniflora Batal.); and *hu tuizi* (Thorny Elaeagnus/Elaeagnus pungens). Reprinted from Li Shizhen, *Bencao gamu* (Nanjing, 1596), illustration by Li Jianyuan, Wellcome Collection.

heat and dispelling poisons, purging fire and relieving restlessness. They can be used to treat heat pain in the stomach, redness of the face and eyes, abscesses and ulcers, distress and oppression in the heart and chest (*xinfan xiongbi*), etc.

The prinsepia nut is round and flat, and the size of a black soya bean. The kernels are used in medicine. They are sweet in sapor, neutral in thermostatic character, and have the medicinal properties of dispelling wind and clearing heat, improving vision and removing nebula from the eye. They can be used to treat redness, pain and swelling of the eye, inflammation of the canthus[6] and watering eyes, dim vision and photophobia.

Thorny Elaeagnus (*hu tuizi*, also known as *ludouzi*) bears a small, elongated fruit similar in appearance to dogwood, with a speckled surface. It is acid in sapor and neutral in thermostatic character. The roots and leaves are used in medicine. This drug stops coughing and bleeding, soothes the throat and relieves pain. It can be used to treat coughs, asthma, coughing or vomiting blood, sore throats, etc.

---

6   *Canthus*: The outer or inner corner of the eye.

A Litany in Time of Plague*

THOMAS NASHE
(English, 1567–ca. 1601)

Cambridge-educated Thomas Nashe was a playwright, but he was also famous for his early novel *The Unfortunate Traveller* and as a prolific writer of pamphlets.[1] His "shewe" (show) *Summer's Last Will and Testament* was probably first performed in 1592 and was published in 1600. Written in England during a period when the bubonic plague, or Black Death, rippled through the country in periodic outbreaks, the work personifies the four seasons and tells us that "the plague reigns in most places in this latter end of summer." The excerpt here appears in the play following the request of the aging Summer, who asks for "some doleful ditty to the Lute / That may complain my near approaching death." It is a song often called "A Litany in Time of Plague," and sometimes also known by its first line, "Adieu, farewell earth's bliss." As you read, consider the narrator's approach to human mortality.

[1] Pamphlets, or short, unbound printed texts, were commonly composed during the early modern period in order to debate contemporary social, religious, or political issues. Sometimes these debates were lengthy and quite heated, breaking out into what were called "Pamphlet Wars" involving two or more impassioned authors.

---

* Reprinted from Thomas Nashe, *A Pleasant Comedie, called Summers last will and Testament* (London: Simon Stafford for Walter Burre, 1600; Folger Shakespeare Library, 2017).

The Song

Adieu, farewell earth's bliss,
This world uncertain is,
Fond are life's lustful joys,
Death proves them all but toys,
None from his darts can fly, [5]
I am sick, I must die.
Lord have mercy on us.

Rich men, trust not in wealth,
Gold cannot buy you health,
Physic himself must fade. [10]
All things, to end are made,
The plague full swift goes high,
I am sick, I must die,
Lord have mercy on us.

Beauty is but a flower, [15]
Which wrinkles will devour,
Brightness falls from the air,
Queens have died young, and fair,
Dust hath closed Helen's Eye.
I am sick, I must die, [20]
Lord have mercy on us.

Strength stoops unto the grave,
Worms feed on Hector brave,
Swords may not fight with fate,
Earth still holds ope her gate, [25]
Come, come, the bells do cry.
I am sick, I must die,
Lord have mercy on us.

              Wit with his wantonness,
              Tasteth death's bitterness,   [30]
                Hell's executioner,
              Hath no ears for to hear,
              What vain art can reply.
                I am sick, I must die,
               Lord have mercy on us.   [35]

            Haste therefore each degree,
                To welcome destiny:
              Heaven is our heritage,
             Earth but a player's stage,
               Mount we unto the sky.   [40]
                I am sick, I must die,
               Lord have mercy on us.

A Brief Discourse of a Disease Called the Suffocation of the Mother*

EDWARD JORDEN
(English, 1569–1632)

Physician Edward Jorden composed this work in part to defend young women accused of witchcraft. In this work, he sought to distinguish between what he understood to be legitimate medical issues and the signs of demonic possession or Satanic influence. His important assertion here is that natural and medical causes are far more common than supernatural ones. The resulting work lays out a physical disorder of the uterus or womb (known also in Jorden's time as "the Mother" or "Matrix") that could cause significant physical distress, sickness, and even coma. Conditions of this kind had been described for centuries and would eventually inform the problematic nineteenth-century diagnostic category of hysteria. As you read these excerpts, consider Jorden's stated reasons for writing the volume, as well his introduction to the nature of—and some symptoms caused by—the "suffocation of the mother."

---

* Reprinted from Edward Jorden, *A Briefe Discourse of a Disease Called the Suffocation of the Mother...* (London: John Windet, 1603), [The Epistle Dedicatorie], chap. 1–2. Google Books.

To the Right Worshipful the President and Fellows of the College of Physicians in London.

As I am desirous to satisfy all indifferent men concerning the occasion and intent of this my discourse: so I thought good to direct the same especially unto this Society,[1] whereof I am a member, to testify how justly or rather necessarily I have been drawn to the undertaking and publishing hereof: as also how willing I am to submit my self to your learned censure; the argument of my writing being such as none can better judge of then yourselves....

Being a physician, and judging in my conscience that these matters have been mistaken by the common people; I thought good to make known the doctrine of this disease, so far forth as may be in vulgar tongue conveniently disclosed, to the end that the unlearned and rash conceits of diverse [individuals], might be thereby brought to better understanding and moderation; who are apt to make every thing a supernatural work which they do not understand,[2] proportioning the bounds of nature unto their own capacities: which might prove and occasions of abusing the name of God, and make us to use holy prayer as ungroundedly as the Papists[3] do their profane tricks; who are ready to draw forth their wooden dagger, if they do but see a maid or woman suffering one the these fits of the Mother,[4] conjuring, and exorcising them as if they were possessed with evil spirits. And for want of work, will oftentimes suborn others that are in health, to counterfeit strange motions and behaviors: as I once saw in the Santo in Padua[5] five or six at one sermon interrupting and reviling

---

1 *This Society*: The Royal College of Physicians, England's oldest professional organization for physicians, was founded in 1518 under Henry VIII, and was responsible for licensing physicians in London. A license signaled that a (male) physician had a classical university education and medical degree.
2 That is, those who assume that there is a supernatural cause for anything they can't themselves explain.
3 *Papists*: A pejorative term for Catholics.
4 *Fits of the Mother*: The condition the book addresses; "The Mother" is one of a range of terms used to refer to the womb or uterus.
5 *Santo in Padua*: The Basilica of Saint Anthony, in Padua, Italy.

the Preacher, until he had put them to silence by the sign of the Cross, and certain powerless spells.

Wherefore it behooves us to be zealous in the truth, so to be wise in discerning truth from counterfeiting and natural causes from supernatural power. I do not deny but that God does in these days work extraordinarily, for the deliverance of his children and for other ends best known unto himself; and that among other, there may be both possessions by the Devil, and obsessions and witchcraft, &c [etc.] and dispossession also through the Prayers and supplications of his servants, which is the only means left unto us for our relief in that case. But Such examples being very rare nowadays, I would in the fear of God advise men to be very circumspect in pronouncing of a possession: both because the impostures be many, and the effects of natural diseases be strange to such as have not looked thoroughly into them.

Chapter 1

That this disease does oftentimes give occasion unto simple and unlearned people, to suspect possession, witchcraft, or some such like supernatural cause.

The passive condition of womankind is subject unto more diseases and of other sorts and natures then men are: and especially in regard of that part[6] from whence this disease which we speak of does arise. For as it has more variety of offices belonging unto it than other parts of the body have,[7] and accordingly is supplied from other parts with whatsoever it has need of for those uses: so it must needs thereby be subject unto more infirmities than other parts are: both by reason of such as are bred in the part it self, and also by reason of such as are communicated unto it from other parts, with which it has correspondence. And as those offices in their proper kinds are more excellent than other; so

---

6 *That part*: The uterus.
7 The author here argues that the uterus serves more purposes and has more functions than do other body parts.

the diseases whereby they are hurt or depraved, are more grievous. But among all the diseases whereunto that sex is obnoxious,[8] there is none comparable unto this which is called The Suffocation of the mother, either for variety, or for strangeness of accidents….

And hereupon the symptoms of this disease are said to be monstrous and terrible to behold, and of such variety as they can hardly be comprehended within any method or bounds. Insomuch as they which are ignorant of the strange affects which natural causes may produce, and of the manifold examples which our possession of Physic[9] does minister in this kind, have sought above the Moon for supernatural causes: ascribing these accidents either to diabolical possession, to witchcraft, or to the immediate finger of the Almighty.

Chapter 2

What this disease is, and by what means it causes such variety of symptoms.

This disease is called by diverse names among our authors. *Passio Hysterica*,[10] *Suffocatio, Prasocatio*, and *Strangulatus uteri, Caducus matricis*,[11] *&c.* In English the Mother, or the Suffocation of the Mother, because most commonly it takes them with choking in the throat: and it is an affect of the Mother or womb wherein the principal parts of the body by consent do suffer diversely according to the diversity of the causes and diseases wherewith the matrix is offended.[12] I call it an affect in a

---

8   *Obnoxious*: Exposed or vulnerable to harm. So here, he means "out of all the diseases which specifically harm women."
9   *Physic*: Medicine. "Physician" means "one who practices physic."
10 *Passio Hysterica*: From the Greek term for womb (ὑστέρα or *hustéra*), this essentially means "suffering caused by the uterus." There was no disorder called hysteria at this time, but by the nineteenth century the word would become associated with (mostly female) psychological neuroses.
11 *Caducus matricis*: The falling of the uterus; another term for uterus was "matrix."
12 The idea here is that the condition of the uterus directly impacts many other body parts, to a degree that depends on the specific uterine issue.

large signification to comprehend both *morbum* and *symptoma*.¹³ For sometimes it is either of them, and sometimes both. For in regard the actions of expulsion or retention in the Mother are hurt. It may be called a *symptoma in actione laesa*:¹⁴ in regard of the humor to be expelled which corrupts and putrifies to a venomous malignity. It is likewise a *Symptom in excremento uteri mutato*.¹⁵ And in regard of the perfrigeration of the Mother, and so of the whole body. It is also a *Symptom in qualitate tangibilis mutata*, not *morbus ex intemperies*:¹⁶ because it is suddenly inflicted & suddenly removed. But in regard of the rising of the Mother whereby it is sometimes drawn upwards or sidewards above his natural seat, compressing the neighbor parts, & so consequently one another.¹⁷ It may be said to be *morbus in situ*,¹⁸ in respect of the compression it self, causing suffocation and difficulty of breathing. In may be *causa morbi in forma*¹⁹ by causing coarctation²⁰ of the instruments of breathing. And sometimes these are complicated and together with a venomous vapor, arising from this corrupt humor unto diverse parts of the body, there will be an evil position of the matrix also: either because the ligaments, veins, and arteries being obstructed: by those vapors are shortened of their wonted length, and so draw up the part higher then it should be; or for that the matrix being grievously annoyed with the malignity of those vapors does contract it self and rise up by a local motion towards the midriff.

I say of the Mother or womb because although the womb many times in this disease do suffer but secondarily, yet the other parts are not

---

13 *Morbum and symptoma*: The disorder and its symptoms.
14 *Symptome in actione laesa*: Deficient action. This symptom causes "the humor to be expelled."
15 *Symptome in excremento uteri mutato*: Spoiled uterine discharge.
16 *Symptom in qualitate tangibilis mutata*, not *morbus ex intemperies*: Translated, this means that the problem is "symptomatic of a tangible change in quality," rather than being "a disorder caused by immoderation."
17 The idea that the uterus could travel around the body, wreaking havoc as it pressed against other organs, is sometimes referred to as the theory of the wandering womb, and debates about whether such a thing was possible date back to ancient Greece.
18 *Morbus in situ*: Disordering of position.
19 *Causa morbi in forma*: Disordering in form.
20 *Coarctation*: Narrowing.

affected in this disease but from the Mother: (*Radix suffocationum uterus*)[21] which finding it self annoyed by some unkind humor, either within it self, or in the vessels adjoining or belonging unto it, does by a natural instinct which is engrafted in every part of the body for his own preservation, endeavor to expel that which is offensive: in which conflict is either the passage be obstructed, or the humor inobedient or malignant, or the functions of the womb in any way depraved, the offense is communicated from whence unto the rest of the body. The principal part of the body are the seats of the three faculties, which do govern the whole body. The brain of the animal, the heart of the vital, the liver of the natural; although some other parts are plentifully endowed with some of these faculties, as the stomach, entrails, veins, spleen, &c. with natural faculties, the instruments of respiration with animal and natural. These parts are affected in this disease, and do suffer in their functions are they are diminished, depraved, or abolished, according to the nature & plenty of the humor, and the temperament and situation of the Mother: and that diversely: For sometimes the instruments of respiration alone does suffer, sometimes the heart alone, sometimes two or three faculties together, sometimes successively one after another, sometimes one part suffers both a resolution and a convulsion in the same fit, or when as it suffers in one part and not in another, as we see oftentimes sense and motion to be taken away and yet hearing to remain, the speech failing and respiration good. Sometimes respiration, sense, and motion do altogether fail, and yet the pulse remain good: So that the variety of these fits is exceeding great, wherein the principal parts of the body do suffer.

---

21 *Radix suffocationem uterus*: The uterus is the root of the suffocation.

Devotions upon Emergent Occasions*

JOHN DONNE
(English, 1572–1631)

Poet John Donne was also a prolific sermon-writer and respected member of the Church of England, who became the Dean of Saint Paul's Cathedral in London in 1621. In 1623, Donne became very sick, and worried he might die. *Devotions upon Emergent Occasions* was completed after his recovery, and published in 1624. The work may be one of the earliest detailed first-person accounts of an extended sickness in English, making it an excellent example of autopathography, or the autobiographical writing of an individual's sickness. *Devotions* follows Donne's experience over twenty-three devotions, each corresponding to a single day in his illness. Each devotion is divided into three smaller sections: a Meditation, an Expostulation, and a Prayer.[1] The excerpts come from the Meditations, which Donne uses to contemplate both "our human condition" and his own individual experience of sickness. As you read, consider Donne's descriptions of the physical and emotional responses to illness and mortality.

---

1 This structure has led many scholars to suggest that the work has been influenced by the Jesuit meditative tradition and by works such as the 1548 *Spiritual Exercises* by Saint Ignatius Loyola (1491–1556), which encouraged spiritual engagement in three stages.

---

* Reprinted from John Donne, *Devotions upon Emergent Occasions, and severall steps in my Sicknes* (London: A. M. for Thomas Jones, 1624; Project Gutenberg, 2007), 7–9, 23–25, 30–32, 35–37, 102–3.

Meditation 1: Insultus Morbi Primus.
The first Alteration, the first Grudging of, the Sickness.

Variable, and therefore miserable condition of Man; this minute I was well, and am ill, this minute. I am surprised with a sudden change, and alteration to worse, and can impute[2] it to no cause, nor call it by any name. We study Health, and we deliberate upon our meats, and drink, and air, and exercises, and we hew, and we polish every stone, that goes to that building; and so our Health is a long and regular work. But in a minute a Cannon batters all, overthrows all, demolishes all; a Sickness unprevented for all our diligence, unsuspected for all our curiosity; nay, undeserved, if we consider only disorder, summons us, seizes us, possesses us, destroys us in an instant.

O miserable condition of Man, which was not imprinted by God, who, as He is immortal Himself, had put a coal, a beam of Immortality into us, which we might have blown into a flame, but blew it out by our first sin; we beggared[3] ourselves by hearkening after false riches, and infatuated ourselves by hearkening after false knowledge. So that now, we do not only die, but die upon the Rack, die by the torment of sickness; nor that only, but are pre-afflicted, super-afflicted with these jealousies and suspicions and apprehensions of Sickness, before we can call it a sickness: we are not sure we are ill; one hand asks the other by the pulse, and our eye asks our own urine, how we do.

O multiplied misery! we die, and cannot enjoy death, because we die in this torment of sickness; we are tormented with sickness and cannot stay till the torment come, but pre-apprehensions and presages[4] prophesy those torments, which induce that death before either come; and our dissolution is conceived in these first changes, quickened in the sickness itself, and born in death, which bears date from these first changes.

Is this the honor which Man has by being a little world,[5] that he has

---

2   *Impute*: Assign, ascribe.
3   *Beggared*: Reduced to poverty.
4   *Presages*: Visions, prophecies.
5   *The honor which Man has by being a little world*: Describing the human body as a little world, or microcosm, was common; this image (sometimes also a philosophical and scientific idea) suggests that humankind represents, in miniature, all the

these earthquakes in himself, sudden shakings; these lightnings, sudden flashes; these thunders, sudden noises; these Eclipses, sudden obfuscations, and darkenings of his senses; these Blazing stars, sudden fiery exhalations; these Rivers of blood, sudden red waters?[6] Is he a world to himself only therefore, that he has enough in himself, not only to destroy, and execute himself, but to presage that execution upon himself; to assist the sickness, to antedate the sickness, to make the sickness the more irremediable by sad apprehensions, and as if he would make a fire the more vehement, by sprinkling water upon the coals, so to wrap a hot fever in cold Melancholy, lest the fever alone should not destroy fast enough, without this contribution, nor perfect the work (which is destruction) except[7] we joined an artificial sickness of our own melancholy, to our natural, our unnatural fever.

O perplexed discomposition,[8] O riddling distemper, O miserable condition of Man!

Meditation 4: Medicusque vocatur. *The Physician is sent for.*

It is too little to call Man a little World; Except God, Man is a diminutive to nothing. Man consists of more pieces, more parts, than the world than the world does; nay, than the world is. And if those pieces were extended, and stretched out in Man, as they in the world, Man would be the Giant, and the World the Dwarf, the World but the Map, and the Man the World. If all the Veins in our bodies were extended to Rivers, and all the Sinews, to Veins of Mines, and all the Muscles that lie upon one another, to Hills, and all the Bones to Quarries of stones, and all the other pieces, to the proportion of those which correspond to them in the world, Air would be too little for this Orb of Man to move in, the firmament[9] would be but enough for this Star....

---

    patterns of the cosmos and was used to draw both metaphorical and literal parallels between humans and the larger world or universe.
6 *Waters*: Urine.
7 *Except*: Unless.
8 *Discomposition*: Inconsistency.
9 *Firmament*: The heavens or outer space.

Enlarge this Meditation upon this great world, Man, so far as to consider the immensity of the creatures this world produces. Our creatures are our thoughts, creatures that are borne Giants; that reach from East to West, from Earth to Heaven, that do not only bestride all the Sea, and Land, but span the Sun and Firmament at once. My thoughts reach all, comprehend all. Inexplicable mystery: I their Creator am in a close prison, in a sick bed; any where, and any one of my Creatures, my thoughts, is with the Sun, and beyond the Sun—overtakes the Sun, and overgoes the Sun in one pace, one step, everywhere.

And then as the other world produces Serpents and Vipers, malignant and venomous creatures, and Worms and Caterpillars that endeavor to devour that world which produces them, and Monsters compiled and complicated of diverse parents, and kinds, so this world, ourselves, produces all these in us, in producing diseases, and sicknesses, of all those sort; venomous, and infectious diseases, feeding and consuming diseases, and manifold and entangled diseases, made up of many several ones. And can the other world name so many venomous, so many consuming, so many monstrous creatures, as we can diseases, of all these kinds? O miserable abundance, O beggarly riches! How much do we lack of having remedies for every disease, when as yet we have not names for them?

But we have a Hercules against these Giants, these Monsters: that is, the Physician. He musters up all the forces of the other world, to succour this, all Nature to relieve Man. We have the Physician, but we are not the Physician. Here we shrink in our proportion, sink in our dignity, in respect of very mean creatures who are Physicians to themselves. The Hart that is pursued and wounded, they say, knows an Herb, which being eaten, throws off the arrow: A strange kind of vomit. The dog that pursues it, though he be subject to sickness even proverbially, knows his grass that recovers him. And it may be true, that the Drugger is as near to Man, as to other creatures, it may be that obvious and present Simples, easy to be had, would cure him; but the Apothecary is not so near him, nor the Physician so near him, as they two are to other creatures.

Man has not that innate instinct, to apply these natural medicines to his present danger, as those inferior creatures have; he is not his own Apothecary, his own Physician, as they are. Call back therefore thy Meditation again, and bring it down; what's become of man's great extent and proportion, when himself shrinks himself, and consumes himself to a handful of dust? What's become of his soaring thoughts, his compassing thoughts, when himself brings himself to the ignorance, to the thoughtlessness of the Grave? His diseases are his own, but the Physician is not; he has them at home, but he must send for the Physician.

Meditation 5: Solus adest. *The Physician comes.*

As Sickness is the greatest misery, so the greatest misery of sickness is solitude. When the infectiousness of the disease deters them, who should assist from coming; even the Physician dares scarce come. Solitude is a torment which is not threatened in hell it self. Mere vacuities[10] the first Agent, God, the first instrument of God, Nature, will not admit; Nothing can be utterly empty, but so near a degree towards Vacuity, as Solitude, to be but one, they love not. When I am dead, and my body might infect, they have a remedy, they may bury me; but when I am but sick, and might infect, they have no remedy but their absence and my solitude. It is an excuse to them that are great, and pretend, and yet are loath to come. It is an inhibition to those who would truly come, because they may be made instruments, and pestiducts[11] to the infection of others, by their coming. And it is an Outlawry, an Excommunication upon the Patient, and separates him from all offices not only of Civility, but of working Charity. A long sickness will weary friends at last, but a pestilential sickness averts them from the beginning....

That is a disease of the mind; as the height of an infectious disease of the body, is solitude, to be left alone. For this makes an infectious bed equal, nay worse, than a grave, that though in both I be equally alone, in my bed I know it, and feel it, and shall not in my grave: and this too, that in my bed, my soul is still in an infectious body, and shall not in my grave be so.

---

10   *Vacuities*: Empty spaces, vacuums.
11   *Pestiducts*: Things that transmit or carry infection.

Meditation 6: Metuit. *He is afraid.*[12]

I observe the Physician with the same diligence as he the disease. I see he fears, and I fear with him; I overtake him, I overrun him in his fear, and I go the faster, because he makes his pace slow. I fear the more, because he disguises his fear, and I see it with the more sharpness, because he would not have me see it. He knows that his fear shall not disorder the practice, and exercise of his Art, but he knows that my fear may disorder the effect, and working of his practice. As the ill affections of the spleen complicate and mingle themselves with every infirmity of the body, so does fear insinuate it self in every action, or passion of the mind.

And as the wind[13] in the body will counterfeit any disease and seem the stone, and seem the Gout, so fear will counterfeit any disease of the Mind: It shall seem love, a love of having, and it is but a fear: a jealous and suspicious fear of losing. It shall seem valor in despising, and undervaluing danger, and it is but fear, in an overvaluing of opinion, and estimation, and a fear of losing that. A man that is not afraid of a Lion is afraid of a Cat; not afraid of starving, and yet is afraid of some joint of meat at the table presented to feed him; not afraid of the sound of Drums, and Trumpets, and Shot, and those which they seek to drown (the last cries of men), and is afraid of some particular harmonious instrument; so much afraid, as that with any of these the enemy might drive this man, otherwise valiant enough, out of the field.

I know not what fear is, nor I know not what it is that I fear now. I fear not the hastening of my death, and yet I do fear the increase of the disease. I should belie Nature if I should deny that I feared this, and if I should say that I feared death, I should belie God. My weakness is from Nature, who has but her Measure; my strength is from God, who possesses and distributes infinitely. As then every cold air is not a dampness, every shivering is not a stupefaction, so every fear is not a fearfulness, every declination is not a running away, every debating

---

12 *He is afraid:* The pronoun is ambiguous; it's not clear whether "He" is Donne or the Doctor.
13 *The wind:* Gas.

is not a resolving, every wish that it were not thus is not a murmuring, nor a dejection though it be thus; but as my Physician's fear puts not him from his practice, neither does mine put me, from receiving from God, and Man, and myself spiritual, and civil, and moral assistance and consolations.

Meditation 16: Et properare meum clamant,
et Turre propinqua, Obstreperae Campanae aliorum
in funere, funus.
Front the Bells of the Church adjoining,
I am daily remembered of my burial in the funerals of others.

…I have lain near a Steeple, in which there are said to be more than thirty Bells; And near another, where there is one so big, as that the Clapper is said to weigh more than six hundred pounds, yet never so affected as here. Here the Bells can scarce solemnize the funeral of any person, but that I knew him, or knew that he was my Neighbor: we dwelt in houses near to one another before, but now he is gone into that house, into which I must follow him. There is a way of correcting the Children of great persons, that other Children are corrected in their behalf, and in their names, and this works upon them, who indeed had more deserved it. And when these Bells tell me, that now one, and now another is buried, must not I acknowledge, that they have the correction due to me, and paid the debt that I owe?…

We scarce hear of any man preferred but we think of our selves, that we might very well have been that Man. Why might not I have been that Man that is carried to his grave now? Could I fit my self, to stand, or sit in any man's place, and not to lie in any man's grave? I may lack much of the good parts of the meanest, but I lack nothing of the mortality of the weakest. They may have acquired better abilities than I, but I was borne to as many infirmities as they. To be an Incumbent by lying down in a grave, to be a Doctor by teaching Mortification by Example, by dying, though I may have seniors, others may be elder than I, yet I have proceeded apace in a good University, and gone a great way in a little time, by the furtherance of a vehement Fever.

And whomsoever these Bells bring to the ground to day, if he and I had been compared yesterday, perchance I should have been thought likelier to come to this preferment then, than he. God has kept the power of death in his own hands, lest any man should bribe death. If man knew the gain of death, the ease of death, he would solicit, he would provoke death to assist him, by any hand, which he might use. But as when men see many of their own professions preferred, it ministers a hope that that may light upon them; so when these hourly Bells tell me of so many funerals of men like me, it presents, if not a desire that it may, yet a comfort whensoever mine shall come.

Meditation 17: *Nunc lento sonitu dicunt, Morieris.*
Now, this Bell tolling softly for another, says to me, "Thou must die."

Perchance he for whom this Bell tolls, may be so ill, as that he knows not it tolls for him. And perchance I may think myself so much better than I am, as that they who are about me, and see my state, may have caused it to toll for me, and I know not that. The Church is catholic, universal, so are all her actions. All that she does, belongs to all. When she baptizes a child, that action concerns me; for that child is thereby connected to that Head which is my Head too, and engrafted into[14] that body, whereof I am a member. And when she buries a Man, that action concerns me: All mankind is of one Author, and is one volume. When one Man dies, one Chapter is not torn out of the book, but translated into a better language, and every Chapter must be so translated. God employs several translators: some pieces are translated by age, some by sickness, some by war, some by justice. But God's hand is in every translation, and his hand shall bind up all our scattered leaves again, for that Library where every book shall lie open to one another: As therefore the Bell that rings to a Sermon, calls not upon the Preacher only, but upon the Congregation to come....

No man is an Island, entire of it self; every man is a piece of the

---

14 *Engrafted into*: Grafted onto, as gardeners do with plants.

Continent, a part of the main; if a Clod be washed away by the Sea, Europe is the less as well as if a Promontory[15] were, as well as if a Manor of thy friends or of thine own were. Any man's death diminishes me, because I am involved in Mankind. And therefore never send to know for whom the bell tolls: It tolls for thee. Neither can we call this a begging of Misery or a borrowing of Misery, as though we were not miserable enough of our selves, but must fetch in more from the next house, in taking upon us the Misery of our Neighbors. Truly it were an excusable covetousness if we did; for affliction is a treasure, and scarce any man has enough of it. No man has affliction enough that is not matured, and ripened by it, and made fit for God by that affliction....

Meditation 19: Oceano tandem emenso, aspicienda resurgit Terra; vident, justis, medici, jam cocta mederi se posse, indiciis.
At last, the Physicians, after a long and stormy voyage, see land; They have so good signs of the concoction of the disease, as that they may safely proceed to purge.

All this while the Physicians themselves have been patients, patiently attending when they should see any land in this Sea, any earth, any cloud, any indication of concoction in these waters. Any disorder of mine, any pretermission[16] of theirs, exalts the disease, accelerates the rages of it; no diligence accelerates the concoction, the maturity of the disease; they must stay till the season of the sickness come, and till it be ripened of it self, and then they may put to their hand, to gather it before it fall off, but they cannot hasten the ripening.

Why should we look for it in a disease, which is the disorder, the discord, the irregularities the commotion, and rebellion of the body? It were scarce a disease, if it could be ordered, and made obedient to our times. Why should we look for that in disorder, in a disease, when we cannot have it in Nature, who is so regular, and so pregnant, so forward

---

15 *Promontory*: An elevated land mass that projects out over a lowland or over water.
16 *Pretermission*: Omission; the act of leaving something out.

to bring her work to perfection, and to light? Yet we cannot awake the July-flowers in January, nor retard the flowers of the spring to autumn. We cannot bid the fruits come in May, nor the leaves to stick on in December. A woman that is weak cannot put off her ninth month to a tenth for her deliveries and say she will stay till she be stronger; nor a Queen cannot hasten it to a seventh, that she may be ready for some other pleasure. Nature (if we look for durable and vigorous effects) will not admit preventions, nor anticipations, nor obligations upon her; for they are precontracts, and she will be left to her liberty. Nature would not be spurred, nor forced to mend her pace; nor power, the power of man; greatness loves not that kind of violence neither.

There are of them that will give, that will do justice, that will pardon, but they have their own seasons for all these, and he that knows not them shall starve before that gift comes, and ruin, before the justice, and die before the pardon save him: some tree bears no fruit, except much dung be laid about it; and Justice comes not from some, till they be richly manured: some trees require much visiting, much watering, much labor; and some men give not their fruits but upon importunity; some trees require incision, and pruning, and lopping; some men must be intimidated and syndicated with Commissions, before they will deliver the fruits of Justice; some trees require the early and the often access of the Sun; some men open not but upon the favors and letters of Court mediation; some trees must be housed and kept within doors; some men lock up, not only their liberality, but their Justice, and their compassion, till the solicitation of a wife, or a son, or a friend, or a servant turns the key. Reward is the season of one man, and importunity[17] of another; fear the season of one man, and favor of another; friendship the season of one man, and natural affection of another; and he that knows not their seasons, nor cannot stay them, must lose the fruits.

As Nature will not, so power and greatness will not be put to change their seasons; and shall we look for this Indulgence in a disease, or think to shake it off before it be ripe? All this while, therefore, we are but upon a defensive war, and that is but a doubtful state; especially where they who are besieged do know the best of their defenses, and do not know

---

17 *Importunity*: Begging or persistent solicitation.

the worst of their enemies power; when they cannot mend their works within, and the enemy can increase his numbers without.

O how many far more miserable, and far more worthy to be less miserable than I, are besieged with this sickness, and lack their Sentinels, their Physicians to watch, and lack their munition, their cordials to defend, and perish before the enemies weakness might invite them to sally, before the disease shows any declination, or admit any way of working upon itself! In me the siege is so far slackened, as that we may come to fight, and so die in the field, if I die, and not in a prison.

Meditation 22: Sit morbi fomes tibi cura.
The Physicians consider the root and occasion, the embers, and coals, and fuel of the disease, and seek to purge or correct that.

How ruinous a farm has man taken, in taking himself! How ready is the house every day to fall down, and how is all the ground overspread with weeds, all the body with diseases! where not only every turf, but every stone, bears weeds; not only every muscle of the flesh, but every bone of the body, has some infirmity; every little flint upon the face of this soil, has some infectious weed, every tooth in our head, such a pain as a constant man is afraid of, and yet ashamed of that fear, of that sense of the pain. How dear, and how often a rent does Man pay for this farm! He pays twice a day, in double meals, and how little time he has to raise his rent! How many holy days to call him from his labor! Every day is half-holy day, half spent in sleep. What reparations, and subsidies, and contributions he is put to, besides his rent! What medicines, besides his diet! and what Inmates he is fain to take in, besides his own families what infectious diseases, from other men! Adam might have had Paradise for dressing and keeping it; and then his rent was not improved to such a labor, as would have made his brow sweat; and yet he gave it over; how far greater a rent do we pay for this farm, this body, who pay ourselves, who pay the farm itself, and cannot live upon it!

Meditation 23: Metusque, relabi.
They warn me of the fearful danger of relapsing.

It is not in man's body, as it is in the City, that when the Bell has rung, to cover your fire, and rake up the embers, you may lie down and sleep without fear. Though you have by physic and diet, raked up the embers of your disease, still there is a fear of a relapse; and the greater danger is in that. Even in pleasures, and in pains, there is a propriety, a *Meum* and *Tuum*;[18] and a man is most affected with that pleasure which is his, his by former enjoying and experience, and most intimidated with those pains which are his, his by a woeful sense of them, in former afflictions. A covetous person, who has preoccupated[19] all his senses, filled all his capacities, with the delight of gathering, wonders how any man can have any taste of any pleasure in any openness, or liberality. So also in bodily pains, in a fit of the stone, the Patient wonders why any man should call the Gout a pain. And he that has felt neither, but the toothache is as much afraid of a fit of that, as either of the other, of either of the other....

It adds to the affliction, that relapses are, (and for the most part justly) imputed to our selves, as occasioned by some disorder in us; and so we are not only passive, but active, in our own ruin; we do not only stand under a falling house, but pull it down upon us; and we are not only executed, (that implies guiltiness) but we are executioners, (that implies dishonor) and executioners of our selves, (and that implies impiety). And we fall from that comfort which we might have in our first sickness, from that meditation, Alas, how generally miserable is Man, and how subject to diseases, (for in that it is some degree of comfort, that we are but in the state common to all) we fall, I say, to this discomfort, and self accusing, and self condemning. Alas, how unprovident, and in that, how unthankful to God and his instruments am I, in making so ill use of so great benefits, in destroying so soon, so long a work, in relapsing, by my disorder, to that from which they had delivered me; and so my meditation is fearfully transferred from the body to the mind,

---

18 *Meum and Tuum*: Mine and yours, in Latin.
19 *Preoccupated*: Preoccupied.

and from the consideration of the sickness to that sin, that sinful carelessness by which I have occasioned my relapse.

And amongst the many weights that aggravate a relapse, this also is one: that a relapse proceeds with a more violent dispatch, and more irremediably, because it finds the Country weakened, and depopulated before. Upon a sickness which as yet appears not, we can scarce fix a fear, because we know not what to fear; but as fear is the busiest, and irksomest affection, so is a relapse (which is still ready to come) into that, which is but newly gone, the nearest object, the most immediate exercise of that affection of fear.

Poems on Sickness and Death*

JOHN DONNE
(English, 1572–1631)

Although most of his poetry was circulated only in manuscript form during his lifetime, John Donne is now often seen as the predominant metaphysical poet of the seventeenth century. The term "metaphysical" originated late in the eighteenth century with English writer and critic Samuel Johnson, and the designation is given to poets who heavily employ metaphor, paradox, and intricacy in the exploration of philosophical or spiritual topics. Included here are two poems that deal in particular with the experience of sickness and mortality. One is a well-known sonnet concerned with human mortality that is part of a series of nineteen poems, called the *Holy Sonnets*. Sonnets are fourteen-line poems that follow carefully defined poetic structures and rhyme schemes, and are most often associated with human desire or romantic love. The other selection is a poem that may have been composed just days before Donne died in 1631 and is structured in six stanzas of five lines each (called quintains). As you read, consider how the poems approach human mortality.

---

* Reprinted from *Poems &c. by John Donne, late dean of St. Pauls*. (London: Printed by T. N. for Henry Herringman, 1669).

Holy Sonnets: Sonnet X (1669)

Death be not proud, though some have called thee
Mighty and dreadful, for, thou art not so,
For, those, whom thou think'st thou dost overthrow,
Die not, poor death, nor yet canst thou kill me.
From rest and sleep, which but thy picture be: [5]
Much pleasure then from thee, much more must flow,
And soonest our best men with thee do go,
Rest of their bones, and souls delivery
Thou art slave to Fate, chance, Kings, and desperate men,
And dost with poison, war and sickness dwell, [10]
And poppy, or charms can make us sleep as well,
And better than thy stroke; why swell's thou then?
One short sleep past, we wake eternally,
And death shall be no more, death thou shalt die.

Hymn to God, my God, in my sickness. (1669)

Since I am coming to that Holy room,
Where, with the Choir of Saints for evermore,
I shall be made thy Music, As I come
I tune the Instrument here at the door,
And what I must do then, think here before. [5]
Whilst my Physicians by their love are grown
Cosmographers, and I their Map, who lie
Flat on this bed, that by them may be shown
That this is my South West discovery
Per fretum febris,[1] by these straights to die. [10]
I joy, that in these straits, I see my West;
For, though those currants yield, return to none,
What shall my West hurt me? As West and East
In all flat Maps (and I am one) are one,

---

1 *Per fretum febris*: Through the strait of fever.

So death doth touch the Resurrection. [15]
Is the Pacific Sea my home; Or are
The Eastern riches? Is Jerusalem?
Anyan, and Magellan, and Gibraltar,
All straights, and none but straights are ways to them,
Whether where Japhet dwelt, or Cham or Sem. [20]
We think that Paradise and Calvary,
Christs Cross, and Adam's tree, stood in one place;
Look Lord, and find both Adams meet in me;
As the first Adam's sweat surrounds my face,
May the last Adam's blood my soul embrace. [25]
So, in his purple wrapp'd receive me Lord,
By these his thorns give me his other Crown'
And as to others souls I preached thy word,
Be this my Text, my sermon to mine own,
Therefore that he may raise the Lord throws down. [30]

On the Art of Surgery and Universal Antidotes

AMBROISE PARÉ
(French, ca. 1510–1590)

Up until the eighteenth century, surgery was seen more as a trade than an art—and often looked down upon by "learned" physicians—throughout much of Europe. It was largely taught by apprenticeship with the barber-surgeons, not university education. French barber-surgeon Ambroise Paré followed this path. Although he had no formal medical training, he nonetheless became the official royal surgeon to four French kings (Henry II, Francis II, Charles IX, and Henry III), advanced surgical knowledge on gunshot wounds and amputation, and designed early versions of surgical instruments that we still use today. Paré published works of surgery and medicine throughout his life. Compilations of these works were frequently reprinted in French, and were translated into other languages, including English. These and other contributions have earned him a place as one of the most important surgeons in European history. The selections here come from a major seventeenth-century translation of Paré's collected works by Thomas Johnson. As you read, consider his view of surgery as a practice and his investigation into the bezoar stone, thought to be a universal antidote to poison.

---

* Reprinted from Ambroise Paré, *The Workes of that famous Chirurgion Ambrose Parey Translated out of Latine and Compared with the French*, trans. Thomas Johnson (London: 1643), 3–5, 809–10, Early English Books Online Text Creation Partnership.

What Surgery Is

Surgery is an Art, which teaches the way by reason, how by the operation of the hand we may cure, prevent, and mitigate diseases, which accidentally happen unto us. Others have thought good to describe it otherwise, as that; it is that part of physic[1] which undertakes the cure of diseases by the sole industry of the hand; as by cutting, burning, sawing off, uniting fractures, restoring dislocations, and performing other works, of which we shall hereafter treat. Surgery also is thus defined by the author of the medicinal definitions; The quick motion of an intrepid hand joined with experience: or an artificial action by the hands used in physic, for some convenient intent. Yet none must think to attain to any great perfection in this art, without the help of the other two parts of physic; I say of diet and pharmacy, and the diverse application of proper medicines, respecting the condition of the causes, diseases, symptoms, and the like circumstances, which comprehended under the names of things natural, not natural, and besides nature[2] (as they commonly call them) we intend to describe in their proper place. But if any reply, that there be many which do the works of surgery, without any knowledge of such like things, who notwithstanding have cured desperate diseases with happy success; let them take this for an answer, that such things happen rather by chance, than by the industry of the art, and that they are not provident that commit themselves to such. Because that for some one happy chance, a thousand dangerous errors happen afterwards, as *Galen* (in diverse places of his *Method*)[3] speaks against the

---

1 *Physic*: Medicine. "Physician" means "one who practices physic."
2 *Things natural, not natural, and besides nature*: Galenic medicine considered the "naturals" to be those things innate to the body, such as physiology, and the "non-naturals" to be external factors to health, such as air, motion and rest (exercise), sleeping and waking, retention (food and drink), excretion, and passion (emotion). These elements could be controlled through careful regimens. Things "beside" or "against" nature were pathologies, including the diseases and their effects.
3 Greek physician Galen of Pergamon (see pp. 41–46) was one of history's most influential physicians. Galenic medicine, based in part on the theory of the four humors, was the dominant model of health for over a millennium and retained some influence until the ascent of germ theory in the late nineteenth century. The work referred to here is *De methodo medendi* ("The Method of Medicine").

Empirics.[4] Wherefore seeing we have set down surgery to be a diligent operation of the hands, strengthened by the assistance of diet and pharmacy, we will now show, what, and of what nature the operations it are.

Of Surgical Operations

Five things are proper to the duty of a surgeon; To take away that which is superfluous; to restore to their places, such things as are displaced; to separate those things which are joined together; to join those which are separated; and to supply the defects of nature. You shall fare more easily and happily attain to the knowledge of these things by long use and much exercise, than by much reading of Books, or daily hearing of Teachers. For speech how perspicuous and elegant soever it be, cannot so vividly express any thing, as that which is subjected to the faithful eyes and hands.

We have examples of taking away that which abounds, in the amputation, or cutting off a finger, if any have six on one hand, or any other monstrous member that may grow out: in the lopping off a putrefied part inwardly corrupted; in the extraction of a dead child, the secundine, mole[5] or such like bodies out of a woman's womb; in taking down of all tumors, as wens, warts, polyps, cancers, and fleshy excrescences of the like nature; in the pulling forth of bullets, of pieces of mail, of darts, arrows, shells, splinters, and of all kind of weapons in what part of the body soever they be. And he takes away that which redounds, which plucks away the hairs of the eye-lids which trouble the eye by their turning in towards it: who cuts away the web, possessing all the *Adnata*,[6] and part of the cornea: who lets forth suppurated matter; who takes out

---

4   The Empiric school of medicine prioritized practical experience over theoretical knowledge and advocated against seeking out hidden or root causes of disease in favor of working with visible symptoms. Empirics were associated with practitioners such as barber-surgeons who weren't "learned" (university trained physicians) and who prioritized observation and experiment over theory.
5   *Mole*: The product of a molar pregnancy, in which a uterine tumor develops and the placenta turns into a mass of cysts.
6   *Adnata*: Coating over the eye.

stones in what part soever of the body they grow; who pulls out a rotten or otherwise hurtful tooth, or cuts a nail that runs into the flesh; who cuts away part of the uvula, or hairs that grow on the eye-lids; who take off a Cataract; who cuts the navel or foreskin of a child newly borne, or the skinny caruncles of women's privates.[7]

Examples of placing those things which are out of their natural site, are manifest in restoring dislocated bones; in replacing of the guts and caul[8] fallen into the cods,[9] or out of the navel or belly by a wound, or of the falling down of the womb, fundament,[10] or great gut, or the eye hanging out of its circle, or proper place.

But we may take examples of disjoining those things which are continued from the fingers growing together, either by some chance, as burning, or by the imbecility of the forming faculty: by the disjunction of the membrane called hymen, or any other troubling the neck of the womb, by the dissection of the ligament of the tongue, which hinders children from sucking and speaking, and of that which hinders the glans from being uncovered of the foreskin; by the division of a varicose vein, or of a half cut nerve or tendon, causing convulsion: by the division of the membrane stopping the auditory passage, the nose, mouth, or fundament, or the stubborn sticking together of the hairs of the eye-lids. Refer to this place all the works done by caustics, the Saw, Trepan, Lancet, Cupping glasses, Incision Knife, Leeches, either for evacuation, derivation or revulsion sake.

The surgeon draws together things separated, which heals wounds by stitching them, by bolstering, binding, giving rest to, and sit placing the part: which repairs fractures; restores luxated[11] parts; who by binding the vessel, stays the violent effusion of blood: who cicatrises[12] cloven lips, commonly called hare-lips; who reduces to equality the cavities of ulcers, and fistulas.

But he repairs those things which are defective, either from the

---

7   *Urethral caruncles*: Common, benign tumors in females.
8   *Caul*: The fatty membrane around the intestines.
9   *Cods*: The scrotum and testicles in males or the ovaries in females.
10 *Fundament*: The rectum.
11 *Luxated*: Dislocated.
12 *Cicatrises*: To heal by inducing the formation of scar tissue.

infancy, or afterwards by accident, as much as Art and Nature will suffer, who sets on an ear, an eye, a nose, one or more teeth; who fills the hollowness of the palate eaten by the Pox, with a thin plate of gold or silver, or such like;[13] who supplies the defect of the tongue in part cut off, by some new addition; who fastens to a hand, an arm or leg with fit ligaments workmanlike: who fits a doublet bombasted,[14] or made with iron plates to make the body straight; who fills a shoe too big with cork, or fastens a stocking or sock to a lame man's girdle to help his gait. We will treat more fully of all these in our following work. But in performing those things with the hands, we cannot but cause pain: (for who can without pain cut off an arm, or leg, divide and tear asunder the neck of the bladder, restore bones put out of their places, open ulcers, bind up wounds, and apply cauteries, and do such like?) notwithstanding the matter often comes to that pass, that unless we use a judicious hand, we must either die, or lead the remnant of our lives in perpetual misery. Who therefore can justly abhor a surgeon for this, or accuse him of cruelty? or desire they may be served, as in ancient times the Romans served Archagatus,[15] who at the first made him free of the City, but presently after, because he did somewhat too cruelly burn, cut and perform the other works of a good surgeon, they drew him from his house into the Campus Martius and there stoned him to death, as we have read it recorded by Sextus Cheroneus Plutarch's[16] niece by his daughter. Truly it was an inhumane kind of ingratitude, so cruelly to murder a man intent to the works of so necessary an art. But the Senate could not approve the act, wherefore to expiate the crime as well as then they could, they made his statue in gold, placed it in Aesculapius[17] his Temple and

---

13 The tertiary stage of syphilis can lead to the tissue of the soft palate and septum to be destroyed. Sufferers often had prosthetics made to cover the damage.
14 *A doublet bombasted*: A jacket padded with a soft material like cotton.
15 *Archagatus*: The Peloponnesian surgeon Archagathus (fl. 219 BCE), who was reportedly the first to establish the practice of surgery as a profession in Rome.
16 *Sextus Cheroneus Plutarche*: More commonly known as Plutarch (46–119 CE), this Greek historian and philosopher wrote biographies of significant Greeks and Romans.
17 *Aesculapius*: Asclepius, Greek god of medicine and son of Apollo (god of the Sun, music, poetry, and healing).

dedicated it to his perpetual memory. For my part I very well like that saying of Celsus;[18] A surgeon must have a strong, stable, and intrepid hand, and a mind resolute and merciless, so that to heal him he takes in hand, he be not moved to make more haste than the thing requires; or to cut less than is needful; but which does all things as if he were nothing affected with their cries; not giving heed to the judgment of the vain common people, who speak ill of surgeons because of their ignorance.

Of Bezoar, and Bezoartic Medicines

...An Antidote or Counterpoison is by the Arabians in their mother tongue termed Bedezahar, as the preservers of life. This word is unknown to the Greeks and Latins, and in use only with the Arabians and Persians, because the thing it self first came from them, as it is plainly shewed by *Garcias ab horto,* Physician to the Vice-Roy of the Indies, in his history of the Spices and Simples of the East-Indies. In Persia (says he) and a certain part of India is a certain kind of goat called Pazain (wherefore in proper speaking, the stone should be termed Pazar, of the word Pazain, that signifies a goat; but we corruptly term it Bezar or Bezoar[19]) the color of this beast is commonly reddish, the height thereof indifferent, in whose stomach concretes the stone called Bezoar; it grows by little and little about a straw or some such like substance in scales like to the scales of an onion, so that when as the first scale is taken off, the next appears more smooth and shining as you still take them away, the which among others is the sign of good Bezoar and not adulterate. This stone is found in sundry shapes, but commonly it resembles an acorn or date-stone; it is sometimes of a sanguine color,[20] and other-whiles of a honey-like or yellowish color, but most frequently of a blackish or dark green, resembling the color of mad apples, or else

---

18 *Celsus*: Aulus Cornelius Celsus (ca. 25 BCE–ca. 50 CE), author of the ancient Roman medical encyclopedia *De Medicina.*
19 *Bezoar*: Indigestible masses of calcified matter formed around a foreign substance, and found in the stomach or intestines of some animals.
20 *Sanguine color*: Reddish brown, akin to dried blood.

of a civet cat. This stone has no heart nor kernel in the midst, but powder in the cavity thereof, which is also of the same faculty. Now this stone is light, & not very hard, but so that it may easily be scraped, or rasped like alabaster, so that it will dissolve, being long macerated in water; at first it was common among us, and of no very great price, because our people who trafficked in Persia, bought it at an easy rate. But after that the faculties thereof were found out, it began to bee more rare and dear, and it was prohibited by an edict from the King of the country, that no body should sell a goat to the stranger merchants, unless he first killed him, and took forth the stone, & brought it to the King. Of the notes by which this stone is tried, (for there are many counterfeits brought hither) the first is already declared; the other is, it may be blown up by the breath, like an ox's hide; for if the wind break through, and do not stay in the density thereof, it is accounted counterfeit....

Some years ago a certain gentleman, who had one of these stones which he brought out of Spain, bragged before King *Charles*[21] then being at Clermont in Auverne, of the most certain efficacy of this stone against all manner of poisons. Then the King asked of me, whether there were any antidote which was equally and in like manner prevalent against all poisons? I answered, that nature could not admit it; for neither have all poisons the like effects, neither do they arise from one cause; for some work from an occult and specific property of their whole nature, others from some elementary quality which is predominant. Wherefore each must be withstood with its proper and contrary Antidote, as to the hot, that which is cold, and to that which assails by an occult propriety of form, another which by the same force may oppugn it, and that it was an easy matter to make trial hereof on such as were condemned to be hanged. The motion pleased the King; there was a cook brought by the jailer who was to have been hanged within a while after for stealing two silver dishes out of his master's house. Yet the King desired first to know of him, whether he would take the poison on this condition, that if the antidote which was predicated to have singular power against all manner of poisons, which should be presently given him after the poison, should free him from death, that then he should have his life saved. The

---

21 *King Charles*: French monarch Charles IX, lived 1550–1574, reigned 1560–1574.

cook answered cheerfully, that he was willing to undergo the hazard, yea, and greater matters, not only for to save his life, but to shun the infamy of the death he was like to be adjudged to. Therefore he then had poison given him by the apothecary that then waited, and presently after the poison, some of the Bezahar brought from Spain, which being taken down, within a while after he began to vomit, and to avoid much by stool with grievous torments, and to cry out that his inward parts were burnt with fire. Wherefore, being thirsty, and desiring water, they gave it him; an hour after, with the good leave of the jailer, I was admitted to him; I find him on the ground going like a beast upon hands and feet, with his tongue thrust forth of his mouth, his eyes fiery, vomiting, with store of cold sweats, and lastly, the blood flowing forth by his ears, nose, mouth, fundament and yard. I gave him eight ounces of oil to drink, but it did him no good, for it came too late. Wherefore at length he died with great torment and exclamation, the seventh hour from the time that he took the poison being scarcely passed. I opened his body in the presence of the jailer and four others, and I found the bottom of his stomach black and dry, as if it had been burnt with a cautery; whereby I understood he had sublimate[22] given him; whose force the Spanish Bezahar could not repress, wherefore the King commanded to burn it.

---

22 *Sublimate*: Likely a reference to corrosive sublimate, or mercuric chloride, a toxic chemical compound used as a medical treatment (especially in the treatment of syphilis) until the development of modern antibiotics.

Theories of Circulation and Reproduction*

WILLIAM HARVEY
(English, 1578–1657)

Physician William Harvey is known for his experimental and observational scientific practices, which led to several major works of anatomy and physiology. He is most famous for accurately identifying how blood circulates through the body, a discovery which he published as *On the Circulation of the Blood Heart and Blood of Animals (Exercitatio Anatomica de Motu Cordis et Sanguinis)* in 1628. The publication initially caused quite a stir, due to its rejection of prevailing belief, and his friend and biographer John Aubrey wrote that people thought he was "crack-brained; and all the physicians were against his opinion."[1] Later, in 1651, he published the seminal *On the Generation of Animals (Exercitationes de generatione animalium)*, which was later translated into English as *Anatomical Exercitations, Concerning the Generation of Living Creatures*. This new work on reproduction and embryology contradicted many previous ideas about the growth of embryos and correctly asserted that *ex ovo, omnia*, which means literally "out of the egg, everything [comes]." Included here are excerpts from each of these major works. As you read, consider his effort to observe physiological phenomena.

1 John Aubrey, *"Brief Lives": Chiefly of Contemporaries, Set Down by John Aubrey, Between the Years 1669 & 1696*, vol. 1. Ed. Andrew Clark, (Oxford: Clarendon Press, 1898), 300.

---

* "On the Circulation of the Blood in Animals" reprinted from William Harvey, *The Works of William Harvey M.D. Translated from the Latin with a life of the author*, trans. Robert Willis (London, 1847; Project Gutenberg, 2019), 64–68; "On Theories of Reproduction" reprinted from William Harvey, *Anatomical Exercitations, Concerning the Generation of Living Creatures* (London, 1653), Preface.

[On the Circulation of the Blood in Animals]

The Third Position is Confirmed: and the Circulation of the Blood is Demonstrated From It

…This I have frequently experienced in my dissections of the veins: if I attempted to pass a probe from the trunk of the veins into one of the smaller branches, whatever care I took I found it impossible to introduce it far any way, by reason of the valves; whilst, on the contrary, it was most easy to push it along in the opposite direction, from without inwards, or from the branches towards the trunks and roots. In many places two valves are so placed and fitted, that when raised they come exactly together in the middle of the vein, and are there united by the contact of their margins; and so accurate is the adaptation, that neither by the eye nor by any other means of examination can the slightest chink along the line of contact be perceived. But if the probe be now introduced from the extreme towards the more central parts, the valves, like the floodgates of a river, give way, and are most readily pushed aside. The effect of this arrangement plainly is to prevent all motion of the blood from the heart and vena cava, whether it be upwards towards the head, or downwards towards the feet, or to either side towards the arms, not a drop can pass; all motion of the blood, beginning in the larger and tending towards the smaller veins, is opposed and resisted by them; whilst the motion that proceeds from the lesser to end in the larger branches is favored, or, at all events, a free and open passage is left for it.

But that this truth may be made the more apparent, let an arm be tied up above the elbow as if for phlebotomy (A, A, fig. 1) [See Illustration 3, fig 1].

At intervals in the course of the veins, especially in laboring people and those whose veins are large, certain knots or elevations (B, C, D, E, F,) will be perceived, and this not only at the places where a branch is received (E, F), but also where none enters (C, D): these knots or risings are all formed by valves, which thus show themselves externally. And now if you press the blood from the space above one of the valves, from H to O, (fig. 2,) [See Illustration 3, fig 2] and keep the point of a finger

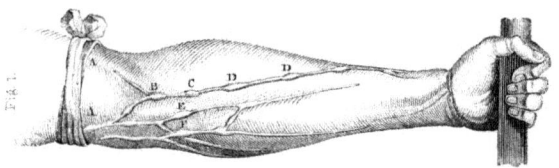

Figure 1.

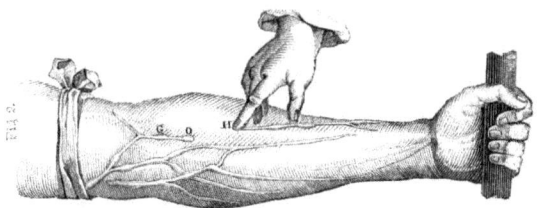

Figure 2.

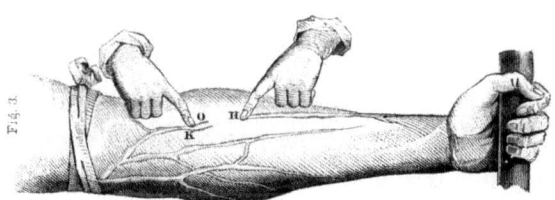

Figure 3.

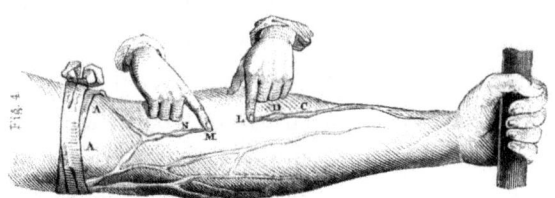

Figure 4.

Illustration 3. Visual depiction of steps in Harvey's observations regarding blood circulation[...], trans. Robert Willis (London, 1847; Project Gutenberg, 2019), 64–68.

upon the vein inferiorly, you will see no influx of blood from above; the portion of the vein between the point of the finger and the valve O will be obliterated; yet will the vessel continue sufficiently distended above that valve (O, G). The blood being thus pressed out, and the vein emptied, if you now apply a finger of the other hand upon the distended part of the vein above the valve O, (fig. 3,) [See Illustration 3, fig 3] and press downwards, you will find that you cannot force the blood through or beyond the valve; but the greater effort you use, you will only see the portion of vein that is between the finger and the valve become more distended, that portion of the vein which is below the valve remaining all the while empty (H, O, fig. 3).

It would therefore appear that the function of the valves in the veins is the same as that of the three sigmoid valves which we find at the commencement of the aorta and pulmonary artery, viz., to prevent all reflux of the blood that is passing over them.

Farther, the arm being bound as before, and the veins looking full and distended, if you press at one part in the course of a vein with the point of a finger (L, fig. 4) [See Illustration 3, fig 4], and then with another finger streak the blood upwards beyond the next valve (N), you will perceive that this portion of the vein continues empty (L N), and that the blood cannot retrograde, precisely as we have already seen the case to be in fig. 2; but the finger first applied (H, fig. 2, L, fig. 4), being removed, immediately the vein is filled from below, and the arm becomes as it appears at D C, fig. 1. That the blood in the veins therefore proceeds from inferior or more remote to superior parts, and towards the heart, moving in these vessels in this and not in the contrary direction, appears most obviously. And although in some places the valves, by not acting with such perfect accuracy, or where there is but a single valve, do not seem totally to prevent the passage of the blood from the center, still the greater number of them plainly do so; and then, where things appear contrived more negligently, this is compensated either by the more frequent occurrence or more perfect action of the succeeding valves or in some other way: the veins, in short, as they are the free and open conduits of the blood returning *to* the heart, so are they effectually prevented from serving as its channels of distribution *from* the heart.

But this other circumstance has to be noted: The arm being bound, and the veins made turgid, and the valves prominent, as before, apply the thumb or finger over a vein in the situation of one of the valves in such a way as to compress it, and prevent any blood from passing upwards from the hand; then, with a finger of the other hand, streak the blood in the vein upwards till it has passed the next valve above, (N, fig. 4,) the vessel now remains empty; but the finger at L being removed for an instant, the vein is immediately filled from below; apply the finger again, and having in the same manner streaked the blood upwards, again remove the finger below, and again the vessel becomes distended as before; and this repeat, say a thousand times, in a short space of time. And now compute the quantity of blood which you have thus pressed up beyond the valve, and then multiplying the assumed quantity by one thousand, you will find that so much blood has passed through a certain portion of the vessel; and I do now believe that you will find yourself convinced of the circulation of the blood, and of its rapid motion. But if in this experiment you say that a violence is done to nature, I do not doubt but that, if you proceed in the same way, only taking as great a length of vein as possible, and merely remark with what rapidity the blood flows upwards, and fills the vessel from below, you will come to the same conclusion.

Conclusion of the Demonstration of the Circulation

And now I may be allowed to give in brief my view of the circulation of the blood, and to propose it for general adoption.

Since all things, both argument and ocular demonstration, show that the blood passes through the lungs and heart by the action of the auricles and ventricles, and is sent for distribution to all parts of the body, where it makes its way into the veins and pores of the flesh, and then flows by the veins from the circumference on every side to the center, from the lesser to the greater veins, and is by them finally discharged into the vena cava and right auricle of the heart, and this in such a quantity or in such a flux and reflux thither by the arteries, hither by the veins, as cannot possibly be supplied by the ingesta,[2] and is much

---

2   *Ingesta*: Things that are ingested for nourishment, such as food and drink.

greater than can be required for mere purposes of nutrition; it is absolutely necessary to conclude that the blood in the animal body is impelled in a circle, and is in a state of ceaseless motion; that this is the act or function which the heart performs by means of its pulse; and that it is the sole and only end of the motion and contraction of the heart.

[On Theories of Reproduction]

The Preface

All physicians, following Galen, teach, that out of the seed of male and female mingled in coition,[3] according to the predominant power of this, or that, the child resembles either this, or that parent, and is also either male or female. And sometimes they pronounce the male's seed to be the efficient cause, and the female's the material; and sometimes again the clean contrary.

But Aristotle (Nature's most diligent searcher) affirms that the male and female are the principles of generation, and that she contributes the matter, and he the form; and that forthwith after coition, there is formed in the womb out of the menstruous blood, the vital principle, and first particle of the future fetus, (namely, the heart, in creatures that have blood.)[4]

But that these are false, and rash assertions, will soon appear; and will like clouds instantly vanish, (when the light of anatomical dissection breaks forth) nor will they require any elaborate confutation, when the reader, instructed by his own eyes, shall discover the contrary by ocular inspection; and shall also understand, how unsafe, and degenerate

---

3   Greek physician Galen (see pp. 41–46) theorized that both males and females produced semen ("seed") and that embryos developed when these two combined.

4   Greek philosopher Aristotle's (384–322 BCE) *On the Generation of Animals* (*De generatione animalium*) was the first recorded work on embryology. His theory that the embryo developed out of the combination of menstrual blood and semen was influential for centuries. Aristotle asserted that menstrual blood served as the material cause of the embryo (the matter it was actually made of) and semen served as the efficient cause (responsible for starting and shaping development).

a thing it is, to be tutored by other men's commentaries, without making trial of the things themselves: especially, since Nature's Book is so open, and legible.

I have therefore exhibited to public view, what in these my Exercitations, I intend to deliver concerning the generation of animals; not only that posterity may thence discern the certain and apparent truth; but also, and that chiefly too, that (by revealing the method I use in searching into things) I might propose to studious men, a new, and (if I mistake not) a surer path to the attainment of knowledge.

For although it be a more new and difficult way, to find out the nature of things, by the things themselves; then by reading of Books, to take our knowledge upon trust from the opinions of Philosophers: yet must it needs be confessed, that the former is much more open, and less fraudulent, especially in the secrets relating to *Natural Philosophy*....

Of the Method to Be Observed in the Knowledge of Generation

Since therefore in the generation of animals (as in all other things of which we covet to know any thing) every inquisition is to be derived from its causes, and chiefly from the material and efficient;[5] it seems fit to me, looking back on perfect animals (namely by what degrees they are begun, and completed) to retreat, as it were, from the end to the beginning: that so at last when there is no place for farther retreat, we may be confident we have arrived at the principles themselves: and then it will appear, out of what first matter, by what efficient, and what procession the plastic power has its original; and then also what progress Nature makes in this work. For both the first, and remoter matter, appears the clearer (being stripped naked as it were) by negation; and whatsoever is first made in generation, that is, as it were, the material cause of that which succeeds. So, for example, a man, was first a boy (because from a boy he grew up to be a man;) before he was a boy, he was an infant; and before an infant, an embryo.

Now we must search farther, what he was in his mother's womb,

---

5   *The material and efficient*: The matter from which something is made and what starts the process of making it.

before he was this embryo, or fetus; whether three bubbles? or some rude and undigested lump? or a conception, or coagulation of mixed seed? or whether any thing else? according to the opinion of writers.

In the same manner, before a hen or cock came to perfection, (and that is called a perfect animal, that can beget its like) there was a chicken; before that chicken, there is seen in the egg an embryo, or fetus; and before that embryo, Hieronymus Fabricius Aquapendens[6] has descried[7] the rudiments of the head, eyes, and spine of the back. But where he affirms, that the bones are made before the muscles, heart, liver, lungs, and all the viscera; and that all the inward parts ought to exist before the outward; he relies upon probability, rather than experience; and laying aside the verdict of sense, which is grounded upon dissections; he flies to petty reasonings borrowed from mechanics: which is very unbeseeming so famous an anatomist. For he ought to have told us what daily changes his own eyes had discovered in the egg, ere ever the fetus came to perfection.[8] Especially seeing he professedly wrote the *History of the Generation of the Chicken out of the Egg*; and has described in pictures what progress is made from day to day. It was, I say, befitting so much diligence, to have acquainted us from the allegation of his own sight, what things in the egg are made first, what last, and what happen together; and not to have confined himself to the example of building of ships, and houses, to render a cloudy conjecture and persuasion only, of the order, and manner of forming the parts.

We therefore (according to the method proposed) will explain, first in an egg, and afterwards in other conceptions of several creatures, what is constituted first, and what last, in a most miraculous order, & with a

---

6   *Hieronymous Fabricius Aquapendens*: Also known as Girolamo Fabrizio (1533–1619), a renowned anatomist and embryologist and Harvey's doctoral advisor. His work influenced Harvey, though Harvey was not, as evidenced here, opposed to critiquing his mentor.
7   *Descried*: Perceived or described.
8   Major embryological debates erupted at this time between "preformationism" (the theory that embryos develop out of preformed material—sometimes even miniature version of the full-grown organism) and "epigenesis" (the theory that embryos develop gradually out of undifferentiated material). Harvey's work generally follows the theory of epigenesis, which he illustrates through the careful observation and detailed description of the day-by-day development of chick embryos.

most inimitable prudence and wisdom, by the great God of nature; and at length we will discover, what we have found out, concerning the first matter out of which, and the first efficient by which, the fetus is made, as also of the order & economy of generation: that thence we may attain to some infallible knowledge of each faculty of the formative and vegetative Soul,[9] by the effects of it; and of the nature of the Soul it self, by the parts, or organs of the body, and their functions.

Now this indeed we could not perform in all kind of animals; because some of them cannot be gotten; and others again are so exceeding small, that our eyes can hardly discern them.

Let it suffice therefore that we have done it in some creatures, which are more known to us; to whose platform, the first originals of all other creatures may be reduced. We have made choice therefore of such, as might render the credit of our experiments less questionable, namely larger, and perfecter creatures, and such as are within our own power. For in the larger creatures, all things are more conspicuous; in the perfecter, more distinct; and in those that are in our own power, & conversant amongst us, more obvious: so that we have liberty (at pleasure) by searching into them, to rescue our observations from wavering hesitation. And of this sort, in the race of oviparous creatures, are hens, geese, pigeons, ducks, shellfish of both kinds (as lobsters, oysters, &c.) fishes that have no shells at all, frogs, serpents: also insects, as bees, wasps, butterflies, silkworms. And of viviparous, sheep, goats, dogs, cats, all cattle that divide the hoof; and in chief, the perfectest of all creatures, man himself.

Having thorough insight & knowledge of these things, we may then contemplate the abstruse nature of the Vegetative Soul; and discern in all creatures what ever, the manner, order, and causes of their generation: because all other creatures agree either generically, or specifically with the fore-cited, or at the least with some of them; and are procreated after the same manner of generation, or else in a manner proportioned to it. For Nature being divine, and perfect, is always consonant to herself

---

9   *Vegetative Soul*: One of three presumed divisions of the soul (along with the sensitive and the rational), the vegetative is the part that powers life itself through nourishment, growth and reproduction.

in the same things. And as her works do either agree or differ (namely in kind, species, or some analogy) so her operation (that is to say, generation or fabric) is the same or different in them. Whoever enters this new, and unfrequented path, and inquires for truth in the vast volume of Nature, by anatomical dissections, and experiments, he meets with such a crowd of observations, and those too in such exotic shapes, that to unfold to others the mysteries himself hath discovered, will be more toil, then the finding of them out: for many things occur which have yet no name; such is the plenty of things, and the dearth of words. So that if a man should clothe them in metaphors, and express his new inventions by old words, and such as are in use: the reader could no more understand them, then canting: and would never be able to comprehend the business, since he never saw it.

And then again to mint up new and fictitious terms, would rather cast a mist, then enlighten. For so he must needs express things unknown, by that which is less known: and the reader would be more afflicted to unriddle the words, then to understand the matter. And therefore Aristotle by unexperimented persons is thought obscure: And this perhaps was the reason, why Fabricius ab Aquapendente chose rather to describe the fabric of the chicken in the egg by tables than words.

Therefore be not offended, courteous reader, if in setting out the history of an egg, and in the description of the generation of the chicken, I make use of a new method, and sometimes of unusual terms; nor think me hereby more desirous of vainglory, then of advantaging others by true experiments, and such as are grounded in Nature's self. To take off that prejudice, know, I tread but the steps of other men who have lighted me the way, and (so far as is fit) I make use of their notions. But in chief, of all the ancients, I follow Aristotle; and of the later writers, Hieronymus Fabricius ab Aquapendente, him as my general, and this as my guide. For as they which find out new plantations, and new shores, call them by names of their own coining, which posterity afterwards accepts and receives; so those that find out new Secrets, have good title to their compellation.[10] And here, methinks, I hear Galen advising; If we consent in the things; contend not about the words.

10 *Compellation*: Naming.

The Midwives Book*

JANE SHARP
(English, born ca. 1641)

In the seventeenth century, female medical practitioners were neither "learned" (they were not educated in universities) nor "licensed" (they were not authorized as elite physicians). However, there were many skilled women working in health-related professions. One such profession was midwifery. For centuries, births happened in the home and with the aid of expert women. Female midwives had a long tradition of practical education and training that helped them successfully guide women through labor. Despite this, printed texts about female health, gynecology, and midwifery practices were written exclusively by men, and male practitioners were beginning to stake a claim on the profession itself (becoming "man-midwives"). They argued that women's supposedly inferior intellect and education made them less suited for the work. Jane Sharp's *The Midwives Book*, published in 1671, is the first English-language midwifery manual written by a woman. Although not much is known about Sharp herself, her book challenges these claims. As you read, consider Sharp's defense of the female midwife against man-midwives and her practical advice to help nursing women.

---

* Reprinted from Jane Sharp, *The Midwives Book, or the whole Art of Midwifery Discovered* (London, 1671), 3–5, 351–352, Early English Books Online Text Creation Partnership.

[Letter to the Midwives of England]

Sisters.

I have often sat down sad in the consideration of the many miseries women endure in the hands of unskillful midwives; many professing the art (without any skill in anatomy, which is the principal part effectually necessary for a midwife) merely for lucre's sake. I have been in great cost in translations for all books, either French, Dutch, or Italian of this kind.[1] All which I offer with my own experience. Humbly begging the assistance of Almighty God to aid you in this great work, and am

Your Affectionate Friend
Jane Sharp

[The Art of Being a Midwife]

As for their [the midwives] knowledge it must be twofold: speculative,[2] and practical. She that wants[3] the knowledge of speculation, is like to one that is blind or wants her sight: she that wants the practice, is like one that is lame and wants her legs, the lame may see but they cannot walk, the blind may walk but they cannot see. Such is the condition of those midwives that are not well versed in both these. Some perhaps may think, that it is not proper for women to be of this profession, because they cannot attain so rarely to the knowledge of things as men may, who are bred up in universities, schools of learning, or serve their apprenticeships for that end and purpose, where anatomy lectures being frequently read, the situation of the parts of both men and women, and other things of great consequence are often made plain to them. But that

---

1. Sharp refers to the range of translated works she used to compile the volume. Although not listed here, English-language midwifery texts may have also influenced her. Sharp seems particularly indebted to the works of Nicholas Culpeper, a prolific author of medical works. See Elaine Hobby, ed., introduction to *The Midwives Book, or the Whole Art of Midwifry Discovered*, by Jane Sharp (New York: Oxford University Press, 1999), xviii.
2. *Speculative*: Theoretical.
3. *Wants*: Lacks.

objection is easily answered, by the former example of the midwives among the Israelites,[4] though we women cannot deny, that men in some things may come to a greater perfection of knowledge than women ordinarily can, by reason of the former helps that women want,[5] yet the holy Scriptures have recorded midwives to the perpetual honor of the female sex. There being not so much as one word concerning men-midwives mentioned there that we can find, it being the natural propriety of women to be much seeing into that art: and though nature be not alone sufficient to the perfection of it, yet farther knowledge may be gained by a long and diligent practice, and be communicated to others of our own sex. I cannot deny the honor due to able physicians and surgeons, when occasion is.[6] Yet we find even that among the Indians, and all barbarous people, where there is no men of learning, the women are sufficient to perform this duty: and even in our own nation, that we need go no farther, the poor country people where there are none but women to assist (unless it be those that are exceeding poor and in a starving condition, and then they have more need of meat than midwives) the women are as fruitful, and as safe and well delivered, if not much more fruitful, and better commonly in childbed[7] than the greatest ladies of the land. It is not hard words that perform the work, as if none understood the art that cannot understand Greek. Words are but the shell, that we ofttimes break our teeth with them to come at the kernel, I mean our brains, to know what is the meaning of them; but to have the same in our mother tongue would save us a great deal of labor. It is commendable for men to employ their spare time in some things of deeper speculation than is required of the female sex; but the art of midwifery chiefly concern us, which, even the best learned men will grant, yielding someone of their own to us, when they are forced to borrow from us the very name they practice by, and to call themselves men-midwives. But to avoid long

---

4   Earlier in the introduction, Sharp cites a biblical example from Exodus 1 about the midwives of Israel as justification for the importance of midwives to humanity.
5   Sharp concedes that men may be able to achieve higher and more complete knowledge than women because they are afforded more "helps" (or assistance), such as access to education.
6   *When occasion is*: When the situation calls for it.
7   *Better commonly in childbed*: Often better during labor.

preambles in a matter so clear and evident, I shall proceed to set down such rules, and method concerning this art as I think needful, and that as plainly and briefly as possibly I can, and with as much modesty in words as the matter will bear: and because it is commonly maintained, that the masculine gender is more worthy than the feminine, though perhaps when men have need of us they will yield the priority to us; that I may not forsake the ordinary method, I shall begin with men, and treat last of my own sex,[8] so as to be understood by the meanest[9] capacity, desiring the courteous reader to use as much modesty in the perusal of it, as I have endeavored to do in the writing of it, considering that such an art as this cannot be set forth, but that young men and maids will have much just cause to blush sometimes, and be ashamed of their own follies, as I wish they may if they shall chance to read it, that they may not convert that into evil that is really intended for a general good.[10]

Directions for Nurses

But there is one consideration more for the nurse before I leave this; and that is, that she may not want[11] good milk in her breasts, for if she do, the child will suffer more than the nurse, because he draws it from her to feed him. Those that are fretful, lean, or sickly, have black livers and stomachs, and ill digestion, that they can have neither much, nor yet good milk, and bad diet hinders much.

Such as want milk should drink milk wherein fennel seed has been soaked, and feed on good nourishment, and drink good drink, barley-water and almond milk are good for hot choleric people; let her

---

8   Sharp's opening section of the book begins with detailed descriptions of the male reproductive anatomy. She describes this as the "ordinary method" because at that time female anatomy was understood as an imperfect version of its male counterpart.
9   *Meanest*: Lowest or most common.
10 Sharp recognizes that her frank and open description of human genitalia and the processes of reproduction might cause some audiences to critique the work as lewd or even pornographic.
11 *Want*: Lack.

eat lettuce, borage, spinach, and lamb sodden, and eaten with vervain, calves' or goat's milk breed milk in the breasts; the eating of aniseed, cumin seeds, caraway seeds or their decoction[12] will help well, all things that increase seed[13] will ripen milk: when you go to bed drink two drams and a half of bruised aniseed in the decoction of coleworts. Use this plaister,[14] take deer's suet half an ounce, parsley herb and root the like quantity, barley meal one ounce and a half, red storax three drams, boil the roots and herbs well, and beat them to pap,[15] and incorporate all with three ounces of oil of sweet almonds, and lay them to the breasts and nipple.

---

12 *Decoction*: An extract, often of plants, used medicinally.
13 *Seed*: This refers both to semen and a seminal fluid sometimes thought to be produced by women.
14 *Plaister*: A medicinal substance, like an ointment, spread on a bandage and then applied to the body, where it adheres.
15 *Pap*: A semiliquid or very soft substance (as in the consistency of porridge).

On Animalcules*

ANTONIE VAN LEEUWENHOEK
(Dutch, 1632–1723)

Microscope technology as we know it today was developed and refined starting in the seventeenth century with the publication of Robert Hooke's *Micrographia* in 1665. Antonie van Leeuwenhoek, a draper (or fabric merchant) from Delft, Holland—now part of the Netherlands—was inspired by this technology. He learned to grind glass lenses and used them to build hundreds of small microscopes, achieving magnification of at least 275 times with just a simple lens. This allowed him to see, for the first time, bacteria and life at the cellular level. His discoveries were composed as letters written to the Royal Society of London for Improving Natural Knowledge, England's first academy of science. They were then published in the associated *Philosophical Transactions*, the oldest and longest running scientific journal in the world.[1] He was inducted into the Royal Society in 1680 and is now known as the founder of microbiology. Included here are two of these letters. As you read, consider Leeuwenhoek's process and his description of "animalcules" (microscopic animals) that we now recognize as spermatozoa and the bacteria that cause dental plaque.

1 Originally compiled from letters sent to the Royal Society, *Philosophical Transactions* was first published in 1665. It has been in continuous publication ever since.

---

* "Animalcules and Frog Reproduction" reprinted from Antonie van Leeuwenhoek, "An Abstract of a Letter from Mr. Anthony Leeuwenhoek of Delft […], *Philosophical Transactions* 13 (1683), 347–355, JSTOR; "Animalcules in the Mouth" reprinted from Antonie van Leeuwenhoek, "An Extract of a Letter from Anth. Van Leeuwenhoek […]," *Philosophical Transactions* 17 (1693), 646–649, JSTOR.

[Animalcules and Frog Reproduction]

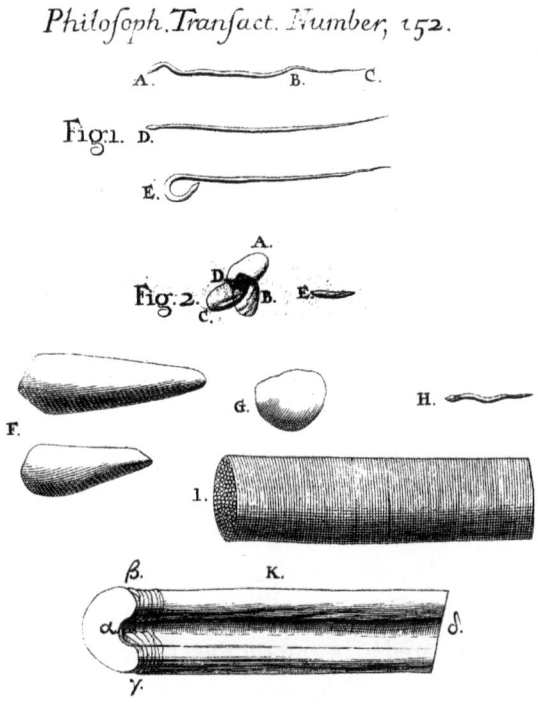

Illustration 4. Leeuwenhoek's illustrations of the various microscopic animalcules witnessed in this experiment, and described in the associated letter. Reprinted fro Antonie van Leeuwenhoek, "An Abstract of a Letter [...]," *Philosophical Transactions* 13 (1683), 347–355. JSTOR

Having been solicitous to examine the generation[2] of frogs, upon the account of their young ones being like a worm, with a round thick body and a short tail: I was surprised to find that the male was not joined to the female in copulation, but that he only sat upon her; and had no

---

2   *Generation*: Reproduction.

membrum masculum:³ that at the same time when the female cast her eggs or spawn, the male also dropped his seed; which is to be spread under the eggs: in like manner as the seed of fished that want the *membrum masculum* is cast under the eggs of the female, that the *animalia in semine*⁴ may conveniently impregnate the eggs.

But on the first of April when frogs were ready to spawn, I took some of the males sitting upon the females, and squeezed their hinder parts that I might get the seed out of the *vasa deferentia*⁵ but the *Animalcules* I then found, moved but little, because the matter they were in was full of salt particles, which made me judge it to be urine.

I then cut open the testicles and there I found an innumerable company of *Animalcules* swimming among a sort of ill-shaped particles, these continued alive till the next day, though there were but a small quantity of liquor to contain them.

I judge the bodies of the *animalcules* to have been of the thickness of 1/1000 part of a hair on my head: If the matter they moved in had not been so thick I should have seen them much plainer, nevertheless they are represented to the best of my skill in *Fig. First* where A B C is an *animalcule* as it lay in the watery matter, and moved itself therein, sometimes the head appeared to be thicker then other times, and often I could see the body but from A to B by reason of the thinness of the Tail BC [See Illustration 4, fig.1]. When the animal moved itself strongly, tho the progress were but little, the motion towards the head was like that of a snake, and the tail was cast into 3 or 4 bows. *Fig D.* is an animalcule lying dead, and stretched out at length, but in this posture I saw but few, for many that were dead lay with the fore part of their body bent in, as in *Fig. E.* Others made as, it were a half circle others had the forepart of their body bent and moved their hinder parts; these last I took to be ready to die.

The number of animalcules in all the seed was so great that I judge there might be 10,000 of them to one of the female's eggs, the same computation I formerly made of the milt of a codfish.

---

3   *Membrum masculum*: Male sexual organ.
4   *Animalia in semine*: Literally, "animals in semen," what we now recognize as sperm.
5   *Vasa deferentia*: The plural of vas deferens, the duct that carries sperm from the testicles to the urethra.

[Animalcules in the Mouth]

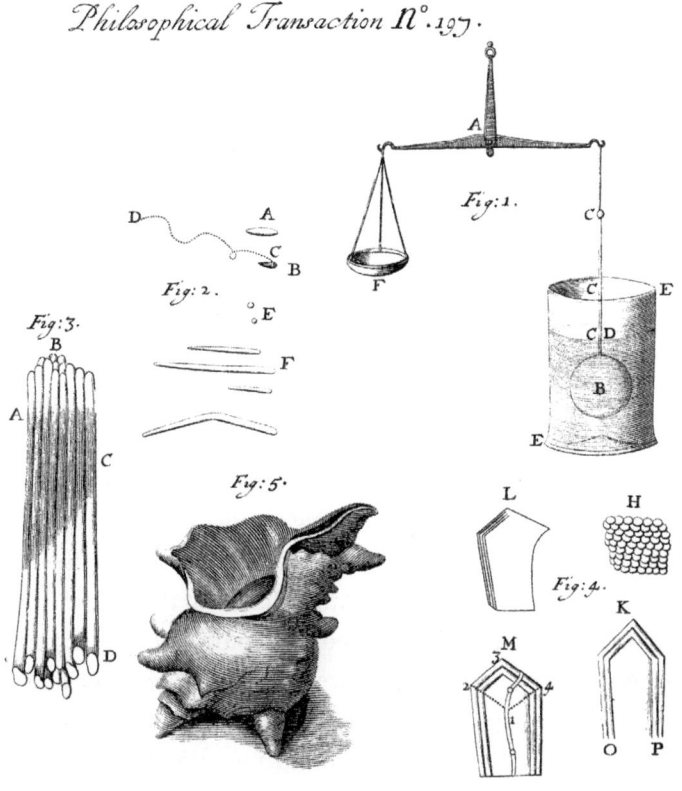

Illustration 5. Leeuwenhoek's illustrations of the microsopic animalcules described in this letter; the excerpt discusses figure 2, depicting what he found between his teeth. Figure 3 depicts a bundle of hair "squeezed out" of his nose; Figure 4 depicts the "scales" of human skin cells and scar tissue; Figures 1 and 5 are not described in the extract. Reprinted from Antonie van Leeuwenhoek, "An Extract of a Letter […]," *Philosophical Transactions* 17 (1693), 646–649, JSTOR.

I have often endeavored to discover animalcules in spittle, but in vain: But examining a kind of gritty matter from between my teeth, and mixing it with sometimes with rain-water, and sometimes with spittle, both which before had no animalcules, I discovered therein with admiration a great number of very small ones moving; the greatest whereof are represented Fig 2.A [See Illustration 5]. They had a very strong and swift motion in the water like eels, of these larger there were not many: a second sort is represented by B. These oft turned themselves round like a top, and moved sometimes as is shewn by the line C.B. These were much more in number. The figure of the third sort I could not well discover, sometimes they appeared oval, and at other times round, they were so small that I could not discern them greater than as a E. They moved swiftly by each other like gnats playing in the air, and of these I discerned thousands in a drop of water they shewed no bigger than a sand, and in the drop, the water was to the animalcules as 9 to 1. But most of the matter I examined, consisted of long slender parts all of a thickness, but differing in length as at F. And one crooked one among the rest; and because I have formerly observed Animalcules of this shape in water, I endeavored to discover if these lived but could not. I have found the same in the matter taken from between the teeth of other persons, as well such as drank wine and smoked tobacco, as of such as did neither, but not in their spittle, in which I found no animalcules. I found the same after I had washed by teeth very well with vinegar, though the vinegar killed them when they were put into it.

Upon the Sight of an Anatomy*

NAHUM TATE
(Irish, 1652–1715)

Author Nahum Tate was educated at Trinity College, Dublin. He is especially known for his playwriting—in particular, for his adaptations and rewrites of Elizabethan-era dramas (including those of William Shakespeare) for late seventeenth-century audiences. "Upon the Sight of an Anatomy" was included in a 1696 volume of poems called *Poems on divine & moral subjects* and was composed in an era when anatomy theaters—indoor amphitheaters built to allow for an audience during dissection—were becoming popular not just for the teaching of anatomy, but for public viewing as well. The term "anatomy" was also used to refer to skeletal remains wired together and put on display in such a space. As you read, consider the description of the remains on display.

---

* Reprinted from Nahum Tate, *Miscellanea Sacra, or, Poems on divine and moral subjects collected by N. Tate* (London, 1696), 40–44, Early English Books Online Text Creation Partnership.

Upon the Sight of an Anatomy

1.
   Nay, start not at that *Skeleton*,
   'Tis your own Picture which you shun;
   Alive it did resemble Thee,
   And thou, when dead, like that shalt be:
   Converse with it, and you will say, [5]
   You cannot better spend the Day;
   You little think how you'll admire
   The Language of those *Bones* and *Wire*.

2.
   The *Tongue* is gone, but yet each Joint
   Reads Lectures, and can speak to th' Point. [10]
   When all your Moralists are read,
   You'll find no Tutors like the Dead.

3.
   If in Truth's Paths those *Feet* have trod,
   'Tis all one whether bare, or shod:
   If us'd to travel to the Door [15]
   Of the Afflicted Sick and Poor,
   Though to the Dance they were estrang'd,
   And ne'er their own rude Motion chang'd;
   Those Feet, now wing'd, may upwards fly,
   And tread the Palace of the Sky. [20]

4.
   Those *Hands*, if ne'er with Murther stain'd,
   Nor fill'd with Wealth unjustly gain'd,
   Nor greedily at Honours graspt,
   But to the *Poor-Man*'s Cry unclaspt;
   It matters not, if in the Myne [25]
   They delv'd, or did with Rubies shine.

5.
   Here grew the *Lips*, and in that Place,
   Where now appears a vacant space,
   Was fix'd the *Tongue*, an Organ, still

    Employ'd extremely well or ill;   [30]
    I know not if it cou'd retort,
    If vers'd i' th' Language of the Court;
    But this I safely can aver,
    That if it was no Flatterer;
    If it traduc'd no Man's Repute,   [35]
    But, where it cou'd not Praise, was Mute:
    If no false Promises it made,
    If it sung Anthems, if it Pray'd,
    'Twas a blest *Tongue*, and will prevail
    When Wit and Eloquence shall fail.   [40]

6.

    If Wise as *Socrates*, that *Skull*,
    Had ever been, 'tis now as dull
    As *Midas*'s; or if its Wit
    To that of *Midas* did submit,
    'Tis now as full of Plot and Skill,   [45]
    As is the Head of *Machiavel*:
    Proud Laurels once might shade that Brow,
    Where not so much as Hair grows now.

7.

    Prime Instances of Nature's Skill,
    The *Eyes*, did once those Hollows fill: [50]
    Were they quick-sighted, sparkling, clear,
    (As those of Hawks and Eagles are,)
    Or say they did with Moisture swim,
    And were distorted, blear'd, and dim;
    Yet if they were from Envy free,   [55]
    Nor lov'd to gaze on Vanity;
    If none with scorn they did behold,
    With no lascivious Glances rowl'd:
    Those Eyes, more bright and piercing grown,
    Shall view the Great Creator's Throne;   [60]
    They shall behold th' *Invisible*,
    And on Eternal Glories dwell.

8.
   See! not the least Remains appear
   To shew where Nature plac'd the *Ear*!
   Who knows if it were Musical, [65]
   Or cou'd not judge of Sounds at all?
   Yet if it were to Council bent,
   To Caution and Reproof attent,
   When the shrill Trump shall rouse the Dead,
   And others hear their Sentence read; [70]
   That *Ear* shall with these Sounds be blest,
   Well done, and, *Enter into Rest.*

The Sham Doctor*

JOSEPH ADDISON
(English, 1672–1719)

Author and politician Richard Steele's *The Tatler* represented a new form of journalism in England, building on the success of news periodicals (which emerged in the sixteenth century) and a shift in culture that made coffeehouses central in English social activity. From 1709 to 1711, the journal published essays relevant to popular culture, fashion, literature, politics, and society. It sought to capture attention and readership by presenting news—real and sensationalized—as gossip. The essays essentially "tattle" on things overheard in coffee shops. One of Steele's partners in this venture was Joseph Addison, poet and member of Parliament, who wrote the *Tatler* essay included here. The essay claims to tell the story of a female doctor—born Margery, but known as Dr. John Young—living and practicing as a man and labeled here as a quack. As you read, consider the attitude toward female practitioners, and the treatment of presumed quackery.

---

* Reprinted from Joseph Addison, *The Tatler: By the Right Honourable Joseph Addison, Esq.* (Glasgow, 1754), 191–95, Early English Online Books Text Creation Partnership.

[The Tatler, Saturday, September 19, 1710]

—Juvenis quondam, nunc Foemina Caeneus,
Rursus et in veterem fato revoluto figuram.—Virg.[1]

From my own apartment, September 18: It is one of the designs of this paper to transmit to posterity an account of every thing that is monstrous in my own times. For this reason I shall here publish to the world the life of a person who was neither man nor woman, as written by one of my ingenious correspondents, who seems to have imitated Plutarch in that multifarious erudition, and those occasional dissertations, which he has wrought into the body of his history. The life I am putting out, is that of Margery, alias John Young, commonly known by the name of Dr. Young, who, as the town very well knows, was a woman that practiced physic[2] in man's clothes, and after having had two wives and several children, died about a month since.

SIR,

I here make bold to trouble you with a short account of the famous doctor Young's life, which you may call, if you please, a second part of the farce of the Sham Doctor. This perhaps will not seem so strange to you, who, if I am not mistaken, have some where mentioned with honor your sister Kirleus,[3] as a practitioner both in physic and astrology: but in the common opinion of mankind, a She-quack[4] is altogether as strange and astonishing a creature as a centaur that practiced physic

---

1 This quote from Virgil's *Aeneid* refers to the Greek myth of Caenis, who demanded to be turned into a man after being raped by Poseidon and was returned to her original sex in the afterlife: "Caeneus, once a youth, now a woman / and returned by Fate to her old form again" (my own translation).
2 *Physic*: Medicine. "Physician" means "one who practices physic."
3 *Kirleus*: Multiple newspapers of the late seventeenth and early eighteenth centuries refer to a Dr. Thomas Kirleus and (later) his wife Mary and daughter Susannah, who advertised their services providing medicinal cures for a variety of ailments.
4 *She-quack*: A female quack. A quack is someone who claims medical skill or credentials they don't have or who manufactures fake treatments. The term is a shortening of the Dutch word *quacksalver*.

in the days of Achilles,[5] or as king Phys in *The Rehearsal*.[6] Asclepius, the great founder of your art,[7] was particularly famous for his beard, as we may conclude from the behavior of a tyrant, who is branded by heathen historians as guilty both of sacrilege and blasphemy, having robbed the statue of Asclepius of a thick bushy golden beard, and then alleged for his excuse, *That it was a shame that the son should have a beard when his father Apollo had none.* This latter instance indeed seems something to favor a female professor, since, as I have been told, the ancient statues of Apollo are generally made with the head and face of a woman: nay I have been credibly informed by those who have seen them both, that the famous Apollo in the Belvidera[8] did very much resemble Dr. Young. Let that be as it will, the doctor was a kind of Amazon in physic, that made as great devastations and slaughters as any of our chief heroes in the art, and was as fatal to the English in these our days, as the famous Joan d' Arc was in those of our forefathers.

I do not find any thing remarkable in the life I am about to write till the year 1695, at which time the doctor being about twenty-three years old, was brought to bed of a bastard child. The scandal of such a misfortune gave so great uneasiness to pretty Mrs. Peggy, (for that was the name by which the doctor was then called) that she left her family, and followed her lover to London, with a fixed resolution some way or other to recover her lost reputation; but instead of changing her life, which one would have expected from so good a disposition of mind, she took it in her head to change her sex. This was soon done by the help of a sword, and a pair of breeches. I have reason to believe, that her first design was to turn man-midwife,[9] having herself had some experience

---

5   A reference to Chiron, a centaur in Greek myth who was famed for his wisdom and skill in medicine and who taught several Greek heroes, including Achilles and the Greek god of medicine Asclepius.

6   George Villiers's satirical play *The Rehearsal* (1671) features a play-within-a-play in which a physician plots to usurp a king.

7   *Asclepius*: The Greek god of medicine.

8   *Apollo in the Belvidera*: A marble statue of Apollo, likely Roman in origin, created ca. 120–140 CE and held in the Belvedere courtyard of the Vatican Museum since the sixteenth century.

9   *Man-midwife*: Through the sixteenth century, child birth was managed almost exclusively by female midwives; however, by the seventeenth century, that role was

in those affairs: but thinking this too narrow a foundation for her future fortune, she at length bought her a gold button coat, and set up for a physician. Thus we see the same fatal miscarriage in her youth made Mrs. Young a doctor, that formerly made one of the same sex a pope.[10]

The doctor succeeded very well in his business at first, but very often met with accidents that disquieted him. As he wanted[11] that deep magisterial voice, which gives authority to a prescription, and is absolutely necessary for the right pronouncing of those words, *Take these pills,* he unfortunately got the nick-name of the Squeaking Doctor. If this circumstance alarmed the Doctor, there was another that gave him no small disquiet, and very much diminished his gains. In short, he found himself run down as a superficial prating quack, in all families that had at the head of them a cautious father, or a jealous husband. These would often complain among one another, that they did not like such a smock-faced[12] physician; though in truth had they known how justly he deserved that name, they would rather have favored his practice, than have apprehended any thing from it.

Such were the motives that determined Mrs. Young to change her condition, and take in marriage a virtuous young woman, who lived with her in good reputation, and made her the father of a very pretty girl. But this part of her happiness was soon after destroyed by a distemper which was too hard for our physician, and carried off his wife. The doctor had not been a widow long, before he married his second lady, with whom also he lived in a very good understanding. It so happened that the doctor was with child at the same time that his lady was; but the little ones coming both together, they passed for twins. The doctor having entirely established the reputation of his manhood, especially by the birth of the boy of whom he had been lately delivered, and who

---

being encroached upon by male practitioners (the controversial "man-midwife"). For a defense of the traditional female midwife, see Jane Sharp's *The Midwives Book* (pp. 143–147).

10 A reference to the legend of Pope Joan who, according to one thirteenth-century account by Martin of Opava, disguised herself as a man and joined the church to be with her lover and served as Pope for two years in the ninth century.

11 *Wanted*: Lacked.

12 *Smock-faced*: Pale, with smooth skin (associated with feminine features).

very much resembles him, grew into good business, and was particularly famous for the cure of venereal distempers; but would had much more practice among his own sex, had not some of them been so unreasonable as to demand certain proofs of their cure, which the doctor was not able to give them. The florid blooming look, which gave the doctor some uneasiness at first, instead of betraying his person, only recommended his physic. Upon this occasion I cannot forbear mentioning what I thought a very agreeable surprise in one of Moliere's plays,[13] where a young woman applies herself to a sick person in the habit of a quack, and speaks to her patient who was something scandalized at the youth of his physician, to the following purpose—*I begun to practice in the reign of Francis I. and am now in the hundred and fiftieth year of my age; but by the virtue of my medicaments, have maintained myself in the same beauty and freshness I had at fifteen.* For this reason Hippocrates lays it down as a rule, that a student in physic should have a sound constitution, and a healthy look; which indeed seems as necessary qualifications for a physician, as a good life, and virtuous behavior, for a divine. But to return to our subject. About two years ago the doctor was very much afflicted with the vapors, which grew upon him to such a degree, that about six weeks since they made an end of him. His death discovered the disguise he had acted under, and brought him back again to his former sex. It is said, that at his burial the pall was held up by six women of some fashion. The doctor left behind him a widow and two fatherless children, if they may be called so, besides the little boy before mentioned. In relation to whom we may say of the doctor, as the good old ballad, about *the children in the wood,* says of the unnatural uncle, that he was father and mother both in one.[14] These are all the circumstances that I could learn of doctor Young's life, which might have given

---

13 *One of Moliere's plays*: Le malade imaginaire (The Imaginary Invalid), which premiered in Paris in 1673.
14 "The Children in the Wood" (or "The Babes in the Woods") was an anonymous broadside ballad that became immensely popular after its publication in 1595. It tells of two children who are murdered by their uncle after being entrusted to his care following the death of their parents. In making the request, the dying father tells his brother "You must be father and mother both, / and uncle all in one: / God knows what will become of them, / when we are dead and gone."

occasion to many obscene fictions: but as I know those would never have gained a place in your paper, I have not troubled you with any impertinence of that nature; having stuck to the truth very scrupulously, as I always do when I subscribe myself,

    SIR,

    Your, *&c.*

On Smallpox Inoculation*

LADY MARY WORTLEY MONTAGU
(English, 1689–1762)

Poet and author Lady Mary Wortley Montagu is perhaps best known for her letters, which she wrote during her travels as the wife of British Ambassador Edward Wortley Montagu (1678–1761). In the letter here, which was written in 1717 and published in 1790, she recounts being in Adrianople, Turkey,[1] while the smallpox epidemic raged through Europe. Montagu, who had herself survived smallpox, writes of the practice of ingrafting, in which active smallpox was injected into veins or rubbed into open wounds. This version of inoculation was the precursor to modern vaccination. Ingrafting was well-established in Turkey, but Montagu's work, and her choice to ingraft her own children, is credited with having introduced the practice to England. As you read, consider her description of smallpox and her advocacy of the Turkish approach to its prevention.

1 *Aprianople*: Modern-day Edirne, Turkey, and once the capital of the Ottoman Empire (369–1453 CE).

---

* Reprinted from Lady Mary Wortley Montague, *Letters of the Right Honourable Lady M—y W—y M—e Written during Her Travels in Europe, Asia and Africa to Persons of Distinction, Men of Letters, &c. in Different Parts of Europe* [...] *Drawn from Sources that have been inaccessible to other Travellers* (London, 1790; Project Gutenberg, 2006), Letter 31.

[The Practice of Ingrafting]

TO MRS S. C.
Adrianople, April 1. O. S.[2]

In my opinion, dear S. I ought rather to quarrel with you, for not answering my Nijmegen letter of August, till December, than to excuse my not writing again till now. I am sure there is on my side a very good excuse for silence, having gone such tiresome land-journeys, though I don't find the conclusion of them so bad as you seem to imagine. I am very easy here, and not in the solitude you fancy me. The great number of Greeks, French, English, and Italians that are under our protection, make their court to me from morning till night; and, I'll assure you, are, many of them, very fine ladies; for there is no possibility for a Christian to live easily under this government, but by the protection of an ambassador—and the richer they are, the greater is their danger.

Those dreadful stories you have heard of the *plague*,[3] have very little foundation in truth. I own, I have much ado to reconcile myself to the sound of a word, which has always given me such terrible ideas; though I am convinced there is little more in it, than in a fever. As a proof of this, let me tell you that we passed through two or three towns most violently infected. In the very next house where we lay, (in one of those places) two persons died of it. Luckily for me I was so well deceived, that I knew nothing of the matter; and I was made believe, that our second cook had only a great cold. However, we left our doctor to take care of him, and yesterday they both arrived here in good health; and I am now let into the secret, that he has had the *plague*. There are many that escape it, neither is the air ever infected. I am persuaded, that it would be as easy a matter to root it out here, as out of Italy and France; but it does so little mischief, they are not very solicitous about it, and are

---

2 O.S.: "Old Style," refers to changes made to the calendrical system of Great Britain and the British American Colonies under the Calendar Act 1750. This Act changed the official calendar of Britain from the Julian Calendar to the Gregorian Calendar (which most of the world uses today) and changed the start of the year from March 25 to January 1. The change resulted in a thirteen-day difference: April 1, Old Style, would be April 13 today.

3 *The plague*: Smallpox.

content to suffer this distemper, instead of our variety, which they are utterly unacquainted with.

A *propos* of distempers, I am going to tell you a thing that will make you wish yourself here. The small-pox, so fatal, and so general amongst us, is here entirely harmless, by the invention of *ingrafting*, which is the term they give it. There is a set of old women, who make it their business to perform the operation, every autumn, in the month of September, when the great heat is abated. People send to one another to know if any of their family has a mind to have the small-pox: they make parties for this purpose, and when they are met (commonly fifteen or sixteen together) the old woman comes with a nutshell full of the matter of the best sort of small-pox,[4] and asks what vein you please to have opened. She immediately rips open that you offer to her, with a large needle, (which gives you no more pain than a common scratch) and puts into the vein as much matter as can lie upon the head of her needle, and after that, binds up the little wound with a hollow bit of shell; and in this manner opens four or five veins. The Grecians have commonly the superstition of opening one in the middle of the forehead, one in each arm, and one on the breast, to mark the sign of the cross; but this has a very ill effect, all these wounds leaving little scars, and is not done by those that are not superstitious, who choose to have them in the legs, or that part of the arm that is concealed. The children or young patients play together all the rest of the day, and are in perfect health to the eighth.[5] Then the fever begins to seize them, and they keep their beds two days, very seldom three. They have very rarely above twenty or thirty in their faces, which never mark;[6] and in eight days time they are as well as before their illness. Where they are wounded, there remain running sores during the distemper, which I don't doubt is

---

4   Also called variolation, ingrafting involved taking a small amount of "matter" (either powdered smallpox scabs or fluid from smallpox sores) and introducing it into small scratches in the skin of a healthy individual, in hopes of promoting mild symptoms followed by immunity.
5   *To the eighth*: Refers to the incubation period of the virus (now recognized to be ten to fourteen days).
6   They rarely have more than twenty or thirty pockmarks on their faces from the smallpox, and those never leave scars.

a great relief to it. Every year thousands undergo this operation; and the French ambassador says pleasantly, that they take the small-pox here by way of diversion, as they take the waters in other countries. There is no example of any one that has died in it; and you may believe I am well satisfied of the safety of this experiment, since I intend to try it on my dear little son.[7] I am patriot enough to take pains to bring this useful invention into fashion in England;[8] and I should not fail to write to some of our doctors very particularly about it, if I knew any one of them that I thought had virtue enough to destroy such a considerable branch of their revenue, for the good of mankind. But that distemper is too beneficial to them, not to expose to all their resentment the hardy wight[9] that should undertake to put an end to it. Perhaps, if I live to return, I may, however, have courage to war with them.

Upon this occasion, admire the heroism in the heart of
Your friend,
&c. &c.

---

7 Montagu followed through on this promise the following year, when her son Edward was five years old.
8 She followed up on this, as well: in 1721, she had her four-year-old daughter Mary variolated; this was the first instance of this method being used in Britain, and it was done in front of witnesses. Both children were successfully inoculated, and the practice rapidly gained in popularity, though Montagu was still seen by some as having recklessly endangered her children's lives.
9 *Wight*: Person (with a suggestion of either contempt or pity).

Historical Account of the Smallpox Inoculated in New England*

ZABDIEL BOYLSTON
(American, 1676–1766)

Because the first North American medical school wasn't founded until a year before he died,[1] Massachusetts-born surgeon Zabdiel Boylston trained informally in medicine.[2] He was the first American-born surgeon to perform operations to remove bladder stones and breast tumors. Perhaps his most critical contribution, however, is to "variolation"—inoculation using the variola virus to immunize individuals against the smallpox virus. The practice, though not uncommon outside Europe (see Lady Mary Wortley Montagu, pp. 163–166), was fraught with controversy when brought to Europe and America, since it required a deliberate infection of an otherwise healthy individual. Urged on by Puritan minister Cotton Mather, who had read of the process, Boylston demonstrated the validity of the method and published his findings in 1726 in his historical account of these inoculations. As you read, consider Boylston's discussion of his experiment, which was conducted first on his own son and two enslaved people, and of the response to that experiment.

1   The first North American medical program was instituted in 1765 at the College of Philadelphia, now the Perelman School of Medicine at the University of Pennsylvania.
2   The author trained first with his own father, who was a surgeon, and later with a Boston physician named John Cutler.

* Reprinted from Zabdiel Boylston, *Historical account of the small-pox inoculated in New-England, upon all sorts of persons, whites, blacks, and of all ages and constitutions.* [...] *Humbly dedicated to Her Royal Highness the Princess of Wales.* (London, 1736; reprinted Boston, 1730), 1–5. Early English Books Online Text Creation Partnership.

Experiments in Inoculation

The *Small-Pox*, which had been a terror to *New-England* since first it paid a visit there, coming into *Boston*, and spreading there in *April*, 1721, put the inhabitants into great consternation and disorder. Dr. *Mather*, in compassion to the lives of the people, transcribed from the *Philosophical Transactions of the Royal Society*, the accounts sent them by Dr. *Timonius* and *Pyllarinus* of inoculating the Small-Pox in the *Levant*,[3] and sent them to the practitioners of the town, for their consideration thereon. Upon reading of which I was very well pleased, and resolved in my mind to try the experiment; well remembering the destruction the Small-Pox made 19 years before, when last in *Boston*; and how narrowly I then escaped with my life. Now, when my wife and many others were gone out of town to avoid the distemper, and all hope given up of preventing the further spreading of it, and the guards were first removed from the doors of infected houses, I began the experiment; and not being able to make it upon my self, (such was my faith in the safety and success of this method) I chose to make it (for example sake) upon my own dear child, and two of my servants.

※

June the 26th, 1721. I inoculated my son *Thomas*, of about six, my negro man, *Jack*, thirty six, and *Jackey*, two and a half years old. They all complained on the 6th day; upon the 7th, the two children were a little hot, dull and sleepy, *Thomas* (only) had twitchings and started in his sleep. The 8th, the children's fevers continued, *Tommy*'s twitchings and startings in sleep increased; and though the fever was gentle and his senses bright, yet as the practice was new, and the clamor, or rather rage of the

---

3   *Dr. Mather:* Cotton Mather, a prominent Puritan minister in Boston and a crusader against the supposed witchcraft that prompted the Salem witch trials, wrote prolifically on topics of history and science. He was published in the academic journal *Philosophical Transactions* (see pp. 148–152 for examples of early journal articles). Boylston here refers to two articles in that same journal, by the Greek physicians Emmanuel Timonis (1669–1720) and Jacob Pylarinus (1659–1718).

people against it so violent,[4] that I was put into a very great fright; and not having any directions from Dr. *Timonius* and *Pyllarinus* concerning this practice, I had nothing to have recourse to but patience, and therefore waited upon Nature for a crisis (neither my fears nor the symptoms abating) until the 9th; when early in the morning I gave him a vomit,[5] upon which the symptoms went off, and the same day, upon him and the black child, a kind and favorable Small-Pox came out, of about a hundred a piece; after which their circumstances became easy, our trouble was over, and they soon were well.

Jack's complaints, in two or three days were over, and though he had but a few pustules about one of his inoculations, I am inclined to think he had had the Small-Pox before.

It was plain and easy to see, (even in these two) with pleasure, the difference between having the Small-Pox this way, and that of having it in the natural way.

And as this practice was new in *Europe*, so it must needs make a strange figure in *New-England*, and more especially so when one or two of our learned *Esculapian* tribe[6] had made the discovery how this practice would produce the plague *viz.* because *Timonius* told them that it sometimes happened that swellings were produced by it in some emunctory of the body; and likewise they caviled and said, that Dr. *Mather* had not given a fair representation from *Timonius* and *Pyllarinus's* accounts. I prayed that they might be read; but Dr. *Douglass*,[7] who owned

---

4   Mather sought Boylston out because of his reputation for undertaking risky medical procedures. Variolation was controversial in Europe and America, labeled "doubtful and dangerous" in part because of the counter-intuitive method of inducing the very illness that is being combated. Amalie M. Kass, "Boston's Historic Smallpox Epidemic," *Massachusetts Historical Review* 14 (2012): 13–14.

5   *Gave him a vomit*: Induced vomiting, either by use of an emetic or through reaching into the mouth. This method was used to purge the system of excess humors that were seen as causing illness.

6   *Learned Esculapian tribe*: Physicians. This refers to those guided by Asclepius, Greek god of medicine.

7   *Dr. Douglass*: William Douglass (ca. 1691–1752) was a Boston-area physician and author who initially opposed the practice of variolation. He claimed to have lent Cotton Mather the *Philosophical Transactions* articles before snatching them back, and the two men remained adversarial even after Douglass conceded the efficacy

them, and had taken them from Dr. *Mather*, refused to have them read, or even afterwards to lend them to the governor to read; such was his extraordinary care, lest the people, in time, should have been reconciled to the practice, and taken the benefit of it.

And upon *July* the 21st, 1721, being a third time called to an account for using this practice by some gentlemen (influenced thereto) who bore authority in *Boston*, I then having seven persons more under inoculation, whose illness were not yet come on: I then gave a public invitation to the practitioners of the town (who were then present) to visit my patients, who were under that practice, and to judge of and report their circumstances as they found them. But Dr. *Lawrence Dalhonde*'s terrible account (see the account at the end)[8] that he then gave of that practice was such, that none of them saw cause to accept my invitation and visit my patients. Instead of this, and reporting their circumstances justly and fairly, as it was their duty, and the people's right, for them to have done, some of them made it their business to invent, collect, and publish idle, unjust, and ridiculous stories and misrepresentations of the people's circumstances under it, and the practice; though none of them had ever been concerned for, or had seen one single person of them in their illness, from the beginning of this practice, to the end of it, except by accident, save Mr. *White* once or twice, or that knew any thing of their circumstances, but that they saw them come well and early abroad after their Small-Pox. And not satisfied with such unjust proceedings in *New-England*, lest the truth should be made known to *Great Britain*, and that our good success might influence them to use this practice, *Douglass* favored them with his pretended wonderful knowledge of things which he knew little of, as may be seen in Dr. *Wagstaff*'s Book against inoculation.[9]

And as for *Dalhonde*'s most surprising instances, the knowing part of mankind now believes as little of them as if he had said that their

---

and relative safety of variolation in 1730.

8   *The account at the end*: Boylston includes, as an appendix, a testimonial by physician Lawrence Dalhonde, in which he claims that variolation was the direct cause of deaths throughout Europe.

9   See William Wagstaff, *A Letter to a Dr. Friend Shewing the Danger and Uncertainty of Inoculating the Smallpox* (London: 1722), Wellcome Collection.

heads had dropped off, or that inoculation had turned men into women, or any other strange thought that might have come into his head.

I have made diligent inquiry in *England*, but could never meet with any one who had heard of any such practice in these parts of *Europe*, until within these five years past, or that believes there ever was, and especially in an army, the most unlikely place to begin it in; and if began there, the most likely place he could have thought of to have made it public to the world. So that if he does not get well-attested proofs from Drs. *Helvetius, Bollatio,* and *Barrera,*[10] of the facts, I doubt, for the future, his affirmation will not have that credit in the world, as an honest man's ought to have.

These were some of the oppositions and difficulties I met with in the beginning of this practice, and which was the means of keeping out hundreds, if not thousands, from coming into the practice of inoculation, which might have saved many valuable lives that were lost by the Small-Pox in the natural way, as may better appear when the success in each way is compared.

---

10 *Drs. Helvetius, Bollatio, and Barrera*: Royal physicians to the Duke of Orleans (Helvetius) and the King of Spain, from whom Dalhonde claimed to have received confirmation of the danger of variolation.

After the Small Pox*

MARY JONES
(English, 1707–1778)

In the eighteenth century, the smallpox pandemic affected nearly every part of the world, with death tolls in the hundreds-of-thousands annually. It was not deadly for everyone, however; those who survived were often left with scarring in the form of pockmarks. Oxford-born poet Mary Jones, whose poem is about a woman who has survived with these marks, was well regarded as a witty writer, skilled at social observation. The poem was first published in 1750 in *Miscellanies in Prose and Verse*. As you read, consider the description of the after effects of the smallpox infection on the survivor's body, mind, and personality.

---

* Reprinted from Mary Jones, "After the Small Pox," *Eighteenth-Century Poetry Archive* 1, no. 4 (Winter 2020/21); From the original text by Mary Jones, *Miscellanies in Prose and Verse* (Oxford: 1750), 79-80; Bodleian Library [Harding C 1723].

After the Small Pox

When skillful traders first set up,
To draw the people to their shop,
They strait hang out some gaudy sign,
Expressive of the goods within.
The Vintner has his boy and grapes, [5]
The Haberdasher thread and tapes,
The Shoemaker exposes boots,
And Monmouth Street old tatter'd suits.

So fares it with the nymph divine;
For what is Beauty but a Sign? [10]
A face hung out, thro' which is seen
The nature of the goods within.
Thus the coquet her beau ensnares
With study'd smiles, and forward airs:
The graver prude hangs out a frown [15]
To strike th' audacious gazer down;
But she alone, whose temp'rate wit
Each nicer medium can hit,
Is still adorn'd with ev'ry grace,
And wears a sample in her face. [20]

What tho' some envious folks have said,
That Stella now must hide her head,
That all her stock of beauty's gone,
And ev'n the very sign took down:
Yet grieve not at the fatal blow; [25]
For if you break a while, we know,
'Tis bankrupt like, more rich to grow.
A fairer sign you'll soon hang up,
And with fresh credit open shop:
For nature's pencil soon shall trace, [30]
And once more finish off your face,
Which all your neighbors shall out-shine,
And of your Mind remain the Sign.

Domestic Medicine*

WILLIAM BUCHAN
(Scottish, 1729–1805)

In the "advertisement" (or preface) of *Domestic Medicine*'s first edition (1769), physician William Buchan announces that "no art ever arrived at any considerable degree of improvement so long as it was kept in the hands of a few," and he criticizes the secrecy around medical knowledge (a sentiment he shares with Sir Thomas Elyot, pp. 84–86). The book aims to make the "medical art more generally useful" to everyone, offering detailed information based on Galenic principles about diseases and their prevention. It was incredibly popular: it went through over 140 English-language editions and was translated into seven other languages. As you read, consider his philosophy and his rules for the nursing and care of children.

---

* Reprinted from William Buchan, *Domestic Medicine: Or, the Family Physician ... Chiefly calculated to recommend a proper attention to Regimen and Simple Medicines* (Edinburgh: Balfour, Auld, and Smellie, 1769), ix, 48–51.

Advertisement

As all men are liable to disease, and equally interested in every thing related to health, it is certainly the duty of physicians to show them what is in their own power both with respect to the cure of the one, and the preservation of the other. Did men take every method to avoid disease, they would seldom need the physician; and would they do what is in their own power when sick, there would be little occasion for medicine. It is hard to say if more lives are not lost by people trusting to medicine, and neglecting their own endeavors, than all that are saved by the help of physic.[1]

[Directions Concerning Children]

As many people can understand the meaning of a short rule, who are not able to attend to a chain of reasoning, we shall reduce the leading principles of nursing under the following general heads.

1. Every mother ought to suckle her own child, if she can do it with safety.
2. A weak, consumptive, nervous, or hysteric mother ought not to give suck, where a healthy nurse can be had.
3. No child should be brought up without the breast, if it be possible to obtain a proper nurse.
4. The clothes of an infant should be soft, light, loose and easy for its body. They ought to be fastened on with strings rather than pins.
5. The cloths of children ought to be kept very clean.
6. A new born infant should not be kept too hot.
7. An infant should be permitted to suck as soon as it shows an inclination for the breast.
8. An infant should neither be crammed with food nor physic as soon as it is born; but permitted to lie quiet for some time, in order to recover the fatigue of the birth, &c.

---

1 *Physic*: Medicine. "Physician" means "one who practices physic."

9. If an infant must have food before it sucks, let it be water-pap[2] mixed with new milk, free of all wines, sugars, spiceries, or the like.

10. While the child sucks, it seldom needs much of any other food. It will however be right, about the third or fourth month, to begin to give it once or twice a-day a little of some food that is light and easy of digestion. This will make the weaning both less troublesome and dangerous.

11. A child should not be weaned all at once, but by degrees; as all sudden changes in the diet of children are dangerous.

12. The food of children ought at all times to be simple, but nourishing. It should consist of a proper mixture of animal and vegetable substances.

13. Children should not be permitted to eat too much fruit, or roots of any kind; but all sorts of green trash ought to be kept from them with the greatest care.

14. Children ought not to be pinched[3] in their food. They require to eat oftener than adults. If their food be simple, and they know that they can have it when hungry, they will seldom or never eat more than enough.

15. As soon as children can take exercise, they ought to be allowed as much as they please; till then it is the business of the nurse to carry and toss them about.

16. A nurse ought not only to carry an infant about, but to divert and amuse it so as to keep it in good humor.

17. An infant should never be suffered to cry long and vehemently.

18. Eruptions, or looseness in children,[4] ought not to be stopped, but with the greatest caution.

19. Nurses should use no means to force children to sleep; but they may always be permitted to take as much as they please.

20. Children ought never to have medicine unless they are diseased.

21. Children should neither be too early set to school, nor confined to any mechanical employment within doors.

---

2   *Water-pap*: A soft, semi-liquid food (like porridge) made with water.
3   *Pinched*: Restricted.
4   *Eruptions, or looseness*: Rashes, or diarrhea; Buchan saw both as typically important in helping to expel dangerous substances (including excess humors) from the body.

22. Schoolmasters, and all who have the care of youth, should allow them plenty of time for exercise and diversions.

23. All children should be nursed and educated in the country, if possible. When that cannot be done, they ought to be carried abroad every day, and kept for a sufficient time in the open air.

24. The children of delicate and diseased parents must be managed with more care than those of the hardy and robust.

25. A mother should never abandon her child solely to the care of a mercenary nurse.

Let no one imagine these matters unworthy of his attention. On the proper management of children depend not only their health and usefulness in life, but likewise the safety and prosperity of the state to which they belong. Effeminacy ever must prove the ruin of any kingdom; and when its foundations are laid in infancy, it can never afterwards be wholly eradicated. We would therefore recommend to all who wish well to their country, to study every method to render their offspring strong and healthy.

> —By arts like these,
> Laconia nurs'd of old her hardy sons;
> And Rome's unconquer'd legions urg'd their way,
> Unhurt, thro' every toil in every clime.[5]

---

5 From John Armstrong's *The Art of Preserving Health: A Poem*, Book III. Exercise (1745).

On the Dissection of a Body*

ANONYMOUS
1770

For most of us today, it feels natural to conceive of the body as a sort of machine or mechanized system of parts. However, this is just one of many metaphors we use for understanding the relationship between body parts. The body-machine metaphor begins to take hold in the seventeenth century, concurrent with innovations in mechanical sciences, advances in anatomical understanding and representation, and new philosophical ideas (including those of Rene Descartes, who compared the healthy body to a clock). It would become increasingly important during the Industrial Revolution, as yet more machines were invented. The poem included here was anonymously published in *The Gentleman's Magazine* in 1770. As you read, consider how the poem works with this metaphor as it discusses "this wonderful machine," the human body.

---

* Reprinted from *The Gentleman's Magazine* 40 (August 1770): 385–386, HathiTrust.

On the Dissection of a Body

Observe this wonderful machine,
View its connection with each part,
Thus furnish'd by the hand unseen,
How far surpassing human art!

Should ablest imitators try, [5]
With utmost skill, to for a like,
Could they so charm the curious eye?
Could they with equal wonder strike?

See how the motion of each part
Upon some other still depends, [10]
When all mutual aid impart,
Conducive to their various ends.

Whilst we th' amazing frame explore,
More secret wonders still we spy,
Yet there remain ten thousand more [15]
Hid from the microscopic eye.

Here may the stupid Atheist see
Convincing proofs—which all combine
To overthrow his wretched plan,
And speak the Maker's hand divine. [20]

What great emoluments accrue to
Those whose Nature's laws obey?
From such instructions in her view,
Ye sons of Esculapius[1] say!

Tho' God has call'd the life he lent, [25]
Each vital function, dormant laid,

---

1   *Esculapius*: Asclepius, the Greek god of medicine.

Here we trace Nature's deep intent,
And see how once the springs were play'd.

These tubes convey'd the purple juice,
Which with new strength supply'd the whole; [30]
And here branch'd forth the nerves, whose use
Was to keep converse with the soul.

This silent preacher points us out
The cause of many a latent ill,
Which, heretofore, lay hid in doubt, [35]
Baffling each effort of our skill.

A Letter to a Lady on the Mode of Conducting Herself during Pregnancy*

SARAH BROWN
(British, ca. late eighteenth century)

Although not much is known about Sarah Brown, the Preface to the letter included here claims that the material was originally written for her two daughters, and made public at the request of another young woman whose own mother had died too young to provide her such advice. Brown's other published works—both apparently published between 1777 and 1779—focus on nursing and child care. Here, we see the guidance not of a practitioner, but rather of one with significant personal experience, since Brown claims to be mother to seven children herself. As you read, consider the nature of her advice for how to behave and care for oneself during pregnancy.

---

* Reprinted from Sarah Brown, *A letter to a lady on the mode of conducting herself during pregnancy: Also on the management of the infant* (London: Baker and Galabin, 1777; Ann Arbor: EEBO-TCP, 2011), i–ii, 3–13, Early English Books Online.

[Managing the Experience of Pregnancy]

Dear Madam,

When I consider how much your present situation demands the advice of a real friend, I shall exert my endeavors, though I fear inadequate to the undertaking, to give you such instructions as I am persuaded will tend much to your relief; you very reasonably imagine, in consequence of the natural courses incident to our sex[1] not appearing at their regular time, that you are breeding;[2] from that circumstance, I readily suppose, you have taken particular notice when nature was last on you;[3] should you continue without any farther alteration, you may begin to reckon from the tenth day after the last time: this method my mother taught me with my first child, and I do assure you that my midwife paid her a very high compliment on the occasion.

Rise at your usual time; and, if you breed sick,[4] (which is usual,) order a cup of chamomile-tea, or pump-water, as soon as you come down stairs in the morning; that will help to keep your body open. If tea does not agree with you, try coffee, chocolate, milk, milk-porridge, water-gruel, balm-tea, or a calf's-foot boiled in milk; some one of which, most likely, will.

Perhaps you may have little or no appetite early in a morning; if so, give a general order to have something brought you at eleven o'clock; should you not be inclined to eat, let it not be removed, for, though it should not be agreeable then, it may a little time afterwards.

By no means ever go out hungry; from that cause the desire of a person, for many things they see, or smell, in general proceeds;[5] to avoid being so, I would wish you to carry a biscuit, or something of that kind, at all times in your pocket. Should you be so unfortunate as to mark the child,[6] be not discouraged, as it will not be of any bad consequence, and, in some cases, a remedy may be applied.

---

1 *The natural courses incident to our sex*: The menstrual period.
2 *Breeding*: Pregnant.
3 *When nature was last on you*: How long it has been since your last menstrual period.
4 *Breed sick*: Have morning sickness.
5 Being hungry leads people to desire everything they see and smell.
6 This, along with the next paragraph, references the theory of maternal impression (see

During your pregnancy, should you chance to meet, or see, any disagreeable object, such as lame, blind, &c. do not suffer it to make any impression on your mind, as you may then rest assured it will have no effect on you or the child.

When you are three months advanced, on no account keep it secret, as many ladies prejudice themselves thereby; should you be hot, or feverish, and frequently sick, it is absolutely necessary you should make your condition known to your midwife, (that he may order you,[7] at that time, to lose a little blood,) otherwise you may depend upon it you will have sore nipples, or your navel start; from both those circumstances I suffered much, with my first child: it therefore behooves you to be particularly careful, to avoid those inconveniences, and, believe me, you cannot do yourself, or midwife, justice to conceal from him or her your condition; a gentleman will understand your meaning at the instant.

Should your body not be regular every day, eat fruit, vegetables, or a few jar-raisins.

When you are five months advanced, put on jumps,[8] wear very broad bandages to your upper and under petticoats; sew an eye to the jumps, that they may hook on; by this method you take the weight off the loins: and at this time you should engage with a nurse.

When turned of six months, should feverish heats, fixed pains in the side, or any inflammatory symptoms appear, lose more blood, which will give you immediate relief. Should you perceive your water warmer than usual, take a table-spoonful of gum arabic twice a-day: be sure, at

---

"What You See: Assumption, Anxiety, and the Appearance of Health," pp. 383–412), which held that women could impress upon (or "mark") their child as a result of strong emotional responses or obsessions, including desire and fear. This impression might manifest physically or psychologically.

7   By the mid-eighteenth century, male midwives were becoming more common and were crowding out women who had previously held the role, but who lacked the clout granted by formal medical education or apprenticeship. This shift was controversial. The man-midwife was more likely to use potentially dangerous surgical implements, was seen as a threat to womanly modesty, and was also viewed as less attentive to the actual experience of women. For a defense of the female midwife, see Jane Sharp, *The Midwives Book* (pp. 143–147).

8   *Jumps*: Soft, unboned (and thus less restrictive than boned corsets and stays) bodices worn as undergarments.

this time, to have your child-bed linen well aired, and put into a large tin-box, in a warm place, for fear of a seven-months child, damp linen being particularly hurtful; strictly observing that napkins are not applied to you, or the child, hot, as they would occasion a violent inflammation in both.

As you find yourself grow weighty, lie down between the blankets at least three times a-day, to alter the posture; from which you will find great relief.

It is necessary to have two motions a-day the two last months; the last fortnight you should drink a glass of mountain,[9] with a table-spoonful of sweet oil in it, as it relaxes, and will be of great service in labor.

Should you, my dear madam, find yourself very uneasy the latter-part of your time, make not yourself unhappy, as it is most probable you will come the quicker and better for it.

As soon as you are taken in labor, comb your hair smooth, have an inch cut off behind and before, or you will find it comb off very much at the month's end. I know several ladies who have lost very fine heads of hair by this omission. The next thing, put on your night-cap, which will prove very comfortable: some ladies will not be persuaded to it, and, by that means, are very much disturbed. Four people about you are quite sufficient, the midwife, nurse, and two assistants; more only heat the room, create confusion, balk your pains, and prevent your taking them as you otherwise would: to prevent flooding, which is too often the case, or the fatigue of raising yourself up, I would recommend a silver sucking-spout, by the assistance of which you may drink without being moved.

A half-shift and body-cloth, with strings, a double napkin to your breasts, and a single waistcoat, with sleeves, to come as low as your elbows, (made by a skillful tailor, as soon as your are with child,) are all that are necessary; when you sit up in your bed, throw a double handkerchief over your neck, and slip on your bed-gown; lie warm, but not hot.

Providence has so ordained it, that a woman, with her first child, has seldom or ever any after-pains; if you are well, and can eat a biscuit,

---

9 *Mountain*: Wine from the mountains of Malaga, in Spain.

or crust of bread, the minute after delivery, it will keep the wind out of your stomach, and strengthen you very much. Be sure to have spermaceti,[10] sugar, and nutmeg, and plenty of very weak brandy and water: and, in a few hours afterwards, a half-pint basin of barley-jelly; but no caudle, on any consideration, till the milk has been at the height, and is quite gone off, so that you have not the least fever; as, by suppressing the milk at that time, according to instructions, you will gain strength very fast.

For the first twelve days, take of sugar and spermaceti about one-third of an ounce frequently; and, every or every other day, take a quarter of an ounce of manna,[11] as you find occasion, one motion a day being sufficient; without which, in all probability, you will have a fever, owing to confinement.

You may eat part of a boiled rabbit, chicken, or such like food, every day for the first week; and, about eleven o'clock, in the forenoon, have some good broth, beef-tea, or calf's-foot jelly, by way of change, with the barley-jelly; after which time (if you follow my directions) you may live as the family do, provided they dine at one o'clock.

If your strength will admit, I would wish you to get up the second day, to have your bed made; about the fourth or fifth put on your jumps, and pin your gown quite close; by attending to that, it will strengthen your back much; and, from that day, endeavor to sit up an hour, and so on by degrees, by which means you will recover your strength sooner than you are aware of: the weak state, ladies in general are reduced to, arises from lying in bed too long.

The fifth day you may drink half a pint of beer, with a glass of mountain in it; and, if you have any desire for cheese, at your dinner, eat a piece the size of a nutmeg, after which drink a glass of port-wine. The seventh or eighth day you may venture to drink beer alone; in that case, at and after dinner, drink a glass of port-wine: some time after lie down between the blankets, for an hour or more; if you can compose yourself to rest, it will be of great service. In this manner you should proceed the

---

10 *Spermaceti*: A fatty substance found in sperm and bottlenose whales and used in medicinal emollients.
11 *Manna*: A plant-based gum rich in mannitol, used as a mild laxative.

first three weeks; during which time always breakfast in bed, and lie two hours after; before you rise be sure to have something warm.

Dine at one o'clock, and by no means drink tea later than five; for, if you do, it will interfere with the undressing your child and getting your supper.

Between your tea and seven o'clock drink a little warm jelly, or a glass of wine with a crust of bread; otherwise, undressing your child and suckling will be too great a fatigue. Sup at nine o'clock, and be in bed by ten; after that time do not suffer any person to come into your room, as it will disturb you, and very likely prevent your sleeping.

Avoid seeing much company; for the weak state you may probably be in will not admit of it: should you be so, attend to this for the first three weeks, by which means you will regain your strength sooner.

When your month is up, and you are able to go abroad, I earnestly recommend you to observe, that if, by any means, you have been prevented suckling for six, eight, or ten, hours, which will sometimes be the case, you will use the Assistant instead of applying the child; should your exercise have thrown you into a perspiration, however gentle, make water,[12] put another cloak on, and drink something warm; the milk then will be fresh and good: should it not have vented itself in such a number of hours, you will be convinced, by its smelling offensively, that it must be hurtful to the infant; and without those preparations the countenance will immediately turn pale, cause it to cry, have a stool, or perhaps both; and then it is the blood gets foul: by this omission I lost a fine boy, four months old. As every disagreeable circumstance injures the milk; if your breasts are hard, and overfull, be assured you have taken cold, which is impossible to be avoided without great precaution; and thus numbers of children, by the foulness of the milk, have been thrown into convulsions.

I have great reason to believe, had I not drawn my breasts at least fourscore times, with each of my two last children, I should not have been able to have reared them, from trouble of mind, fatigue, and cold.

---

12 *Make water*: Urinate.

An Inquiry into the Causes and Effects of the Variolæ Vaccinæ*

EDWARD JENNER
(English, 1749–1823)

Folk medicine in the late eighteenth-century English countryside held that those infected with cowpox, only a minor illness in humans, could not later be infected with smallpox. With this knowledge, physician Edward Jenner set to work. In 1796, he deliberately infected human subjects with vaccinia (the cowpox virus) beginning with the eight-year-old son of his gardener. Jenner chose the boy, James Phipps, because he was healthy and, presumably, close at hand. Jenner's experiments were risky and controversial, but Western medicine at the time had no strong ethical rules in place about informed consent. Phipps had a strong immune response to cowpox, with nine days of discomfort, and recovered. Six weeks later, Jenner infected him with smallpox, but the risk paid off: the child was indeed immune. From this set of experiments, Jenner became known as the founder of vaccination—and we refer to all such treatments as vaccines (see also Zabdiel Boylston, pp. 167–171, and Lady Mary Wortley Montagu, pp. 163–166). Included here are excerpts from Jenner's description of these experiments, published in 1798. As you read, consider his description of cowpox and his case studies from these early vaccination efforts.

---

* Reprinted from Edward Jenner, *An Inquiry Into the Causes and Effects of the Variolæ Vaccinæ, A Disease Discovered in Some of the Western Counties of England [...] Known by the Name of the Cow Pox* (London, 1798), 1–7, Google Books.

[On the Cow Pox]

The deviation of man from the state in which he was originally placed by Nature seems to have proved to him a prolific source of diseases. From the love of splendor, from the indulgences of luxury, and from his fondness for amusement, he has familiarized himself with a great number of animals, which may not originally have been intended for his associates.

The wolf, disarmed of ferocity, is now pillowed in the lady's lap.[1] The cat, the little tiger of our island, whose natural home is the forest, is equally domesticated and caressed. The cow, the hog, the sheep, and the horse, are all, for a variety of purposes, brought under his care and dominion.

There is a disease to which the Horse, from his state of domestication, is frequently subject. The farriers have termed it *the Grease*.[2] It is an inflammation and swelling in the heel, from which issues matter possessing properties of a very peculiar kind, which seems capable of generating a disease in the human body (after it has undergone the modification which I shall presently speak of), which bears so strong a resemblance to the Small Pox, that I think it highly probable it may be the source of that disease.

In this dairy country a great number of cows are kept, and the office of milking is performed indiscriminately by men and maid servants. One of the former having been appointed to apply dressings to the heels of a horse affected with *the Grease*, and not paying due attention to cleanliness, incautiously bears his part in milking the cows, with some particles of the infectious matter adhering to his fingers. When this is the case, it commonly happens that a disease is communicated to the cows, and from the cows to the dairy-maids, which spreads through the farm until most of the cattle and domestics feel its unpleasant

---

1   [Jenner's note: The late Mr. John Hunter proved, by experiments, that the Dog is the Wolf in a degenerated state.]
2   *The Grease*: Also known as "mud fever," "dew poisoning," and "pastern dermatitis," and caused by a bacterial or fungal infection of the skin, this causes dermatitis and inflammation in the lower legs of horses.

consequences. This disease has obtained the name of the Cow Pox. It appears on the nipples of the cows in the form of irregular pustules. At their first appearance they are commonly of a palish blue, or rather of a color somewhat approaching to livid, and are surrounded by an erysipelatous inflammation. These pustules, unless a timely remedy be applied, frequently degenerate into phagedenic ulcers, which prove extremely troublesome.[3] The animals become indisposed, and the secretion of milk is much lessened. Inflamed spots now begin to appear on different parts of the hands of the domestics employed in milking, and sometimes on the wrists, which quickly run on to suppuration, first assuming the appearance of the small vesications[4] produced by a burn. Most commonly they appear about the joints of the fingers, and at their extremities; but whatever parts are affected, if the situation will admit, these superficial suppurations put on a circular form, with their edges more elevated than their center, and of a color distantly approaching to blue. Absorption takes place, and tumors appear in each axilla.[5] The system becomes affected–the pulse is quickened; and shiverings succeeded by heat, with general lassitude and pains about the loins and limbs, with vomiting, come on. The head is painful, and the patient is now and then even affected with delirium. These symptoms, varying in their degrees of violence, generally continue from one day to three or four, leaving ulcerated sores about the hands, which, from the sensibility of the parts, are very troublesome, and commonly heal slowly, frequently becoming phagedenic,[6] like those from whence they sprung. The lips, nostrils, eyelids, and other parts of the body, are sometimes affected with sores; but these evidently arise from their being heedlessly rubbed or scratched with the patient's infected fingers. No eruptions on the skin have followed the decline of the feverish symptoms in any instance that has come under my inspection, one only excepted, and in

---

3   [Jenner's note: They who attend sick cattle in this country find a speedy remedy for stopping the progress of this complaint in those applications which act chemically upon the morbid matter, such as the solutions of the Vitriolum Zinci, the Vitriolum Cupri, &c.]
4   *Vesications*: Blisters.
5   *Axilla*: Armpit.
6   *Phagedenic*: Ulcerous.

this case a very few appeared on the arms: they were very minute, of a vivid red color, and soon died away without advancing to maturation; so that I cannot determine whether they had any connection with the preceding symptoms.

Thus the disease makes its progress from the horse to the nipple of the cow, and from the cow to the human subject.

Morbid matter of various kinds, when absorbed into the system, may produce effects in some degree similar; but what renders the Cow-pox virus so extremely singular, is, that the person who has been thus affected is for ever after secure from the infection of the Small Pox; neither exposure to the variolous effluvia,[7] nor the insertion of the matter into the skin, producing this distemper.

In support of so extraordinary a fact, I shall lay before my reader a great number of instances....

CASE II

Sarah Portlock, of this place, was infected with the Cow-Pox, when a servant at a farmer's in the neighborhood, twenty-seven years ago.[8]

In the year 1792, conceiving herself, from this circumstance, secure from the infection of the Small Pox, she nursed one of her own children who had accidentally caught the disease, but no indisposition ensued. During the time she remained in the infected room, variolous matter was inserted into both her arms, but without any further effect than in the preceding case.

---

7   *Variolus effluvia*: Smallpox discharge (smallpox is caused by the variola virus).
8   [Jenner's note: I have purposely selected several cases in which the disease had appeared at a very distant period previous to the experiments made with variolous matter, to shew that the change produced in the constitution is not affected by time.]

CASE IX

Although the Cow Pox shields the constitution from the Small Pox, and the Small Pox proves a protection against its own future poison, yet it appears that the human body is again and again susceptible of the infectious matter of the Cow Pox, as the following history will demonstrate:

William Smith, of Pyrton in this parish, contracted this disease when he lived with a neighboring farmer in the year 1780. One of the horses belonging to the farm had sore heels, and it fell to his lot to attend him. By these means the infection was carried to the cows, and from the cows it was communicated to Smith. On one of his hands were several ulcerated sores, and he was affected with such symptoms as have been before described.

In the year 1791 the Cow Pox broke out at another farm where he then lived as a servant, and he became affected with it a second time; and in the year 1794 he was so unfortunate as to catch it again. The disease was equally as severe the second and third time as it was on the first.[9]

In the spring of the year 1795 he was twice inoculated, but no affection of the system could be produced from the variolous matter; and he has since associated with those who had the Small Pox in its most contagious state without feeling any effect from it.

CASE XXI

April 5th. Several children and adults were inoculated from the arm of William Pead. The greater part of them sickened on the 6th day, and were well on the 7th, but in three of the number a secondary indisposition arose in consequence of an extensive erysipelatous inflammation[10]

---

9 [Jenner's note: This is not the case in general—a second attack is commonly very slight, and so, I am informed, it is among the cows.]

10 *Erysipelatous inflammation*: Once commonly known as St. Anthony's Fire, *erysipelas* is a bacterial skin disease caused by *streptococcus pyogenes* that causes red, raised patches of skin and may lead to extreme pain, fever, chills, and vomiting.

which appeared on the inoculated arms. It seemed to arise from the state of the pustule, which spread out, accompanied with some degree of pain, to about half the diameter of a six-pence. One of these patients was an infant of half a year old. By the application of mercurial ointment[11] to the inflamed parts (a treatment recommended under similar circumstances in the inoculated Small-pox) the complaint subsided without giving much trouble....

[Conclusion]

Although I presume it may be unnecessary to produce further testimony in support of my assertion "that the Cow-pox protects the human constitution from the infection of the Small-pox," yet it affords me considerable satisfaction to say, that Lord Somerville, the President of the Board of Agriculture, to whom this paper was shown by Sir Joseph Banks,[12] has found upon inquiry that the statements were confirmed by the concurring testimony of Mr. Dolland, a surgeon, who resides in a dairy country remote from this, in which these observations were made. With respect to the opinion adduced "that the source of the infection is a peculiar morbid matter arising in the horse," although I have not been able to prove it from actual experiments conducted immediately under my own eye, yet the evidence I have adduced appears sufficient to establish it.

They who are not in the habit of conducting experiments may not be aware of the coincidence of circumstances necessary for their being managed so as to prove perfectly decisive; nor how often men engaged in professional pursuits are liable to interruptions which disappoint them almost at the instant of their being accomplished: however, I feel no room for hesitation respecting the common origin of the disease, being well convinced that it never appears among the cows (except it

---

11 *Mercurial ointment*: Ointments and topical treatments including mercury were long used for treating conditions that affected the skin (most famously, syphilis).

12 Sir Joseph Banks (1743–1820), naturalist and botanist, was the president of England's academy of scientific inquiry, The Royal Society, for 41 years.

can be traced to a cow introduced among the general herd which has been previously infected, or to an infected servant), unless they have been milked by some one who, at the same time, has the care of a horse affected with diseased heels....

Thus far have I proceeded in an inquiry, founded, as it must appear, on the basis of experiment; in which, however, conjecture has been occasionally admitted in order to present to persons well situated for such discussions, objects for a more minute investigation. In the mean time I shall myself continue to prosecute this inquiry, encouraged by the hope of its becoming essentially beneficial to mankind.

Medical Ethics*

THOMAS PERCIVAL
(English, 1740–1804)

English physician Thomas Percival's *Medical Ethics* (1803) is lauded as the first systematic and expansive code of ethics for those in the medical profession. The work emerged at the same time as the modern hospital began to develop, with its trained medical practitioners and more specialized care. Where previous ethical models (like those of Sushruta, Hippocrates, and Guy de Chauliac in this volume) offered expectations of individual physicians and surgeons, Percival proposes a wide-ranging set of principles for use across hospitals and for all practitioners. His work spans ethical concerns for collegiality and patient care, etiquette, record-keeping and legal matters, setting up not just a physician's oath but also a network of ethical standards. As you read, consider his approach to the physician's role in relation to patients and other physicians and his thoughts on hospital management.

---

* Reprinted from Thomas Percival, *Medical Ethics; Or, a Code of Institutes and Precepts, Adapted to the Professional Conduct of Physicians and Surgeons* (Manchester: S. Russell, 1803), 9–5, 20–27, Google Books.

Chapter I. *Of Professional Conduct, Relative to Hospitals, or other medical charities.*

1. Hospital physicians and surgeons should minister to the sick, with due impressions of the importance of their office; reflecting that the ease, the health, and the lives of those committed to their charge depend upon their skill, attention, and fidelity. They should study, also, in their deportment, so to unite tenderness with steadiness, and condescension with authority, as to inspire the minds of their patients with gratitude, respect, and confidence.

2. The choice of a physician or surgeon cannot be allowed to hospital patients, consistently with the regular and established succession of medical attendance. Yet personal confidence is not less important to the comfort and relief of the sick-poor, than of the rich under similar circumstances: And it would be equally just and humane, to inquire into and to indulge their partialities, by occasionally calling into consultation the favorite practitioner. The rectitude and wisdom of this conduct will be still more apparent, when it is recollected that patients in hospitals not infrequently request their discharge, on a deceitful plea of having received relief; and afterwards procure another recommendation, that they may be admitted under the physician or surgeon of their choice. Such practices involve in them a degree of falsehood; produce unnecessary trouble; and may be occasion of irreparable loss of time in the treatment of diseases.

3. The feelings and emotions of the patients, under critical circumstances, require to be known and attended to, no less than the symptoms of their diseases. Thus, extreme timidity, with respect to venesection, contraindicates its use, in certain areas and constitutions. Even prejudices of the sick are not to be contemned,[1] or opposed with harshness. For though silenced by authority, they will operate secretly and forcibly on the mind, creating fear, anxiety, and watchfulness.

4. As misapprehension may magnify real evils, or create imaginary ones, no discussion concerning the nature of the case should be entered into before the patients, either with the house surgeon, the pupils of the hospitals, or any medical visitor.

---

1 *To be contemned*: To be treated with contempt.

5. In the large wards of an infirmary the patients should be interrogated concerning their complaint, in a tone of voice which cannot be overheard. Secrecy, also, when required by peculiar circumstances, should be strictly observed. And females should always be treated with the most scrupulous delicacy. To neglect or to sport with their feelings is cruelty; and every wound thus inflicted tends to produce a callousness of mind, a contempt of decorum, and an insensibility to modesty and virtue. Let these considerations be forcibly and repeatedly urged on the hospital pupils....

9. The medical gentlemen of every charitable institution are, in some degree, responsible for, and the guardians of, the honor of each other. No physician or surgeon, therefore should reveal occurrences in the hospital, which may injure the reputation of any one of his colleagues; except under the restriction contained in the succeeding article.

10. No professional charge should be made by a physician or surgeon, either publicly or privately, against any associate, without previously laying the complaint before the gentlemen of the faculty belonging to the institution, that they may judge concerning the reasonableness of its grounds, and the measures to be adopted....

14. Hospital registers usually contain only a simple report of the number of patients admitted and discharged. By adopting a more comprehensive plan, they might be rendered subservient to medical science, and beneficial to mankind. The following sketch is offered, with deference, to the gentlemen of the faculty. Let the register consist of three tables; the first specifying the number of patients admitted, cured, relieved, discharged, or dead; the second the several diseases of the patients, with their events; the third the sexes, ages, and occupations of the patients. The ages should be reduced into classes; and the tables adapted to the four divisions of the year. By such an institution, the increase or decrease of sickness; the attack, progress, and cessation of epidemics; the comparative healthiness of different situations, climates, and seasons; the influences of particular trades and manufactures on health and life; with many other curious circumstances, not more interesting to physicians than to the community, would be ascertained with sufficient precision....

22. Due notice should be given of a consultation, and no person

admitted to it, except the physicians and surgeons of the hospital, and the house-surgeon, without the unanimous consent of the gentlemen present. If an examination of the patient be previously necessary, the particular circumstances of danger or difficulty should be carefully concealed from him, and every just precaution used to guard him from anxiety or alarm.

23. No important operation should be determined upon, without a consultation of the physicians and surgeons, and the acquiescence of a majority of them. Twenty-four hours notice should be given of the proposed operation, except in dangerous accidents, or when peculiar circumstances occur, which may render delay hazardous. The presence of a spectator should not be allowed during an operation, without the express permission of the operator. All extra-official interference in the management of it should be forbidden. A decorous silence ought to be observed. It may be humane and salutary, however, for one of the attending physicians or surgeons to speak occasionally to the patient; to comfort him under his sufferings; and to give him assurance, if consistent with the truth, that the operation goes on well, and promises a speedy and successful termination.

As a hospital is the best school for practical surgery, it would be liberal and beneficial to invite, in rotation, two surgeons of the town, who do not belong to the institution, to be present at each operation.

24. Hospital consultations ought not to be held on Sundays, except in cases of urgent necessity; and on such occasions an hours should be appointed, which does not interfere with attendance on public worship.

25. It is an established usage, in some hospitals, to have a stated day in the week for the performance of operations. But this may occasion improper delay, or equally unjustifiable anticipation. When several operations are to take place in succession, one patient should not have his mind agitated by the knowledge of the sufferings of another. The surgeon should change his apron, when besmeared; and the table or instruments should be freed from all marks of blood, and every thing that may excite terror....

27. Hospitals, appropriated to particular maladies, are established in different places, and claim both the patronage and the aid of the gentlemen of the faculty. To an asylum for female patients, laboring under

syphilis, it is to be lamented that discouragements have been too often and successfully opposed. Yet whoever reflects on the variety of diseases to which the human body is incident, will find that as considerable part of them are derived from immoderate passions, and vicious indulgences. Sloth, intemperance, and irregular desires are the great sources of those evils, which contract the duration, and embitter the enjoyment of life. But humanity, whilst she bewails the vices of mankind, incites us to alleviate the miseries which flow from them. And it may be proved that a lock hospital[2] is an institution founded on the most benevolent principles, consonant to sound policy, and favorable to reformation and to virtue. It provides relief for a painful and loathsome distemper, which contaminates, in its progress, the innocent as well as the guilty, and extends its baneful influence to future generations. It restores to virtue and to religion those votaries whom pleasure has seduced, or villainy betrayed; and who now feels, by sad experience, that ruin, misery, and disgrace are the wages of sin. Over such objects pity sheds the generous tear; austerity softens into forgiveness; and benevolence expands at the united pleas of frailty, penitence, and wretchedness.

No peculiar rules of conduct are requisite in the medical attendance on lock hospitals. But as these institutions must, from the nature of their object, be in a great measure shut from the inspection of the public, it will behoove the faculty to consider themselves as responsible, to an extraordinary degree, for their right government; that the moral, no less than the medical purposes of such establishments may be fully answered. The strictest decorum should be observed in the conduct towards the female patients; no young pupils should be admitted into the house; every ministering office should be performed by nurses properly instructed; and books adapted to the moral improvement of the patients should be put into their hands, and given them on their discharge. To provide against the danger of urgent want, a small sum of money, and decent clothes should at this time be dispensed to them; and, when

---

2   *Lock hospital*: In Britain and its colonies, a medical facility dedicated specifically to the treatment of sexually transmitted diseases. In some cases, police were deputized to round up prostitutes and women who were thought to have these diseases. The women were taken to the lock hospital and forcibly held for treatment.

practicable, some mode should be pointed out of obtaining a reputable livelihood.

28. Asylums for insanity possess accommodations and advantages, of which the poor must, in all circumstances, be destitute; and which no private family, however opulent, may provide. Of these schemes of benevolence all classes of men may have equal occasion to participate the benefits; for human nature itself becomes the mournful object of such institutions. Other diseases leave man a rational and moral agent, and sometimes improve both the faculties of the head, and the affections of the heart. But lunacy subverts the whole rational and moral character; extinguishes every tender charity; and excludes the degraded sufferer from all the enjoyments and advantages of social intercourse. Painful is the office of a physician, when he is called upon to minister to such humiliating objects of distress. Yet great must be his felicity, when he can render himself instrumental, under providence, in the restoration of reason, and in the renewal of the lost image of God. Let no one, however, promise himself this divine privilege, if he be not deeply skilled in the philosophy of human nature. For though casual success may sometimes be the result of empirical practice, the *medicina mentis*[3] can only be administered with steady efficacy by him, how, to a knowledge of the animal economy, and of the physical causes which regulate or disturb its movements, unites an intimate acquaintance with the laws of association; the control of fancy over judgment; the force of habit; the direction and comparative strength of opposite passions; and the reciprocal dependence and relations of the moral and intellectual powers of man.

---

3 *Medicina mentis*: Medicine of the mind.

On Mediate Auscultation*

RENÉ LAËNNEC
(French, 1781–1826)

During René Laënnec's university study in France, he learned common practices for diagnosing conditions of the chest, like percussion using fingers or placing an ear directly on the chest itself (direct auscultation). This was a useful, if impractical and sometimes invasive, method, especially in the case of treating female patients. It was considered important to maintain and respect ideals of feminine modesty, which would limit access to a woman's bare chest. Laënnec devised a solution in 1816 while working with a woman whose build did not permit percussive tests: to allow for indirect (or "mediate") auscultation, he invented the stethoscope. Included here is the introduction of his treatise explaining this process, *On Mediate Auscultation* (*De l'Auscultation Médiate*), published in 1819. As you read, consider his account of making this discovery and invention.

---

* Reprinted from René Laënnec, *A Treatise on the Diseases of the Chest and on Mediate Auscultation*, 4th ed., trans. John Forbes (London, 1834), 3–5, Google Books.

[The Invention of the Stethoscope]

The percussion of the chest, according to the method of the ingenious observer just mentioned,[1] is one of the most valuable discoveries ever made in medicine. By means of it, several diseases which had hitherto been cognizable by general and equivocal signs only, are brought within the immediate sphere of our perceptions, and their diagnosis, consequently, rendered both more easy and more certain. It is not to be concealed, however, that this mode of exploration is very incomplete. Confined, in great measure, to the indication of *fullness* or *emptiness*, it is only applicable to a limited number of organic lesions; it does not enable us to discriminate some which are very different in their nature or seat; it scarcely affords any indication except in extreme cases, and cannot therefore enable us to detect, or even to suspect, diseases in their very commencement. It is more particularly in diseases of the heart that we regret the insufficiency of this method, and wish for something more precise. The general symptoms of disease in this organ greatly resemble those produced by many nervous complaints, and by the diseases of other organs. The application of the hand affords some indications as to the extent, strength, and rhythm of the heart's motions; but these in general are by no means distinct, while, in cases of considerable fatness or anasarca,[2] they become very obscure, or are altogether imperceptible. Within these few years some physicians have, in those cases, attempted to gain further information by the application of the ear to the cardiac region. In this way, the pulsations of the heart, perceived at once by the ear and touch, become, no doubt, more distinct. But even this method comes far short of what might be expected from it. Bayle[3] was the first to my knowledge who had recourse to it, at the time when we were attending the lectures of Corvisart.[4] This great man himself never used it:

---

1 Leopold Auenbrugger (1722–1809), Austrian physician who pioneered the use of percussion for the diagnosis of conditions of the thorax and abdomen.
2 *Anasarca*: Another term for edema, or the swelling of the body caused by tissues retaining fluid.
3 Gaspard Laurent Bayle (1774–1816), French physician, known for research into cancer and tuberculosis.
4 Jean-Nocilas Corvisart (1755–1821), a renowned French cardiologist.

he says only that he had several times heard the pulsation of the heart in *listening very close to the chest*. We shall afterwards find that this phenomenon is different from auscultation, properly so called, and is only observable in some particular cases. But neither Bayle nor any other of our fellow-students, who with myself might, in imitation of him, employ this immediate auscultation, (of which, by the way, the first notion is derived from Hippocrates,) obtained any other result from it than that of perceiving more distinctly the action of the heart, in the cases where this was not very perceptible to the touch. The reason of this limited application will be stated hereafter. But, independently of its deficiencies, there are other objections to its use: it is always inconvenient both to the physician and patient; in the case of females it is not only indelicate but often impracticable; and in that class of person found in hospitals it is disgusting.[5] For these various reasons this measure can but rarely be had recourse to, and cannot therefore become practically useful; since it is only by numerous observations and the comparison of numerous facts of the same kind, that we can ever, in medicine, separate the truth from the errors which are constantly derived from the inexperience of the observer, from the varying fitness of his perceptive powers, the illusions of his senses, and the inherent difficulties of the method of exploration which he employs. Observations made after long intervals can never overcome difficulties of this kind. Nevertheless, I had been in the habit of using this method for a long time, in obscure cases, and where it was practicable; and it was the employment of it which led me to the discovery of one much better.

In 1816, I was consulted by a young woman laboring under general symptoms of a diseased heart, and in whose case percussion and the application of the hand were of little avail on account of the great degree of fatness. The other method just mentioned being rendered inadmissible by the age and sex of the patient, I happened to recollect a simple and well-known fact in acoustics, and fancied it might be turned to some use on the present occasion. The fact I allude to is the great distinctness

---

5   The medical profession in France was instrumental in shaping the nature of the modern hospital, but in the early nineteenth century many hospitals were troubled by poor conditions, inadequate space, and improper sanitation.

with which we hear the scratch of a pin at one end of a piece of wood, on applying our ear to the other. Immediately, on this suggestion, I rolled a quire of paper into a kind of cylinder and applied on end of it to the region of the heart and the other to my ear, and was not a little surprised and please, to find that I could thereby perceive the action of the heart in a manner much more clear and distinct than I had ever been able to do by the immediate application of the ear. From this moment I imagined that the circumstance might furnish means for enabling us to ascertain the character, not only of the action of the heart, but of every species of sound produced by the motion of the thoracic viscera, and, consequently, for the exploration of respiration, the voice, the *rhonchus*, and perhaps even the fluctuation of fluid extravasated in the pleura or the pericardium. With this conviction, I forthwith commenced at the Hospital Necker[6] a series of observations from which I have been able to deduce a set of new signs of diseases of the chest, for the most part certain, and prominent, and calculated, perhaps, to render the diagnosis of the diseases of the lungs, heart, and pleura, as decided and circumstantial, as the indications furnished to the surgeon by the introduction of the finger or sound, in the complaints wherein they are used.

6   *The Hospital Necker*: The Necker-Enfants Malades Hospital, founded in 1778 in Paris, France.

Sketches in Bedlam;
Or, Characteristic Traits of Insanity*

BY A CONSTANT OBSERVER
1823

Originally founded in London in 1247, the Bethlem Royal Hospital later became infamous as an asylum for people who were considered insane. Over the next several centuries, it developed into an asylum, taking in the incapacitated and "mad"—and in doing so, led to the coining of the word "bedlam" to mean "chaos." Bedlam—the hospital—earned mentions in a number of popular plays and written works as well as in art. Conditions were often reported to be wretched. The troubled hospital was relocated to new facilities in 1815, and by 1823 *Sketches in Bedlam; or, Characteristic Traits of Insanity* was published. The book, apparently written by a hospital insider (the "Constant Observer"), offers a picture of some of the hospital's procedures and practices, followed by 140 patient profiles. These include some of the hospital's more lurid tales and famous occupants, as well as more humanizing portraits. As you read, consider the description of the facility and its rules, and the characterization of its patients.

---

* Reprinted from *Sketches in Bedlam; or Characteristic Traits of Insanity, as Displayed in the Cases of One Hundred and Forty Patients of Both Sexes, now, or recently, Confined in New Bethlem* (London: Sherwood, Jones & Co., 1823), xx, xxxiv–xxxv, 46–48, 49–50, 76, 91, 262, 267–268, 270–271, Google Books.

Regulations

The patients rise every morning in summer at six o'clock, and in winter at seven. They breakfast at eight in summer, and in winter at half past eight. They dine daily at one, sup at six, and retire to bed at eight, when they are locked up. Each patient has a separate room. The bedsteads are of iron, with common sacking[1] bottoms; the bedding a good flock mattress, a pillow, three blankets, a pair of sheets, and a rug. The sheets are regularly changed every fortnight, or oftener if necessary.

In the basement gallery, where the disorderly patients are, there are no sheets, and they sleep on straw, which is changed every morning if requisite....

Instructions for Persons Applying for the Admission of Patients into Bethlem Hospital

All lunatics who are not disqualified by the following regulations may be admitted into this hospital at all seasons of the year, and will be provided with every thing necessary for their complete recovery, provided the same can be effected within twelve months from the time of their admission, upon payment of £2,[2] if the patient is sent by relatives or friends; and of £4 if such patient is a parish pauper, or has received alms or support from any body in the community; which sums are not returnable, unless the patient dies or is discharged within one month after admission, nor in any case where deception has been practiced upon the hospital by a false statement.

The following cases are inadmissible:

---

1 *Sacking*: Closely woven material used to make sturdy sacks; often made from jute, flax, or hemp.
2 £2 in 1823 would be worth roughly £240 (or $333 in US dollars). In addition to charging to take patients in, Bethlem officials also allowed for a kind of tourism: visitors could "donate" to the hospital to enter.

1. Those lunatics who are possessed of property sufficient for their decent support in a private asylum, and also those whose near relations are capable of affording such support.
2. Those who have been insane for more than twelve months.
3. Those who have been discharged uncured from any other hospital for the reception of lunatics.
4. Female lunatics who are with child, or who have been discharged from this hospital in consequence of their pregnancy having been discovered.
5. Lunatics in a state of idiocy, afflicted with palsy, or with epileptic or convulsive fits.[3]
6. Lunatics having the venereal disease or the itch.
7. Those who are so weakened by age or by disease as to require the attendance of a nurse, or to threaten the speedy dissolution of life, or who are so lame as to require the assistance of a crutch.

[Selected Case Studies]

Charles Goldney

Aged near seventy. This poor old man has been confined at Sir Jonathan Miles's, in Old Bethlem,[4] and here, altogether between thirty

---

3   Although not legally distinguished from the mentally ill until the "Idiots Act" of 1886 (which established distinct facilities for the long term care of those deemed to have developmental, intellectual, or cognitive disabilities), Bethlem Hospital was actively committed to only treating patients who were thought to have curable mental conditions. Permanent disabilities, incurable physical conditions (like epilepsy), and contagious physical diseases were outside the purview of this commitment.

4   *Old Bethlem*: The hospital has stood on several different sites in the London area since its founding in 1247 (when it was just outside the wall of the medieval city in Bishopsgate). "Old Bethlem" was the second site, rebuilt to the north of the city in Moorfields in 1676. This old facility fell into disrepair within just over a hundred years, and was rebuilt again in Southwark, just south of the Thames River. This third building was completed in 1816 and is the facility referred to in this volume. The hospital currently stands on a fourth site, finished in 1930.

and forty years; and was many of those years restrained in irons at Old Bethlem.

But his derangement is not abated. He has the strangest notions imaginable: he believes himself to be a man of immense property; he says he gave his son, in Somersetshire, a fortune of £400,000; but they murdered him, and built monuments, churches, and canals with the money. He has, by his own account, a hundred coaches running in London at this day. As an amusement he has charge of the ducks, and assists, as well as his age permits, the cutter of provisions. He is particularly tender about the ducks and pigs; the ducks, he believes, are of a very high breed, between a cock pheasant and a game hen; some are double high, some treble high cross breed. When a duck is to be killed it must be done without his knowledge: he soon, however, misses it, and exclaims, "Ah! So they have been at their damnable work again, have they? I'll make them pay for it." During the very cold weather in January this year, when the pond was frozen over, all the ducks died but four, and Goldney swore they had all been poisoned. He is equally exasperated with a pig is killed: he believes ducks and pigs, Bethlem, and all belonging to it, are his own property, and says they know it, but they want to keep him out of it if they can, but it must come to him after all, when the time comes. A pig was lately killed, which he says he would not take any money for: he bought its mother in France thirty-six years ago, and gave eighteen pounds twenty-eight shillings and fourteen-pence, for her. He says he is but forty-six years old, and has been confined forty-two years, but his present body is the third he has had, the former two bodies were worn out many years ago: the present one is forty-six years old. He chews a quantity of tobacco, and when speaking to any one seriously, he turns his quid, winks his eyes or shuts both, gives you a touch with his elbow, in a sort of knowing way, and says, "all will be well with him very soon, he knows all about it, but he keeps quiet and peaceable: he don't let them know that he knows anything about it, but they can't deceive him." In the last summer he swore that air-pumps were employed to pump fleas into his neck, with a view of devouring him alive: he believes that they (God knows who) would give £500,000,000 of money if he was dead, but they will be deceived, he assures them. He does some trifling jobs about the house, which employ his mind; the exercise is conducive to his health. His appetite is good, but age creeps on the poor fellow apace. He is perfectly harmless, and may be trusted with safety any where; is punctual and attentive in all his little works, and offensive to no one....

William Killiner

Aged near sixty, admitted about six years since. This unfortunate man comes from London, and was convicted of firing a loaded gun indiscriminately amongst a crowd of people, who were assembled around his house. It appeared that he had repeatedly desired them to go away, which they refused to do; and at length he, in a rage, fired amongst them, but providentially no mischief was done. He was, however, convicted of the criminal intent, but his derangement at the time of the act was fully proved, and he was sent here.[5] He seems at present perfectly calm, rational, cleanly, and well behaved, and has many respectable friends.

Francis Wilkes

A Welshman, aged twenty-seven, admitted about five years since. He was before a patient in Old Bethlem when a boy, and was discharged cured: but at more advanced years he became again deranged; and having in a paroxysm of frenzy murdered his mother, was sent here, where he is constantly confined in the criminal wing.

He is extremely vicious and dangerous while the paroxysms of his disorder continue (which do not very frequently occur), and then he would murder indiscriminately all he met, friends or strangers; but in his tranquil intervals he is generally quiet and well-conducted. He is handy and industrious, and can make and mend the clothes of other patients, for which he is regularly paid....

---

5   Throughout much of England's history, those who were acquitted of criminal charges on the basis of insanity were often released back into the community. However, in 1800, the Criminal Lunatics Act established that these people, the "criminally insane," were to be indefinitely committed to an institution like Bethlem Hospital.

John Paling

Aged about forty-five. This man was tried and convicted of the willful murder of a young woman who was his sweetheart, and a suspicion of her inconstancy was said to have prompted him to the horrid act. But he was found to be insane in his intellects, and was sent here upwards of five years since. He is of a sullen and morose disposition, and it requires, of course, much caution to avoid offending him; but in general he is tolerably well-behaved, and evinces no obvious symptoms of insanity.

Charlotte Dully

Aged forty-five, belonged to Putney, and was transferred hither from Old Bethlem: she is a married woman, and mother of a family. This poor woman has contracted a most singular persuasion: she fancies herself to be a man, and sometimes styles herself a boy; and, when spoken to, she bows, scrapes, and puts her hand to her head in every respect like a footman.

She is particularly attached to the matron, whom she calls her beauty, and is quite uneasy every day until she sees her.

There is nothing else particularly remarkable in her manner; she is orderly, cleanly in her person and habits, and perfectly quiet and harmless....

Christiana Ross

Aged... This is a Scotchwoman, and was one of those unfortunate females that nightly infest the streets of the metropolis. In one of her professional excursions she fell in with a butcher, and before she parted with him robbed him of £20.

She appears more simple than mad. She says that Mr. Capper robbed her of all her rings and jewels, muff, and all her fine things, when she was first apprehended. She still preserves a broach, and a shilling, which she carefully keeps wrapped up in a number of papers; which shilling, she says, is to pay for a lodging, the first night she obtains her liberty. She takes snuff, and although she feels much in want of it sometimes, she is so scrupulously careful of her shilling, that she will beg, borrow, or go without the exhilarating powder altogether, rather than break upon this last remnant of her cash.

Jane Cook

Aged…, London. This is a married woman, and was servant in a family in London. The family being out of town, she one night set fire to the house in the following manner. She had seen her husband, on the night alluded to, with whom she had very high words,[6] on what account is not known, but, mortified and driven to desperation, she resolved on her own destruction. With this view she procured a quantity of laudanum and gin mixed together: she then went to rest, doubly intoxicated, having first placed a lighted candle underneath the bed.

She soon became insensible. The bed and furniture caught fire, and the flames spread. The watchman on his post observing it, obtained assistance, broke into the house, repaired to the room on fire, where he found the unfortunate woman in a state of complete insensibility, and much burnt. She was taken out; but the house and furniture received considerable damage. She remained ill a long time, from the double effects of poison and fire, and was ultimately found to be deranged.

She betrays no symptoms of insanity, attends divine service, is orderly and regular, and conducts herself very well, but does not recollect setting fire to her master's house….

Elizabeth Burrowes

London. This wretched woman was found guilty of destroying one of her children, and, being deranged, was sent to Bethlem. She appears to be perfectly sensible of the crime she has committed, and is in consequence extremely disconsolate, desponding,[7] and dejected. She has no particular insane ideas, but her mind appears to be continually on the rack, most probably on reflections at what she has done.

---

6   *High words*: Angry words, or a verbal fight.
7   *Desponding*: Despairing.

The History of Mary Prince, a West Indian Slave*

MARY PRINCE
(Afro-Caribbean, 1788–ca. 1833)

Mary Prince was born into enslavement in Bermuda, which had been colonized by the English early in the seventeenth century. After being bought and sold multiple times, she was brought to England by enslaver John Adams Wood in 1828. Wood refused to allow Prince to purchase her own freedom, and when he eventually wrote a letter allowing her to leave, that letter also actively discouraged anyone from hiring her. She found freedom by seeking out London's Anti-Slavery Society, and eventually took paid work with Thomas Pringle, the secretary of the society. *The History of Mary Prince, a West Indian Slave* (1831) is her autobiography. Because enslaved people were rarely taught to read and write, the book was transcribed for her by abolitionist Susanna Strickland (later Moody) and brought to press by Pringle. The book was very popular, going through multiple printings in its first year, and was influential in the movement to abolish slavery. In this excerpt, Prince mixes autopathography (a personal illness narrative) with more traditional biographical narrative. As you read, consider her description of her experience with rheumatism and the treatment she faced while enduring it.

---

* Reprinted from Mary Prince, *The History of Mary Prince, A West Indian Slave. Related By Herself* (London: F. Westley and A.H. Davis, Stationers' Hall Court, 1831; Project Gutenberg, 2006), 14–15, 18–22.

[On Sickness and Slavery]

During the time I worked there, I heard that Mr. John Wood was going to Antigua. I felt a great wish to go there, and I went to Mr. D—, and asked him to let me go in Mr. Wood's service. Mr. Wood did not then want to purchase me; it was my own fault that I came under him, I was so anxious to go. It was ordained to be, I suppose; God led me there. The truth is, I did not wish to be any longer the slave of my indecent master.

Mr. Wood took me with him to Antigua, to the town of St. John's, where he lived. This was about fifteen years ago. He did not then know whether I was to be sold; but Mrs. Wood found that I could work, and she wanted to buy me. Her husband then wrote to my master to inquire whether I was to be sold? Mr. D— wrote in reply, "that I should not be sold to any one that would treat me ill." It was strange he should say this, when he had treated me so ill himself. So I was purchased by Mr. Wood for 300 dollars, (or £100 Bermuda currency.)[1]

My work there was to attend the chambers and nurse the child, and to go down to the pond and wash clothes. But I soon fell ill of the rheumatism,[2] and grew so very lame that I was forced to walk with a stick. I got the Saint Anthony's fire,[3] also, in my left leg, and became quite a cripple. No one cared much to come near me, and I was ill a long long time; for several months I could not lift the limb. I had to lie in a little old out-house, that was swarming with bugs and other vermin, which tormented me greatly; but I had no other place to lie in. I got the rheumatism by catching cold at the pond side, from washing in the fresh

---

1 Roughly £7,000, or $9,700USD.
2 *Rheumatism*: Any of a number of chronic, painful conditions of the joints and connective tissue. Currently, rheumatic disorders fall into ten major categories and comprise over 200 conditions, including some types of arthritis, gout, and bursitis.
3 *Saint Anthony's Fire*: This can refer to three different medical conditions, all of which can impact the legs: ergotism (or ergot poisoning) can cause dry gangrene in the feet and hands; erysipelas (often caused by *streptococcus pyogenes*) causes edema and blistering and can lead to necrosis of the skin; and shingles (a reactivation of *varicella zoster*, the virus that causes chicken pox) causes painful skin rashes, blisters, and nerve pain in localized areas.

water; in the salt water I never got cold. The person who lived in next yard, (a Mrs. Greene,) could not bear to hear my cries and groans. She was kind, and used to send an old slave woman to help me, who sometimes brought me a little soup. When the doctor found I was so ill, he said I must be put into a bath of hot water. The old slave got the bark of some bush that was good for the pains, which she boiled in the hot water, and every night she came and put me into the bath, and did what she could for me: I don't know what I should have done, or what would have become of me, had it not been for her.—My mistress, it is true, did send me a little food; but no one from our family came near me but the cook, who used to shove my food in at the door, and say, "Molly,[4] Molly, there's your dinner." My mistress did not care to take any trouble about me; and if the Lord had not put it into the hearts of the neighbors to be kind to me, I must, I really think, have lain and died.

It was a long time before I got well enough to work in the house. Mrs. Wood, in the meanwhile, hired a mulatto woman to nurse the child; but she was such a fine lady she wanted to be mistress over me. I thought it very hard for a colored woman to have rule over me because I was a slave and she was free. Her name was Martha Wilcox; she was a saucy woman, very saucy; and she went and complained of me, without cause, to my mistress, and made her angry with me. Mrs. Wood told me that if I did not mind what I was about, she would get my master to strip me and give me fifty lashes: "You have been used to the whip," she said, "and you shall have it here." This was the first time she threatened to have me flogged; and she gave me the threatening so strong of what she would have done to me, that I thought I should have fallen down at her feet, I was so vexed and hurt by her words. The mulatto woman was rejoiced to have power to keep me down. She was constantly making mischief; there was no living for the slaves—no peace after she came.

I was also sent by Mrs. Wood to be put in the cage one night, and was next morning flogged, by the magistrate's order, at her desire; and this all for a quarrel I had about a pig with another slave woman. I was flogged on my naked back on this occasion: although I was in no fault after all; for old Justice Dyett, when we came before him, said that I was

---

4   *Molly*: A diminutive form of Mary.

in the right, and ordered the pig to be given to me. This was about two or three years after I came to Antigua.

When we moved from the middle of the town to the Point, I used to be in the house and do all the work and mind the children, though still very ill with the rheumatism. Every week I had to wash two large bundles of clothes, as much as a boy could help me to lift; but I could give no satisfaction. My mistress was always abusing and fretting after me. It is not possible to tell all her ill language.—One day she followed me foot after foot scolding and rating[5] me. I bore in silence a great deal of ill words: at last my heart was quite full, and I told her that she ought not to use me so;—that when I was ill I might have lain and died for what she cared; and no one would then come near me to nurse me, because they were afraid of my mistress. This was a great affront. She called her husband and told him what I had said. He flew into a passion: but did not beat me then; he only abused and swore at me; and then gave me a note and bade me go and look for an owner. Not that he meant to sell me; but he did this to please his wife and to frighten me. I went to Adam White, a cooper,[6] a free black, who had money, and asked him to buy me. He went directly to Mr. Wood, but was informed that I was not to be sold. The next day my master whipped me.

Another time (about five years ago) my mistress got vexed with me, because I fell sick and I could not keep on with my work. She complained to her husband, and he sent me off again to look for an owner. I went to a Mr. Burchell, showed him the note, and asked him to buy me for my own benefit; for I had saved about 100 dollars, and hoped, with a little help, to purchase my freedom. He accordingly went to my master:— "Mr. Wood," he said, "Molly has brought me a note that she wants an owner. If you intend to sell her, I may as well buy her as another." My master put him off and said that he did not mean to sell me. I was very sorry at this, for I had no comfort with Mrs. Wood, and I wished greatly to get my freedom….

I had not much happiness in my marriage, owing to my being a slave. It made my husband sad to see me so ill-treated. Mrs. Wood was

---

5   *Rating*: Berating or scolding.
6   *Cooper*: A craftsman who specializes in making and repairing wooden vessels like casks and buckets.

always abusing me about him. She did not lick me herself, but she got her husband to do it for her, whilst she fretted the flesh off my bones. Yet for all this she would not sell me. She sold five slaves whilst I was with her; but though she was always finding fault with me, she would not part with me. However, Mr. Wood afterwards allowed Daniel[7] to have a place to live in our yard, which we were very thankful for.

After this, I fell ill again with the rheumatism, and was sick a long time; but whether sick or well, I had my work to do. About this time I asked my master and mistress to let me buy my own freedom. With the help of Mr. Burchell, I could have found the means to pay Mr. Wood; for it was agreed that I should afterwards, serve Mr. Burchell a while, for the cash he was to advance for me. I was earnest in the request to my owners; but their hearts were hard—too hard to consent. Mrs. Wood was very angry—she grew quite outrageous—she called me a black devil, and asked me who had put freedom into my head. "To be free is very sweet," I said: but she took good care to keep me a slave. I saw her change color, and I left the room.

About this time my master and mistress were going to England to put their son to school, and bring their daughters home; and they took me with them to take care of the child. I was willing to come to England: I thought that by going there I should probably get cured of my rheumatism, and should return with my master and mistress, quite well, to my husband. My husband was willing for me to come away, for he had heard that my master would free me,—and I also hoped this might prove true; but it was all a false report.

The steward of the ship was very kind to me. He and my husband were in the same class in the Moravian Church. I was thankful that he was so friendly, for my mistress was not kind to me on the passage; and she told me, when she was angry, that she did not intend to treat me any better in England than in the West Indies—that I need not expect it. And she was as good as her word.

---

7 *Daniel*: Daniel James, Prince's husband. Formerly enslaved, he worked as a cooper and a carpenter, and they married in 1826. They were permanently separated just two years later, when Wood brought Prince to England. Had she attempted to return to her husband, she would have been re-enslaved.

When we drew near to England, the rheumatism seized all my limbs worse than ever, and my body was dreadfully swelled. When we landed at the Tower,[8] I shewed my flesh to my mistress, but she took no great notice of it. We were obliged to stop at the tavern till my master got a house; and a day or two after, my mistress sent me down into the wash-house to learn to wash in the English way. In the West Indies we wash with cold water—in England with hot. I told my mistress I was afraid that putting my hands first into the hot water and then into the cold, would increase the pain in my limbs. The doctor had told my mistress long before I came from the West Indies, that I was a sickly body and the washing did not agree with me. But Mrs. Wood would not release me from the tub, so I was forced to do as I could. I grew worse, and could not stand to wash. I was then forced to sit down with the tub before me, and often through pain and weakness was reduced to kneel or to sit down on the floor, to finish my task. When I complained to my mistress of this, she only got into a passion as usual, and said washing in hot water could not hurt any one;—that I was lazy and insolent, and wanted to be free of my work; but that she would make me do it. I thought her very hard on me, and my heart rose up within me. However I kept still at that time, and went down again to wash the child's things; but the English washerwomen who were at work there, when they saw that I was so ill, had pity upon me and washed them for me.

After that, when we came up to live in Leigh Street, Mrs. Wood sorted out five bags of clothes which we had used at sea, and also such as had been worn since we came on shore, for me and the cook to wash. Elizabeth the cook told her, that she did not think that I was able to stand to the tub, and that she had better hire a woman. I also said myself, that I had come over to nurse the child, and that I was sorry I had come from Antigua, since mistress would work me so hard, without compassion for my rheumatism. Mr. and Mrs. Wood, when they heard this, rose up in a passion against me. They opened the door and bade me get out. But I was a stranger, and did not know one door in the street from another, and was unwilling to go away. They made a dreadful uproar, and from that day they constantly kept cursing and abusing me. I was

---

8   *The Tower*: The Tower of London, which is on the banks of the Thames River.

obliged to wash, though I was very ill. Mrs. Wood, indeed once hired a washerwoman, but she was not well treated, and would come no more.

My master quarreled with me another time, about one of our great washings, his wife having stirred him up to do so. He said he would compel me to do the whole of the washing given out to me, or if I again refused, he would take a short course with me: he would either send me down to the brig in the river, to carry me back to Antigua, or he would turn me at once out of doors, and let me provide for myself. I said I would willingly go back, if he would let me purchase my own freedom. But this enraged him more than all the rest: he cursed and swore at me dreadfully, and said he would never sell my freedom—if I wished to be free, I was free in England, and I might go and try what freedom would do for me, and be d—d. My heart was very sore with this treatment, but I had to go on. I continued to do my work, and did all I could to give satisfaction, but all would not do.

Shortly after, the cook left them, and then matters went on ten times worse. I always washed the child's clothes without being commanded to do it, and any thing else that was wanted in the family; though still I was very sick—very sick indeed. When the great washing came round, which was every two months, my mistress got together again a great many heavy things, such as bed-ticks,[9] bed-coverlets, &c. for me to wash. I told her I was too ill to wash such heavy things that day. She said, she supposed I thought myself a free woman, but I was not; and if I did not do it directly I should be instantly turned out of doors. I stood a long time before I could answer, for I did not know well what to do. I knew that I was free in England, but I did not know where to go, or how to get my living; and therefore, I did not like to leave the house. But Mr. Wood said he would send for a constable to thrust me out; and at last I took courage and resolved that I would not be longer thus treated, but would go and trust to Providence. This was the fourth time they had threatened turn me out, and, go where I might, I was determined now to take them at their word; though I thought it very hard, after I had lived with them for thirteen years, and worked for them like a horse, to

---

9 *Bed-ticks*: A large bag or case that can be stuffed with feathers, hair, or straw to make a bed.

be driven out in this way, like a beggar. My only fault was being sick, and therefore unable to please my mistress, who thought she never could get work enough out of her slaves; and I told them so: but they only abused me and drove me out. This took place from two to three months, I think, after we came to England.

When I came away, I went to the man (one Mash) who used to black the shoes of the family, and asked his wife to get somebody to go with me to Hatton Garden to the Moravian Missionaries: these were the only persons I knew in England. The woman sent a young girl with me to the mission house, and I saw there a gentleman called Mr. Moore. I told him my whole story, and how my owners had treated me, and asked him to take in my trunk with what few clothes I had. The missionaries were very kind to me—they were sorry for my destitute situation, and gave me leave to bring my things to be placed under their care. They were very good people, and they told me to come to the church.

When I went back to Mr. Wood's to get my trunk, I saw a lady, Mrs. Pell, who was on a visit to my mistress. When Mr. and Mrs. Wood heard me come in, they set this lady to stop me, finding that they had gone too far with me. Mrs. Pell came out to me, and said, "Are you really going to leave, Molly? Don't leave, but come into the country with me." I believe she said this because she thought Mrs. Wood would easily get me back again. I replied to her, "Ma'am, this is the fourth time my master and mistress have driven me out, or threatened to drive me—and I will give them no more occasion to bid me go. I was not willing to leave them, for I am a stranger in this country, but now I must go—I can stay no longer to be so used." Mrs. Pell then went up stairs to my mistress, and told that I would go, and that she could not stop me. Mrs. Wood was very much hurt and frightened when she found I was determined to go out that day. She said, "If she goes the people will rob her, and then turn her adrift." She did not say this to me, but she spoke it loud enough for me to hear; that it might induce me not to go, I suppose. Mr. Wood also asked me where I was going to. I told him where I had been, and that I should never have gone away had I not been driven out by my owners. He had given me a written paper some time before, which said that I had come with them to England by my own desire; and that was true. It said also that I left them of my own free will, because I was a free woman in England; and that I was idle and would not do my work—which was not true. I gave this paper afterwards to a gentleman who inquired into my case.

I went into the kitchen and got my clothes out. The nurse and the servant girl were there, and I said to the man who was going to take out my trunk, "Stop, before you take up this trunk, and hear what I have to say before these people. I am going out of this house, as I was ordered; but I have done no wrong at all to my owners, neither here nor in the West Indies. I always worked very hard to please them, both by night and day; but there was no giving satisfaction, for my mistress could never be satisfied with reasonable service. I told my mistress I was sick, and yet she has ordered me out of doors. This is the fourth time; and now I am going out."

And so I came out, and went and carried my trunk to the Moravians. I then returned back to Mash the shoe-black's house, and begged his wife to take me in. I had a little West Indian money in my trunk; and they got it changed for me. This helped to support me for a little while. The man's wife was very kind to me. I was very sick, and she boiled nourishing things up for me. She also sent for a doctor to see me, and he sent me medicine, which did me good, though I was ill for a long time with the rheumatic pains. I lived a good many months with these poor people, and they nursed me, and did all that lay in their power to serve me. The man was well acquainted with my situation, as he used to go to and fro to Mr. Wood's house to clean shoes and knives; and he and his wife were sorry for me.

About this time, a woman of the name of Hill told me of the Anti-Slavery Society, and went with me to their office, to inquire if they could do any thing to get me my freedom, and send me back to the West Indies. The gentlemen of the Society took me to a lawyer, who examined very strictly into my case; but told me that the laws of England could do nothing to make me free in Antigua[10] However they did all they could for me: they gave me a little money from time to time to keep me from

---

10 [Original note: She came first to the Anti-Slavery Office in Aldermanbury, about the latter end of November 1828; and her case was referred to Mr. George Stephen to be investigated.]

want; and some of them went to Mr. Wood to try to persuade him to let me return a free woman to my husband; but though they offered him, as I have heard, a large sum for my freedom, he was sulky and obstinate, and would not consent to let me go free.

This was the first winter I spent in England, and I suffered much from the severe cold, and from the rheumatic pains, which still at times torment me. However, Providence was very good to me, and I got many friends—especially some Quaker ladies, who hearing of my case, came and sought me out, and gave me good warm clothing and money. Thus I had great cause to bless God in my affliction.

When I got better I was anxious to get some work to do, as I was unwilling to eat the bread of idleness. Mrs. Mash, who was a laundress, recommended me to a lady for a charwoman. She paid me very handsomely for what work I did, and I divided the money with Mrs. Mash; for though very poor, they gave me food when my own money was done, and never suffered me to want.

In the spring, I got into service with a lady, who saw me at the house where I sometimes worked as a charwoman. This lady's name was Mrs. Forsyth. She had been in the West Indies, and was accustomed to Blacks, and liked them. I was with her six months, and went with her to Margate. She treated me well, and gave me a good character[11] when she left London.

After Mrs. Forsyth went away, I was again out of place, and went to lodgings, for which I paid two shillings a week, and found coals and candle. After eleven weeks, the money I had saved in service was all gone, and I was forced to go back to the Anti-Slavery office to ask a supply, till I could get another situation. I did not like to go back—I did not like to be idle. I would rather work for my living than get it for nothing. They were very good to give me a supply, but I felt shame at being obliged to apply for relief whilst I had strength to work.

At last I went into the service of Mr. and Mrs. Pringle, where I have been ever since, and am as comfortable as I can be while separated from my dear husband, and away from my own country and all old friends and connections. My dear mistress teaches me daily to read the word of

---

11 *A good character*: A character reference.

God, and takes great pains to make me understand it. I enjoy the great privilege of being enabled to attend church three times on the Sunday; and I have met with many kind friends since I have been here, both clergymen and others. The Rev. Mr. Young, who lives in the next house, has shown me much kindness, and taken much pains to instruct me, particularly while my master and mistress were absent in Scotland. Nor must I forget, among my friends, the Rev. Mr. Mortimer, the good clergyman of the parish, under whose ministry I have now sat for upwards of twelve months. I trust in God I have profited by what I have heard from him. He never keeps back the truth, and I think he has been the means of opening my eyes and ears much better to understand the word of God. Mr. Mortimer tells me that he cannot open the eyes of my heart, but that I must pray to God to change my heart, and make me to know the truth, and the truth will make me free.

To the Siamese Twins*

HANNAH FLAGG GOULD
(American, 1789–1865)

Poet Hannah Flagg Gould was born in Massachusetts and began her writing career in her thirties. She was interested in a wide range of topics, including the natural sciences and contemporary marvels: she has poems on automata (early versions of robots, designed to look like humans or animals) and a mummified female discovered in a cave in Kentucky.[1] The poem included here, which was published in 1832, is addressed "To the Siamese Twins"[2] and was written after the conjoined twins Chang and Eng Bunker had become media sensations. The twins were the subjects of endless medical study and exploited as curiosities in "freak shows," traveling sideshows featuring living creatures with biological anomalies. Chang and Eng's first stop in their American tour had been to Boston in 1829. As you read, consider how conjoined twins are imagined and described in the poem.

1 Archaeology developed significantly as a field in the nineteenth century, and archaeological discoveries have always been a source of fascination and excitement.

2 The title of the poem is reminiscent of a letter to the editors of the *Salem Gazette* published August 16, 1831, entitled "To the Public." The letter was written by Elbridge Gerry, who accused the twins and their manager James W. Hale of assaulting him during a recreational visit to Lynnfield, Massachusetts. Accounts of the incident varied, but *Salem Gazette*'s earlier report suggests that the twins faced significant harassment from the locals.

* Reprinted from Hannah Flagg Gould, *Poems by Miss H.F. Gould* (Boston: Hilliard, Gray, Little, and Wilkins, 1832), 48–49, Google Books.

To the Siamese Twins

Mysterious tie by the Hand above,
Which nothing below must part!
Thou visible image of faithful love,
Firm union of heart and heart;
The mind to her utmost bound may run, [5]
And summon her light in vain
To scan the *twain* that must still be *one*;
The *one* that will still be *twain*!

The beat of this bosom forbears to reach
Where the other distinctly goes; [10]
Yet, the stream that empurples the veins of each
Through the breast of his brother flows!
One grief must be felt by this two-fold mark,
As the points of a double dart;
And the joy lit up by a single spark [15]
Is sunshine in either heart.

O wonder, to baffle poor human skill
In clay of the human mold!
But a greater mystery all must still,
In the union of souls, behold. [20]
Ye are living harps, by your silken strings
In a heavenly concord bound;
And who o'er one but a finger flings
Awakens you both to sound.

But, what do you do when your slumbers come, [25]
When ye've sweetly sunken to rest?
Do your spirits, side by side, fly home,
Still linked, to your mother's breast?
Did ye ever dream that your bond was broke;
That ye were asunder thrown? [30]
And how did ye feel at the severing stroke,
When each was forever alone?

No—ye would not think of yourselves apart,
Even in fancy's wildest mood,
For each would seem but a broken heart, [35]
And the world but a solitude!
Dear youths, may your lives be a flowery way,
And, watched by your Maker's eye,
May both, at the close, one call over
To shine as twin stars on high! [40]

The Masque of the Red Death*

EDGAR ALLAN POE
(American, 1809–1849)

Author Edgar Allan Poe is especially renowned for works with macabre subjects and a dash (or more) of horror. Poems like "The Raven" and tales like "The Fall of the House of Usher" employ dark themes and engage with elements of the gothic. Gothic literature of the nineteenth century often relies on suspense or even outright terror, sensational or supernatural plots, and a grim outlook on the (frequently medieval) past. Poe brings this gothic sensibility to "The Masque of the Red Death," as well. This short story, first published in *Graham's Magazine* in 1842, takes place during an epidemic.[1] The setting is a party (the "masque," or masquerade, of the title) hosted by the wealthy Prince Prospero, who has cut himself and his friends off from the common people of the town. The group of friends is well stocked and prepared to wait out the plague. As you read, consider the disruption of the masqueraders' revelry and comfort by the arrival of a mysterious stranger.

1 The Red Death is not definitively linked to any one disease, though the name is evocative of the Black Death (or bubonic plague).

---

* Reprinted from Edgar Allan Poe, "The Masque of the Red Death," *Graham's Magazine* 20, no. 5 (May 1842): 257–259. Project Gutenberg, 2010/2020.

The Masque of the Red Death

The "Red Death" had long devastated the country. No pestilence had ever been so fatal, or so hideous. Blood was its Avatar[2] and its seal—the redness and the horror of blood. There were sharp pains, and sudden dizziness, and then profuse bleeding at the pores, with dissolution. The scarlet stains upon the body and especially upon the face of the victim, were the pest ban which shut him out from the aid and from the sympathy of his fellow-men. And the whole seizure, progress and termination of the disease, were the incidents of half an hour.

But the Prince Prospero was happy and dauntless and sagacious. When his dominions were half depopulated, he summoned to his presence a thousand hale and lighthearted friends from among the knights and dames of his court, and with these retired to the deep seclusion of one of his castellated abbeys. This was an extensive and magnificent structure, the creation of the prince's own eccentric yet august taste. A strong and lofty wall girdled it in. This wall had gates of iron. The courtiers, having entered, brought furnaces and massy hammers and welded the bolts. They resolved to leave means neither of ingress nor egress to the sudden impulses of despair or of frenzy from within. The abbey was amply provisioned. With such precautions the courtiers might bid defiance to contagion. The external world could take care of itself. In the meantime it was folly to grieve, or to think. The prince had provided all the appliances of pleasure. There were buffoons, there were improvisatori, there were ballet-dancers, there were musicians, there was Beauty, there was wine. All these and security were within. Without was the "Red Death."

It was towards the close of the fifth or sixth month of his seclusion, and while the pestilence raged most furiously abroad, that the Prince Prospero entertained his thousand friends at a masked ball of the most unusual magnificence.

It was a voluptuous scene, that masquerade. But first let me tell of the rooms in which it was held. These were seven—an imperial suite. In many palaces, however, such suites form a long and straight vista,

---

2 *Avatar*: A manifestation in human form of something non-human.

while the folding doors slide back nearly to the walls on either hand, so that the view of the whole extent is scarcely impeded. Here the case was very different, as might have been expected from the duke's love of the *bizarre*. The apartments were so irregularly disposed that the vision embraced but little more than one at a time. There was a sharp turn at every twenty or thirty yards, and at each turn a novel effect. To the right and left, in the middle of each wall, a tall and narrow Gothic window looked out upon a closed corridor which pursued the windings of the suite. These windows were of stained glass whose color varied in accordance with the prevailing hue of the decorations of the chamber into which it opened. That at the eastern extremity was hung, for example in blue—and vividly blue were its windows. The second chamber was purple in its ornaments and tapestries, and here the panes were purple. The third was green throughout, and so were the casements. The fourth was furnished and lighted with orange—the fifth with white—the sixth with violet. The seventh apartment was closely shrouded in black velvet tapestries that hung all over the ceiling and down the walls, falling in heavy folds upon a carpet of the same material and hue. But in this chamber only, the color of the windows failed to correspond with the decorations. The panes here were scarlet—a deep blood color. Now in no one of the seven apartments was there any lamp or candelabrum, amid the profusion of golden ornaments that lay scattered to and fro or depended from the roof. There was no light of any kind emanating from lamp or candle within the suite of chambers. But in the corridors that followed the suite, there stood, opposite to each window, a heavy tripod, bearing a brazier of fire, that projected its rays through the tinted glass and so glaringly illumined the room. And thus were produced a multitude of gaudy and fantastic appearances. But in the western or black chamber the effect of the fire-light that streamed upon the dark hangings through the blood-tinted panes, was ghastly in the extreme, and produced so wild a look upon the countenances of those who entered, that there were few of the company bold enough to set foot within its precincts at all.

It was in this apartment, also, that there stood against the western wall, a gigantic clock of ebony. Its pendulum swung to and fro with a dull, heavy, monotonous clang; and when the minute-hand made the circuit of the face, and the hour was to be stricken, there came from the brazen lungs of the clock a sound which was clear and loud and deep and exceedingly musical, but of so peculiar a note and emphasis that, at each lapse of an hour, the musicians of the orchestra were constrained to pause, momentarily, in their performance, to hearken to the sound; and thus the waltzers perforce ceased their evolutions; and there was a brief disconcert of the whole gay company; and, while the chimes of the clock yet rang, it was observed that the giddiest grew pale, and the more aged and sedate passed their hands over their brows as if in confused reverie or meditation. But when the echoes had fully ceased, a light laughter at once pervaded the assembly; the musicians looked at each other and smiled as if at their own nervousness and folly, and made whispering vows, each to the other, that the next chiming of the clock should produce in them no similar emotion; and then, after the lapse of sixty minutes, (which embrace three thousand and six hundred seconds of the Time that flies,) there came yet another chiming of the clock, and then were the same disconcert and tremulousness and meditation as before.

But, in spite of these things, it was a gay and magnificent revel. The tastes of the duke were peculiar. He had a fine eye for colors and effects. He disregarded the *decora* of mere fashion. His plans were bold and fiery, and his conceptions glowed with barbaric luster. There are some who would have thought him mad. His followers felt that he was not. It was necessary to hear and see and touch him to be *sure* that he was not.

He had directed, in great part, the movable embellishments of the seven chambers, upon occasion of this great *fête*; and it was his own guiding taste which had given character to the masqueraders. Be sure they were grotesque. There were much glare and glitter and piquancy and phantasm—much of what has been since seen in *Hernani*.[3] There were arabesque figures with unsuited limbs and appointments. There were delirious fancies such as the madman fashions. There were much

---

3   *Hernani*: *Hernani, ou l'Honneur Castillan*, a play by the French author Victor Hugo (known for *Les Misérables* and *The Hunchback of Notre-Dame*), which premiered in 1830. The play inspired Giuseppe Verdi's Italian opera *Ernani* (1844) and is perhaps most notable for inciting a riot on the night of its premiere over its abandonment of classical plot structure.

of the beautiful, much of the wanton, much of the *bizarre*, something of the terrible, and not a little of that which might have excited disgust. To and fro in the seven chambers there stalked, in fact, a multitude of dreams. And these—the dreams—writhed in and about taking hue from the rooms, and causing the wild music of the orchestra to seem as the echo of their steps. And, anon, there strikes the ebony clock which stands in the hall of the velvet. And then, for a moment, all is still, and all is silent save the voice of the clock. The dreams are stiff-frozen as they stand. But the echoes of the chime die away—they have endured but an instant—and a light, half-subdued laughter floats after them as they depart. And now again the music swells, and the dreams live, and writhe to and fro more merrily than ever, taking hue from the many tinted windows through which stream the rays from the tripods. But to the chamber which lies most westwardly of the seven, there are now none of the maskers who venture; for the night is waning away; and there flows a ruddier light through the blood-colored panes; and the blackness of the sable drapery appalls; and to him whose foot falls upon the sable carpet, there comes from the near clock of ebony a muffled peal more solemnly emphatic than any which reaches *their* ears who indulged in the more remote gaieties of the other apartments.

But these other apartments were densely crowded, and in them beat feverishly the heart of life. And the revel went whirlingly on, until at length there commenced the sounding of midnight upon the clock. And then the music ceased, as I have told; and the evolutions of the waltzers were quieted; and there was an uneasy cessation of all things as before. But now there were twelve strokes to be sounded by the bell of the clock; and thus it happened, perhaps, that more of thought crept, with more of time, into the meditations of the thoughtful among those who reveled. And thus too, it happened, perhaps, that before the last echoes of the last chime had utterly sunk into silence, there were many individuals in the crowd who had found leisure to become aware of the presence of a masked figure which had arrested the attention of no single individual before. And the rumor of this new presence having spread itself whisperingly around, there arose at length from the whole company a buzz, or murmur, expressive of disapprobation and surprise—then, finally, of terror, of horror, and of disgust.

In an assembly of phantasms such as I have painted, it may well be supposed that no ordinary appearance could have excited such sensation. In truth the masquerade license of the night was nearly unlimited; but the figure in question had out-Heroded Herod, and gone beyond the bounds of even the prince's indefinite decorum. There are chords in the hearts of the most reckless which cannot be touched without emotion. Even with the utterly lost, to whom life and death are equally jests, there are matters of which no jest can be made. The whole company, indeed, seemed now deeply to feel that in the costume and bearing of the stranger neither wit nor propriety existed. The figure was tall and gaunt, and shrouded from head to foot in the habiliments of the grave. The mask which concealed the visage was made so nearly to resemble the countenance of a stiffened corpse that the closest scrutiny must have had difficulty in detecting the cheat. And yet all this might have been endured, if not approved, by the mad revelers around. But the mummer had gone so far as to assume the type of the Red Death. His vesture was dabbled in *blood*—and his broad brow, with all the features of the face, was besprinkled with the scarlet horror.

When the eyes of the Prince Prospero fell upon this spectral image (which, with a slow and solemn movement, as if more fully to sustain its role, stalked to and fro among the waltzers) he was seen to be convulsed, in the first moment with a strong shudder either of terror or distaste; but, in the next, his brow reddened with rage.

"Who dares,"—he demanded hoarsely of the courtiers who stood near him—"who dares insult us with this blasphemous mockery? Seize him and unmask him—that we may know whom we have to hang, at sunrise, from the battlements!"

It was in the eastern or blue chamber in which stood the Prince Prospero as he uttered these words. They rang throughout the seven rooms loudly and clearly, for the prince was a bold and robust man, and the music had become hushed at the waving of his hand.

It was in the blue room where stood the prince, with a group of pale courtiers by his side. At first, as he spoke, there was a slight rushing movement of this group in the direction of the intruder, who at the moment was also near at hand, and now, with deliberate and stately step, made closer approach to the speaker. But from a certain nameless awe with which the mad assumptions of the mummer had inspired the whole party, there were found none who put forth hand to seize him; so that, unimpeded, he passed within a yard of the prince's person; and, while the vast assembly, as if with one impulse, shrank from the centers of the rooms to the walls, he made his way uninterruptedly, but with the same solemn and measured step which had distinguished him from the first, through the blue chamber to the purple—through the purple to the green—through the green to the orange—through this again to the white—and even thence to the violet, ere a decided movement had been made to arrest him. It was then, however, that the Prince Prospero, maddening with rage and the shame of his own momentary cowardice, rushed hurriedly through the six chambers, while none followed him on account of a deadly terror that had seized upon all. He bore aloft a drawn dagger, and had approached, in rapid impetuosity, to within three or four feet of the retreating figure, when the latter, having attained the extremity of the velvet apartment, turned suddenly and confronted his pursuer. There was a sharp cry—and the dagger dropped gleaming upon the sable carpet, upon which, instantly afterwards, fell prostrate in death the Prince Prospero. Then, summoning the wild courage of despair, a throng of the revelers at once threw themselves into the black apartment, and, seizing the mummer, whose tall figure stood erect and motionless within the shadow of the ebony clock, gasped in unutterable horror at finding the grave cerements and corpse-like mask, which they handled with so violent a rudeness, untenanted by any tangible form.

And now was acknowledged the presence of the Red Death. He had come like a thief in the night. And one by one dropped the revelers in the blood-bedewed halls of their revel, and died each in the despairing posture of his fall. And the life of the ebony clock went out with that of the last of the gay. And the flames of the tripods expired. And Darkness and Decay and the Red Death held illimitable dominion over all.

Lecture on the First Surgical Operations under Ether*

CRAWFORD WILLIAMSON LONG
(American, 1815–1878)

Prior to the nineteenth century, anesthetic options were scarce. Not until the 1840s did Western medicine begin fully exploring ether as an option for general anesthesia. Produced by heating a mixture of ethyl alcohol and sulfuric acid, ether had been periodically recognized for its analgesic properties throughout the centuries, but Crawford Williamson Long, a Georgia physician, is now credited with discovering its potential use for surgical practice. Long conducted his first operations in late 1841, but he wouldn't publish his findings until 1849, a delay that led to a dispute over who made the discovery. William T. G. Morton, an American dentist and physician, independently realized ether's anesthetic potential and used it during surgery in 1846, temporarily claiming the innovation as his own. Long's account was presented as a lecture in 1852 and was published in 1853. As you read, consider Long's narration of the discovery, which began with the observation of bruises appearing after recreational use of ether—known at the time as an "ether frolic."

---

* Reprinted from Hugh H. Young, "Long: The Discoverer of Anesthesia. A Presentation of His Original Documents" *Johns Hopkins Historical Bulletin* 77–78 (1897): Appendix I, U.S. National Library of Medicine, National Institutes for Health.

[On Discovering Ether as an Anesthetic]

In the month of December, 1841, or January, 1842, the subject of the inhalation of nitrous oxide gas was introduced in a company of young men assembled at night in this village, (Jefferson,) and several persons present desired me to prepare some for their use. I informed them that I had no apparatus for preparing or preserving the gas, but that I had a medicine (sulfuric ether) which would produce equally exhilarating effects; that I had inhaled it myself, and considered it as safe as the nitrous oxide gas. One of the company stated, that he had inhaled ether while at school, and was then willing to inhale it. The company were all anxious to witness its effects. The ether was introduced: I gave it first to the gentleman who had previously inhaled it, then inhaled it myself, and afterwards gave it to all persons present. They were so much pleased with the exhilarating effects of ether, that they afterwards inhaled it frequently, and induced others to do so, and its inhalation soon became quite fashionable in this county, and in fact extended from this place through several counties in this part of Georgia.

On numerous occasions I have inhaled ether for its exhilarating properties, and would frequently, at some short time subsequent to its inhalation, discover bruised or painful spots on my person, which I had no recollection of causing, and which I felt satisfied were received while under the influence of ether. I noticed, my friends, while etherized, received falls and blows, which I believed were sufficient to produce pain on a person not in a state of anesthesia, and on questioning them, they uniformly assured me that they did not feel the least pain from these accidents. These facts are mentioned, that the reasons may be apparent why I was induced to make an experiment in etherization.

The first patient to whom I administered ether in a surgical operation, was Mr. James M. Venable, who then resided within two miles of Jefferson, and at present lives in Cobb county, Ga. Mr. Venable consulted me on several occasions in regard to the propriety of removing two small tumors situated on the back part of his neck, but would postpone from time to time having the operations performed, from dread of pain. At length I mentioned to him the fact of my receiving bruises while under the influence of the vapor of ether, without suffering, and as I knew him to be fond of, and accustomed to inhale ether, I suggested to him the probability that the operations might be performed without pain, and proposed operating on him while under its influence. He consented to have one tumor removed, and the operation was performed the same evening. The ether was given to Mr. Venable on a towel; and when fully under its influence I extirpated the tumor. It was encysted, and about half an inch in diameter. The patient continued to inhale ether during the time of the operation: and when informed it was over, seemed incredulous, until the tumor was shown him. He gave no evidence of suffering during the operation, and assured me, after it was over, that he did not experience the slightest degree of pain from its performance. This operation was performed on the 30th March, 1842.

The second operation I performed upon a patient etherized was on the 6th June, 1842, and was on the same person, for the removal of another small tumor. This operation required more time than the first, from the cyst of the tumor having formed adhesions to the surrounding parts. The patient was insensible to pain during the operation, until the last attachment of the cyst was separated, when he exhibited signs of slight suffering, but asserted, after the operation was over, that the sensation of pain was so slight as scarcely to be perceived. In this operation, the inhalation of ether ceased before the first incision was made: since that time I have invariably desired patients, when practicable, to continue its inhalation during the time of the operation.

Notes on Nursing*

FLORENCE NIGHTINGALE
(British, 1820–1910)

Social reformer and nurse Florence Nightingale is now known as the founder of modern nursing. Prior to her efforts, most training for nurses was informal and could be inconsistent. Her works on hospital management and nursing laid down clear and precise principles for medical practice. *Notes on Nursing: What It Is, and What It Is Not* (1859) is the first manual composed specifically for nurses and was written to instruct women tasked with caretaking (especially in the home). The year after it was published, in 1860, Nightingale founded the first school in England designed to train medically qualified nurses. Following its success, hundreds of new nursing schools were founded in the United Kingdom and United States, and in 1909, the University of Minnesota began the now-standard practice of providing this training in colleges and universities. As you read, consider Nightingale's definitions of nursing and disease and her ideas about sanitation and treatment—some of which we still employ, and even take for granted, today.

---

* Reprinted from Florence Nightingale, *Notes on Nursing: What It Is, and What It Is Not* (London: Harrison and Sons, 1859; Project Gutenberg, 2005), 3, 5–8, 52–54.

Preface

The following notes are by no means intended as a rule of thought by which nurses can teach themselves to nurse, still less as a manual to teach nurses to nurse. They are meant simply to give hints for thought to women who have personal charge of the health of others. Every woman, or at least almost every woman, in England has, at one time or another of her life, charge of the personal health of somebody, whether child or invalid, —in other words, every woman is a nurse. Every day sanitary knowledge, or the knowledge of nursing, or in other words, of how to put the constitution in such a state as that it will have no disease, or that it can recover from disease, takes a higher place. It is recognized as the knowledge which every one ought to have[1]—distinct from medical knowledge, which only a profession can have.

If, then, every woman must, at some time or other of her life, become a nurse, *i.e.*, have charge of somebody's health, how immense and how valuable would be the produce of her united experience if every woman would think[2] how to nurse.

I do not pretend to teach her how, I ask her to teach herself, and for this purpose I venture to give her some hints.

Notes on Nursing: What It Is, and What It Is Not

Shall we begin by taking it as a general principle—that all disease, at some period or other of its course, is more or less a reparative process, not necessarily accompanied with suffering: an effort of nature to remedy a process of poisoning or of decay, which has taken place weeks, months, sometimes years beforehand, unnoticed, the termination of the disease being then, while the antecedent process was going on, determined?

If we accept this as a general principle we shall be immediately met

---

1 This refers to the basic rules of nursing (as caretaking, not as career) as something everyone should know.
2 *Think*: Understand.

with anecdotes and instances to prove the contrary. Just so if we were to take, as a principle—all the climates of the earth are meant to be made habitable for man, by the efforts of man—the objection would be immediately raised, —Will the top of Mont Blanc ever be made habitable? Our answer would be, it will be many thousands of years before we have reached the bottom of Mont Blanc in making the earth healthy. Wait till we have reached the bottom before we discuss the top.

In watching disease, both in private houses and in public hospitals, the thing which strikes the experienced observer most forcibly is this, that the symptoms or the sufferings generally considered to be inevitable and incident to the disease are very often not symptoms of the disease at all, but of something quite different—of the want[3] of fresh air, or of light, or of warmth, or of quiet, or of cleanliness, or of punctuality and care in the administration of diet, of each or of all of these. And this quite as much in private as in hospital nursing.

The reparative process which Nature has instituted and which we call disease has been hindered by some want of knowledge or attention, in one or in all of these things, and pain, suffering, or interruption of the whole process sets in.

If a patient is cold, if a patient is feverish, if a patient is faint, if he is sick after taking food, if he has a bed-sore, it is generally the fault not of the disease, but of the nursing.

I use the word nursing for want of a better. It has been limited to signify little more than the administration of medicines and the application of poultices. It ought to signify the proper use of fresh air, light, warmth, cleanliness, quiet, and the proper selection and administration of diet—all at the least expense of vital power to the patient.

It has been said and written scores of times, that every woman makes a good nurse. I believe, on the contrary, that the very elements of nursing are all but unknown.

By this I do not mean that the nurse is always to blame. Bad sanitary, bad architectural, and bad administrative arrangements often make it impossible to nurse. But the art of nursing ought to include such arrangements as alone make what I understand by nursing, possible.

---

3   *Want*: Lack.

The art of nursing, as now practiced, seems to be expressly constituted to unmake what God had made disease to be, viz., a reparative process.

To recur to the first objection. If we are asked, Is such or such a disease a reparative process? Can such an illness be unaccompanied with suffering? Will any care prevent such a patient from suffering this or that? —I humbly say, I do not know. But when you have done away with all that pain and suffering, which in patients are the symptoms not of their disease, but of the absence of one or all of the above-mentioned essentials to the success of Nature's reparative processes, we shall then know what are the symptoms of and the sufferings inseparable from the disease.

Another and the commonest exclamation which will be instantly made is—Would you do nothing, then, in cholera, fever, &c.? —so deep-rooted and universal is the conviction that to give medicine is to be doing something, or rather everything; to give air, warmth, cleanliness, &c., is to do nothing. The reply is, that in these and many other similar diseases the exact value of particular remedies and modes of treatment is by no means ascertained, while there is universal experience as to the extreme importance of careful nursing in determining the issue of the disease.

II. The very elements of what constitutes good nursing are as little understood for the well as for the sick. The same laws of health or of nursing, for they are in reality the same, obtain among the well as among the sick. The breaking of them produces only a less violent consequence among the former than among the latter, —and this sometimes, not always.

It is constantly objected,—"But how can I obtain this medical knowledge? I am not a doctor. I must leave this to doctors."

Oh, mothers of families! You who say this, do you know that one in every seven infants in this civilized land of England perishes before it is one year old? That, in London, two in every five die before they are five years old? And, in the other great cities of England, nearly one out of two? "The life duration of tender babies" (as some Saturn,[4] turned ana-

---

4 *Saturn*: Roman god of generation (or reproduction); often conflated with the Greek god Cronus, who ate five of his own children to prevent a prophecy that one would overthrow him. It didn't work: Cronus's son Zeus was born in secret and grew up to

lytical chemist, says) "is the most delicate test" of sanitary conditions. Is all this premature suffering and death necessary? Or did Nature intend mothers to be always accompanied by doctors? Or is it better to learn the piano-forte than to learn the laws which subserve the preservation of offspring?

Macaulay[5] somewhere says, that it is extraordinary that, whereas the laws of the motions of the heavenly bodies, far removed as they are from us, are perfectly well understood, the laws of the human mind, which are under our observation all day and every day, are no better understood than they were two thousand years ago.

But how much more extraordinary is it that, whereas what we might call the coxcombries of education[6]—*e.g.*, the elements of astronomy—are now taught to every school-girl, neither mothers of families of any class, nor school-mistresses of any class, nor nurses of children, nor nurses of hospitals, are taught anything about those laws which God has assigned to the relations of our bodies with the world in which He has put them. In other words, the laws which make these bodies, into which He has put our minds, healthy or unhealthy organs of those minds, are all but unlearned. Not but that these laws—the laws of life—are in a certain measure understood, but not even mothers think it worth their while to study them—to study how to give their children healthy existences. They call it medical or physiological knowledge, fit only for doctors.

We are constantly told, — "But the circumstances which govern our children's health are beyond our control. What can we do with winds? There is the east wind. Most people can tell before they get up in the morning whether the wind is in the east."

To this one can answer with more certainty than to the former objections. Who is it who knows when the wind is in the east? Not the Highland drover,[7] certainly, exposed to the east wind, but the young lady who is worn out with the want of exposure to fresh air, to sunlight,

---

    defeat his father, free his siblings, and become king of the Greek pantheon.
5 *Macaulay*: Thomas Babington Macaulay (1800–1859), British historian and politician.
6 *Coxcombries*: Foolish, faddish, or pretentious educational pursuits.
7 *Drover*: One who drives herds of livestock (or "droves").

&c. Put the latter under as good sanitary circumstances as the former, and she too will not know when the wind is in the east.

Personal Cleanliness

In almost all diseases, the function of the skin is, more or less, disordered; and in many most important diseases nature relieves herself almost entirely by the skin. This is particularly the case with children. But the excretion, which comes from the skin, is left there, unless removed by washing or by the clothes. Every nurse should keep this fact constantly in mind, —for, if she allow her sick to remain unwashed, or their clothing to remain on them after being saturated with perspiration or other excretion, she is interfering injuriously with the natural processes of health just as effectually as if she were to give the patient a dose of slow poison by the mouth. Poisoning by the skin is no less certain than poisoning by the mouth—only it is slower in its operation.

The amount of relief and comfort experienced by sick after the skin has been carefully washed and dried, is one of the commonest observations made at a sick bed. But it must not be forgotten that the comfort and relief so obtained are not all. They are, in fact, nothing more than a sign that the vital powers have been relieved by removing something that was oppressing them. The nurse, therefore, must never put off attending to the personal cleanliness of her patient under the plea that all that is to be gained is a little relief, which can be quite as well given later.

In all well-regulated hospitals this ought to be, and generally is, attended to. But it is very generally neglected with private sick.

Just as it is necessary to renew the air round a sick person frequently, to carry off morbid effluvia from the lungs and skin, by maintaining free ventilation, so is it necessary to keep the pores of the skin free from all obstructing excretions. The object, both of ventilation and of skin-cleanliness, is pretty much the same, to wit, removing noxious matter from the system as rapidly as possible.

Care should be taken in all these operations of sponging, washing, and cleansing the skin, not to expose too great a surface at once, so as to check the perspiration, which would renew the evil in another form.

The various ways of washing the sick need not here be specified, — the less so as the doctors ought to say which is to be used.

In several forms of diarrhea, dysentery, &c., where the skin is hard and harsh, the relief afforded by washing with a great deal of soft soap is incalculable. In other cases, sponging with tepid soap and water, then with tepid water and drying with a hot towel will be ordered.

Every nurse ought to be careful to wash her hands very frequently during the day. If her face too, so much the better.

One word as to cleanliness merely as cleanliness.

Compare the dirtiness of the water in which you have washed when it is cold without soap, cold with soap, hot with soap. You will find the first has hardly removed any dirt at all, the second a little more, the third a great deal more. But hold your hand over a cup of hot water for a minute or two, and then, by merely rubbing with the finger, you will bring off flakes of dirt or dirty skin. After a vapor bath you may peel your whole self clean in this way. What I mean is, that by simply washing or sponging with water you do not really clean your skin. Take a rough towel, dip one corner in very hot water, —if a little spirit be added to it it will be more effectual,—and then rub as if you were rubbing the towel into your skin with your fingers. The black flakes which will come off will convince you that you were not clean before, however much soap and water you have used. These flakes are what require removing. And you can really keep yourself cleaner with a tumbler of hot water and a rough towel and rubbing, than with a whole apparatus of bath and soap and sponge, without rubbing. It is quite nonsense to say that anybody need be dirty. Patients have been kept as clean by these means on a long voyage, when a basin full of water could not be afforded, and when they could not be moved out of their berths, as if all the appurtenances of home had been at hand.

Washing, however, with a large quantity of water has quite other effects than those of mere cleanliness. The skin absorbs the water and becomes softer and more perspirable.[8] To wash with soap and soft water is, therefore, desirable from other points of view than that of cleanliness.

---

8   *Perspirable*: More capable of appropriate perspiration.

In Hospital*

WILLIAM ERNEST HENLEY
(British, 1849–1903)

William Ernest Henley was a poet, critic, and editor in the latter half of the nineteenth century and is best known for the poem "Invictus" with its final lines, "I am the master of my fate, / I am the captain of my soul." Henley had his lower leg amputated in the late 1860s because of an infection of tuberculosis of the bone. To save the other leg, he sought out the surgeon James Lister in Edinburgh, Scotland. The poem sequence *In Hospital* was written during an extended hospital stay between 1873 and 1875 (and originally published in 1898) while he was undergoing Lister's treatment. The narrator in his poems offers a vivid glimpse at the experience of being a patient in twenty-eight short poems. As you read, consider the narrator's descriptions and emotions, from arriving at the hospital through being anesthetized for surgery.

---

* Reprinted from William Ernest Henley, *Poems*, 3rd ed. (London: David Nutt, 1898; Project Gutenberg, 2015), 3–4, 6–7.

I. Enter Patient

The morning mists still haunt the stony street;
The northern summer air is shrill and cold;
And lo, the Hospital, grey, quiet, old,
Where Life and Death like friendly chafferers meet.
Thro' the loud spaciousness and draughty gloom [5]
A small, strange child—so agèd yet so young!—
Her little arm besplinted and beslung,
Precedes me gravely to the waiting-room.
I limp behind, my confidence all gone.
The grey-haired soldier-porter waves me on, [10]
And on I crawl, and still my spirits fail:
A tragic meanness seems so to environ
These corridors and stairs of stone and iron,
Cold, naked, clean—half-workhouse and half jail.

II. Waiting

A square, squat room (a cellar on promotion),
Drab to the soul, drab to the very daylight;
Plasters astray in unnatural-looking tinware;
Scissors and lint and apothecary's jars.

Here, on a bench a skeleton would writhe from, [5]
Angry and sore I wait to be admitted:
Wait till my heart is lead upon my stomach,
While at their ease two dressers do their chores.

One has a probe—it feels to me a crowbar.
A small boy sniffs and shudders after bluestone.[1] [10]

---

1 *Bluestone*: Copper sulfate, also known as blue vitriol, once used as an emetic (before its toxicity was fully recognized) and an antiseptic; still in use as a fungicide and as an ingredient in styptic powders (to stop bleeding).

A poor old tramp explains his poor old ulcers.
Life is (I think) a blunder and a shame.

IV. Before

Behold me waiting—waiting for the knife.
A little while, and at a leap I storm
The thick, sweet mystery of chloroform,
The drunken dark, the little death-in-life.
The gods are good to me: I have no wife,   [5]
No innocent child, to think of as I near
The fateful minute; nothing all-too dear
Unmans me for my bout of passive strife.
Yet I am tremulous and a trifle sick,
And, face to face with chance, I shrink a little: [10]
My hopes are strong, my will is something weak.
Here comes the basket? Thank you. I am ready.
But, gentlemen my porters, life is brittle:
You carry Caesar and his fortunes—steady!

V. Operation

You are carried in a basket,
Like a carcase[2] from the shambles,
To the theatre, a cockpit
Where they stretch you on a table.

Then they bid you close your eyelids,   [5]
And they mask you with a napkin,
And the anesthetic reaches
Hot and subtle through your being.

---

2   *Carcase*: An alternate spelling of carcass.

And you gasp and reel and shudder
In a rushing, swaying rapture,   [10]
While the voices at your elbow
Fade—receding—fainter—farther.

Lights about you shower and tumble,
And your blood seems crystallizing—
Edged and vibrant, yet within you   [15]
Racked and hurried back and forward.

Then the lights row fast and furious,
And you hear a noise of waters,
And you wrestle, blind and dizzy,
In an agony of effort,   [20]

Till a sudden lull accepts you,
And you sound an utter darkness…
And awaken…with a struggle…
On a hushed, attentive audience.

Selected Poems*

EMILY DICKINSON
(American, 1830–1886)

Now recognized as one of the greatest poets of the nineteenth century, Emily Dickinson was not a famous writer in her own time. Only a handful of her nearly 1,800 poems were published in her lifetime, and only anonymously. Instead, she shared them with family and friends, drafting some poems multiple times (often on scraps of paper). Dickinson's poetic style is distinctive, with dashes and unusual grammatical structure. This style was largely edited away in the earliest published versions, but is clear in her handwritten manuscripts and has been restored in some modern editions. The poems have been edited with reference to manuscript copies to help retain her unique voice. Dickinson suffered bouts of physical illness throughout her life (including an eye condition and possible tuberculosis infection), and gradually became a recluse. Some of her work shows the influence of this experience. As you read these short poems, consider her approach to issues of physical and mental health.

---

* "Surgeons must be very careful" and "Is Heaven a physician?" reprinted from *Poems by Emily Dickinson*, eds. T. W. Higginson and Mabel Loomis Todd (Boston: Little, Brown, and Company, 1910), 38, 43, Google Books; "Much madness is divinest sense" and "Pain has an element of blank" reprinted from *Poems by Emily Dickinson*, eds. Mabel Loomis Todd and T. W. Higginson, 11th ed. (Boston: Roberts Brothers, 1892), 24, 33, Google Books; Edited by the author with reference to manuscript copies from the Emily Dickinson Archive.

Surgeons must be very careful

Surgeons must be very careful
When they take the knife!
Underneath their fine incisions
Stirs the Culprit—Life!

Is Heaven a Physician?

Is Heaven a Physician?
They say that He can heal—
But Medicine Posthumous
Is unavailable—
Is Heaven an Exchequer? [5]
They speak of what we owe—
But that negotiation
I'm not a Party to—

Much Madness is divinest Sense

Much Madness is divinest Sense
To a discerning Eye—
Much Sense—the starkest Madness—
'Tis the Majority
In this, as All, prevails— [5]
Assent—and you are sane—
Demur—you're straightway dangerous—
And handled with a Chain—

Pain has an Element of Blank

Pain—has an Element of Blank—
It cannot recollect
When it began—or if there were
A time when it was not.

It has no Future—but itself— [5]
Its Infinite contain
Its Past—Enlightened to perceive
New Periods—of Pain.

Memoirs of a Civil War Nurse[*]

EMILY ELIZABETH PARSONS
(American, 1824–1880)

When the American Civil War broke out in 1861, Massachusetts-born Emily Elizabeth Parsons began training as a nurse in Boston so that she could volunteer for the United States military. In 1862 she was briefly stationed at Fort Schuyler on Long Island Sound in New York, but she struggled with her own health and eventually left for New York City. In 1863, she was granted a position at Lawson Hospital in St. Louis, Missouri, where she gained a prominent position as head nurse of a Mississippi-River steamship. Throughout her time as a nurse, she kept up correspondence with her family, and after her death in 1880, her father collected some of her wartime letters into a memoir. As you read, consider her account of the working conditions and people she encountered, as well as the general experience of wartime nursing.

---

[*] Reprinted from Emily Elizabeth Parsons, *Memoir of Emily Elizabeth Parsons* (Boston: Little, Brown, 1880), 26–35, 133–4, 136–7, Google Books.

Letter II

Fort Schuyler Hospital, November 1

Dear Mother,—It is evening; I am obliged to write now, for I have no time in the day, as a general thing, nor much at night. Today my ward was washed from one end to the other; I superintend and assist in various ways; just think of moving fifty-one beds out and in again! After supper I had to give out clean under-clothing to all the patients. I wonder what a mother, who thinks it is something to look after two or three, would say to forty-four; I said so to one of my patients; the idea, differently expressed, amused him. I am told that the ward will be filled to its utmost capacity presently. There are fifty-one beds in it now, and there can be more, though I hope not; fifty-one wounded men are about enough for one ward. Several of the forty-four now here are convalescent, but some suffer very much. I go round at night seeing to them, covering them up, and the other night I came to one poor boy, badly wounded and sick; as I laid the clothes over him he half opened his eyes to see who it was, and when he saw me, gave such a pleasant smile it quite went to my heart; he laid his head down again as if entirely satisfied. He does not get well very fast, and I am afraid he is going to have more trouble. His wound is a musket-shot in the shoulder, and the Doctor is obliged to take out pieces of diseased bone or splinters of bone: I dread the sight of the instruments; he is a mere boy. They seem so much pleased when they wake and find me bending over them, – it is not much I can do, but that is something. These wounds are trying[1] to the poor fellows. I have all sorts of characters, and several nations in my ward. The Doctor came to my door just now to make his night's tour among the patients; I attend him, candle in hand. My ward is now arranged for the night, and I am going to make my last round.

Sunday morning. My ward is all in order, waiting for the inspectors who are performing operations elsewhere. After it was in order I sat down and read a little while; now I am writing for a few minutes. I do

---

1 *Trying*: Distressing or painful.

not want anything done on Sundays that can be helped; that is the reason I am able to sit down a little while.

The Doctor spoke hopefully of my worst case this morning, and I am now in hopes he will save his arm, but he suffers a great deal; this morning, when I was washing it for the surgeon to apply the dressings, he could hardly bear the sponge, the arm was so sensitive; three ball-shots through it. He is very patient and good; I took him some Cologne the other day and it refreshed him very much. Mrs. Sampson Reed, and Mrs. Worcester asked me to apply to them for what I needed; will you ask them if they would like to send me some Cologne water; when the men are faint and sick after the surgeon has left them, it is very refreshing. I have sent my orderlies for dinner, and am expecting it every minute.

Afternoon. Instead of dinner, they sent me two cases from the operating room; they put a damper on *my* dinner. The poor fellows are quite new, considering what they have gone through. One of them was suffering extremely; a fever-heat had come on in the wounded arm; I put a cold water compress on, and in a few minutes he felt better, and then fell asleep; so I sat by him to keep the flies off, and presently in came the surgeon. I had to assist him in dressing one of the men, then he left, and the work went on. I feel very much afraid of failing at some point, it is such a responsibility, and, as one of the ladies remarked to me, we were never "out at service" before. I have two charming friends here, Miss Spaulding and Miss Mary Hill. I enjoy them very much; they are the only friends I have here with whom I have any intimacy; I am so busy that I have no time to go out to see any one, so they come to see me, when they can. I have plenty of fresh air from windows and doors, to say nothing of cracks which are to be boarded in by and by. My dinner consists of government soup, bread, and perhaps a little rice, or sometimes there are more Isabella grapes than my patients can eat. Breakfast and supper, bread and milk; my breakfast has to be taken in such a hurry that I do not eat more than is necessary. I take supper a little more leisurely. You have hardly a conception of the wants of a ward full of patients. And then the ward must be kept in such a state of order, – the beds must all be made after one particular order and pattern; then they must all be EXACTLY in a line or my surgeon finds it out; he stands in one end of the ward and looks down, if one bed is in the least projecting an orderly has to fly down and push it in. Then they every now and then find some new way of making the beds a little more symmetrical than the previous; I have been taught my third arrangement to-day. Imagine arranging the covers of forty-four beds. As my Doctor is a man of genius he may think of another way before the week is out. Some of the men make their own beds, but I have to arrange them afterwards, also examine them in search of contraband articles of food under the pillows; I found a quantity of cheese under one. The Doctor immediately confiscated it in great indignation, it not being good for sick people. Close by me is Miss Spaulding's ward; between her Doctor and mine is quite a rivalry as to which ward looks the best. We do not care an atom, and so we have a great deal of amusement over it. The two doctors survey each other's wards, and then each declares his own the best looking. I have not had time to see my friend's yet, but am going some day; in the mean time she comes in and reports to me the remarks of our two housekeepers, as we call them.

We are having a very high wind, and the barn-like building rocks like a cradle, or rather creaks like one. We had a tempest the other day and night; my friends asked me the next day if I was not afraid the building would blow over; I told them, no, I did not think that anything would be allowed to happen to so many helpless people; so I slept in peace, feeling that they took care of me and I of them, under Higher Power.

Letter III

Fort Schuyler Hospital, November 8

Dear Mother,—I hoped to have continued my journal this week, but it has not been possible. Early in the week I had a new patient, – a young man who had reamputation of the arm performed on Sunday. He was brought into my ward as it was more comfortable than the one he was in; he was so ill that there was little chance of his life; you may imagine the charge he was to me: all the day I kept in the ward either directly nursing him or keeping my eye on him while about my work; in the evening sat by his side till relieved by the watcher who took charge of him during the night; so all my writing time was taken.

I am the only nurse in the ward, so that when the surgeon was not in, the case fell on me. I allowed no one else to touch his bed or his food; the surgeon sometimes pours out his porter, but it is handed me to give. He is doing well now, though great care is necessary; I am writing near his bed. They will not let me work day and night both, so at ten I am ordered off to bed. I have been fighting the weather lately. The snow came in at the open slats on the roof, and we were nearly frozen, and wet into the bargain. I grew desperate, and when the ward-master came in, insisted upon something being done. I got possession of a ladder, one of my men mounted up, tied slats together, and wound up by nailing one of my sheets, torn in strips, over crevices that could be stopped in no other way; we finally got ahead of the deluge, and I commenced drying bed-clothes by installments round the stoves; by half-past-nine, evening, they were mostly dry, and the floor of the ward drying also. I went about all day in my water-proof cloak, hood over my head; I wear my India-rubber shoes all the time to help keep my poor feet warm. We are not warm, for there are so many cracks in these unfinished buildings that a regiment of stoves could hardly make them really warm. I only wish the contractor had been here the other day; I would have put him under the biggest hole. My health is good, so I conclude this primitive way of life suits me; at any rate, I shall stay by my sick men while I can. If it is right for me to be here I shall have strength given me. My little spirit-lamp[2] is a great comfort to me; when I boil my milk over it, it warms me a good deal: I also heat up tepid bowls of government soup. If you have another box to come to me, please send me some more alcohol, and also, may I have your white aprons, unless you would prefer making me some, – I have not enough to keep clean. The box arrived to-day; I wanted to embrace it. I fell into a rapture over the bandages, – they are beauties. Somebody sent me some Scripture cards and pictures; the men were very much pleased with them; I shall give them the books to-morrow. My candlesticks are loves, I have one on the table now. We

---

2 *Spirit-lamp*: A lamp that uses alcohol or methylated spirits as fuel, usually used for heating or cooking rather than light.

want bandages more than anything except old linen and cotton, – we cannot have too much of that; squares of linen or old damask, hemmed for pocket-kerchiefs, are very acceptable; the soldiers are very glad of a clean handkerchief at hand. I hoped to have written to-morrow, but I am to have three operation cases to attend to. The poor fellows dread it; I have been trying to give them comfort; two are rather bad cases. Tomorrow is inspection day also, as my surgeon reminded me to-night; he says he is coming at eight o'clock.

I am within two yards of a stove and am cold; one of the surgeons agreed with me to-day that we would never, *never* go to the North Pole. I did so enjoy your letter tonight; if you knew the pleasure it gave you would write often and tell me what you are going to do, so that then I may imagine you. I was assisting the surgeon when your letter came; I was so glad when I was able to sit down and read it. Sarah came to see me this week and brought me some flannel shirts for my men. I was very grateful for them; I went round that cold stormy day putting them on my men: I have to help the poor lame fellows to dress.

I hope these buildings will be finished up soon. I have sent all my men to bed and am waiting the visit of the surgeon, and then to bed, I hope.

Tuesday. I am now trying to finish my letter. We did not have operations on Sunday on account of the chilly rain, *some* of which penetrated through; thanks to my energetic efforts on Saturday, not much. Today is lovely – quite mild, and the patients able to go out in the sunshine and smoke their darling, horrid pipes.

This morning we were ordered to prepare for an inspection by the surgeon general of the State. After being made nearly frantic by the efforts to be in wonderful order he never came! My very sick patient is a little better, I have just been washing his face and one poor hand. I asked him when I had done, if he felt any better, "Oh yes," he replied, with such a grateful look. I take the whole care of him, except dressing the wound; I wait upon the surgeon, and assist, if necessary. I sit by him all the evening; he was very restless last evening; I stroked his head and his hair, and quieted him at intervals, but he did not get much quieter till the Doctor came and gave him morphine. He is obliged to take morphine every night.

I love my ward better and better; and if some things are rough and trying, why that is a reason for staying and trying to make them better, not for running away. It would be poor soldiering to run when the enemy appeared.

I lose several of my patients this week; three go back to the regiments; six others go home, too much disabled to fight any more. I hope my ward will not be filled up till all the carpenter-work is done, the noise is so trying to patients. The most useful width for bandages is one and three-fourths inches, two and a half inches, three inches, – the two and a half most used; we do not use thread lint, but a good deal of that scraped with a knife; squares of old linen for handkerchiefs are useful. The slippers you sent are very useful; they are on the feet of two wearers who admire them very much.

Evening. – I have had such a piece of work this evening! My three ward stoves taken down and two much better ones put up in their place; consequently, a new arrangement of beds, which I could not put off till morning; it is all right now, and the Doctor has just been in and expressed his admiration. I am finishing my letter, and then must go to bed, as my night-watch has orders to call me at quarter before six; when I come home, I am going to sleep for a week steady; I have perhaps enough sleep now, but I am obliged to improve my time to get it. The bugle has just sounded, and I am going the round of my beds. Good night, dear mother.

Letter XXXVI

Benton Barracks Hospital, March 16

Dear Kittie,—I thought you would like to hear from me once in a while. I am busy among the sick, both colored[3] and white. The white are pretty sick, but hardly so much as the colored. We have had many cases of the small-pox and erysipelas. I found a case of small-pox and

---

3   *Colored*: A Black person; often used in nineteenth- and early twentieth-century writing and speech. Today, the term is considered dated and only used in historical documents.

one of varioloid[4] this morning the first ward I entered. The poor man with small-pox looked up so sadly at me as I covered him up. The colored people are very grateful for all that is done for them. I have a great many smiles as I go round among them. We are trying to train colored women as nurses among the black; it is a difficult task, but one worth trying. We put them under white nurses, two or more colored women to one white nurse. In regard to the latter we hold to our old rule of employing for nurses only women of character and respectable position. They are more responsible than others, and a person cannot know too much for a nurse. It is a very serious position. We have one large child ward, or rather building, devoted to women and children. The children are generally well, being taken in as accompaniments to their mammas; there are nineteen pickaninnies[5] in this ward. Ask mother if she would like one. Some are very pretty; I can have as many as I want. The men are trying hard to learn to read and write, though the latter accomplishment is confined to few. One woman came this morning bringing her baby; it had a harelip and I have asked Dr. Russell to operate on it upon tomorrow morning. He says he will. I suppose I shall assist. I wonder what I shall do next. I asked the mother's permission, telling her the baby would look as pretty as she did! She looked pleased, and consented. She is quite good-looking. We are whitewashing, and expect that will check some of the diseases; it also makes everything look nice and clean.

Letter XXXVIII

Benton Barracks Hospital, March 21

Darling Mother,—I felt a little lonely to-night, so thought I would write a line to you. I do not go out evenings on account of pneumonia; the

---

4   *Varioloid*: A mild form of smallpox occurring in a person who has been inoculated against the disease (either through previous infection or vaccination).
5   *Pickaninnies*: Likely derived from a Portuguese-based pidgin language associated with the slave trade, an infantilizing term for a child of color (in America, it would have referred almost exclusively to Black children).

Doctor is afraid of my having it. I get very tired in the day-time and am glad to rest when night comes. Is there any news with you? Do tell me how your wrist is, and how you and father are generally. I feel already as if I have drifted far off away from you all. I work over our poor colored soldiers, and they are so grateful for our care. They are as pleasant to take care of as white soldiers, and the wards are as nice, with regard to comfort and order. We have water enough, the Mississippi has not yet given out, and the reservoir has been cleaned. We have a new arrangement here now; the great amphitheater is to be what is called a general hospital, that is a hospital that takes in any patients that the military government sends. The outside wards, or buildings, are mostly for the post hospital; that is, they only take the soldiers from the adjacent military post of Benton Barracks. The general hospital is to be entirely for colored soldiers. It is to be the colored hospital; we shall probably have colored soldiers from down the river. There are over seventy thousand colored soldiers in the Western army. There is a great interest excited here with regard to their care and treatment. Some of the most influential men at the West are taking up the matter. This hospital is doing a great work, not merely by taking care of their bodies, but by bringing around them noble, devoted men and women who give the blacks the place which freedmen should have, and treat them rightly and make others treat them rightly. There is too much of a feeling among many here that they must be treated like inferior beings; they are only inferior from neglect, that is, in many respects; I hope I shall see my way clear to do my duty by them and all. If you have any thoughts about it in any way, let me have them, for you always help me.

American Nervousness: Its Causes and Consequences*

GEORGE MILLER BEARD
(American, 1839–1883)

Late nineteenth-century America saw a nearly 230 percent growth in population, large-scale urbanization as people swarmed to cities across the country, and massive technological changes. This period also witnessed the onset among (largely) well-to-do Americans of a condition called "neurasthenia." A diagnostic term popularized by neurologist George Miller Beard, neurasthenia was defined as a nervous exhaustion (literally, a depletion of energy in the central nervous system) that led to depression, fatigue, digestive problems, and a range of other somewhat vaguely defined symptoms. Men were considered more likely to develop the condition from working in business and banking. Women could develop it from a hectic office job, excessive social activity, or in response to the stress of attending a modern, coed college. Neurasthenia, according to Beard, resulted from the stressors of urban life. In this excerpt, Beard offers an overview of his theory, as published in 1881. As you read, consider the description of what he deemed a distinctly American brand of mental illness and its causes.

---

* Reprinted from George M. Beard, *American Nervousness: Its Causes and Consequences; a supplement to Nervous Exhaustion (Neurasthenia)* (New York: G. P. Putnam's Sons, 1881), vi–ix, Google Books.

Preface

To those who are beginning this study of this interesting theme the following epitome of the philosophy of this work may be of assistance, as a preliminary to a detailed examination.

First. Nervousness is strictly deficiency or lack of nerve-force.[1] This condition, together with all the symptoms of diseases that are evolved from it, has developed mainly within the nineteenth century, and is especially frequent and severe in the Northern and Eastern portions of the United States. Nervousness, in the sense here used, is to be distinguished rigidly and systematically from simple excess of emotion and from organic disease.

Secondly. The chief and primary cause of this development and very rapid increase of nervousness is *modern civilization*, which is distinguished from the ancient by these five characteristics: steam-power, the periodical press, the telegraph, the sciences, and the mental activity of women.

Civilization is the one constant factor without which there can be little or no nervousness, and under which in its modern form nervousness in its many varieties must arise inevitably. Among the secondary and tertiary causes of nervousness are climate, institutions—civil, political, and religious, social, and business—personal habits, indulgence of appetites and passions.

Third. These secondary and tertiary causes are of themselves without power to induce nervousness, save when they supplement and are interwoven with the modern forms of civilization.

Fourth. The sign and type of functional nervous diseases that are evolved out of this general nerve sensitiveness is, neurasthenia (nervous exhaustion), which is in close and constant relation with such functional nerve maladies as certain physical forms of hysteria, hay-fever,

---

1 *Nerve-force*: The energy-producing power of nerves, which people supposedly had only in limited amounts, according to physicians of the period. In addition to causing nervousness, a depletion of nerve-force could eventually lead to being completely incapacitated.

sick-headache, inebriety,[2] and some phases of insanity; is, indeed, a branch whence at early or later stages of growth these diseases may take their origin.

Fifth. The greater prevalence of nervousness in America is a complex resultant of influences, the chief of which are dryness of the air, extremes of heat and cold, civil and religious liberty, and the great mental activity made necessary and possible in a new and productive country under such climatic conditions.

A new crop of diseases has sprung up in America, of which Great Britain until lately knew nothing, or but little. A class of functional diseases of the nervous system, now beginning to be known everywhere in civilization, seem to have first taken root under an American sky, whence their seed is being distributed.

All this is modern, and originally American; and no age, no country, and no form of civilization, not Greece, nor Rome, nor Spain, nor the Netherlands, in the days of their glory, possessed such maladies. Of all the facts of modern sociology, this rise and growth of functional nervous disease in the northern part of America is one of the most stupendous, complex, and suggestive; to solve it in all its interlacings, to unfold its marvelous phenomena and trace them back to their sources and forward to their future developments, is to solve the problem of sociology itself.

But although nervousness, and the functional nervous diseases derived from it, are most frequent in America, and were here first observed and first systematically studies, they are now and for some time have been, becoming more and more frequent in Europe.

Sixth. Among the signs of American nervousness specifically worthy of attention are the following: The nervous diathesis;[3] susceptibility to stimulants and narcotics and various drugs, and consequent necessity of temperance; increase of the nervous diseases inebriety and neurasthenia (nervous exhaustion), hay fever, neuralgia, nervous dyspepsia, asthenopia[4] and allied diseases and symptoms; early and rapid decay

---

2   *Inebriety*: Habitual drunkenness.
3   *The nervous diathesis*: A tendency to suffer from nervous conditions.
4   *Asthenopia*: Eye strain.

of teeth; premature baldness; sensitiveness to cold and heat; increase of diseases not exclusively nervous, as diabetes and certain forms of Bright's disease of the kidneys and chronic catarrhs; unprecedented beauty of American women; frequency of trance and muscle-reading; the strain of dentition, puberty, and change of life; American oratory, humor, speech, and language; change in type of disease during the past half century, and the greater intensity of animal life on this continent.

Seventh. Side by side with this increase of nervousness, and partly as a result of it, longevity has increased, and in all ages brain-workers have, on the average, been long-lived, the very greatest geniuses being the longest-lived of all. In connection with this fact of longevity of brain-workers is to be noted also, the law of the relation of age to work, by which it is shown that original brain-work is done mostly in youth and early and middle life, the latter decades being reserved for work requiring simply experience and routine.

Eighth. The evil of American nervousness, like all other evils, tends within certain limits, to correct itself; and the physical future of the American people has a bright as well as a dark side; increasing wealth will bring increasing calm and repose; the friction of nervousness shall be diminished by various inventions; social customs with the needs of the times, shall be modified, and as a consequence strength and vigor shall be developed at the same time with, and by the side of debility and nervousness.

Specimen Days*

WALT WHITMAN
(American, 1819–1892)

New York-born Walt Whitman changed the face of poetry with his volume *Leaves of Grass* (1855), which used free verse (poetry without regular rhyme or meter) and took up subjects such as nature, humanity, and sexuality in unconventional ways. He was nearly forty-two when the American Civil War broke out in 1861. When a name mentioned in a listing of fallen soldiers seemed to refer to his brother George, Whitman headed south to find him. Fortunately, Whitman found his brother unharmed. He then volunteered as a nurse in the field hospitals for the army. Whitman's experiences with the atrocities of the war and as a nurse inspired a book of poetry, *Drum Taps* (1865), and the notes that would eventually make their way into *Specimen Days*, a largely autobiographical collection published in 1882 and promptly banned in Boston due to content that some reviewers labeled obscene. The excerpts provided here present Whitman's experience caring for the wounded in a narrative that feels casual and conversational. As you read, consider his approach to the role of caretaker and his interactions with his patients.

---

* Reprinted from Walt Whitman, *Complete Prose Works: Specimen Days and Collect, November Boughs and Goodbye My Fancy* (Boston: Small, Maynard, & Company, 1898), 23–24, 27–28, 31–32, 35–36, 47, 61, 70, Google Books.

Fifty Hours Left Wounded on the Field

Here is a case of a soldier I found among the crowded cots in the Patent-office. He likes to have some one to talk to, and we will listen to him. He got badly hit in his leg and side at Fredericksburg that eventful Saturday, 13th of December. He lay the succeeding two days and nights helpless on the field, between the city and those grim terraces of batteries; his company and regiment had been compell'd to leave him to his fate. To make matters worse, it happen'd he lay with his head slightly down hill, and could not help himself. At the end of some fifty hours he was brought off, with other wounded, under a flag of truce. I ask him how the rebels treated him as he lay during those two days and nights within reach of them—whether they came to him—whether they abused him? He answers that several of the rebels, soldiers and others, came to him at one time and another. A couple of them, who were together, spoke roughly and sarcastically, but nothing worse. One middle-aged man, however, who seem'd to be moving around the field, among the dead and wounded, for benevolent purposes, came to him in a way he will never forget; treated our soldier kindly, bound up his wounds, cheer'd him, gave him a couple of biscuits and a drink of whiskey and water; asked him if he could eat some beef. This good secesh,[1] however, did not change our soldier's position, for it might have caused the blood to burst from the wounds, clotted and stagnated. Our soldier is from Pennsylvania; has had a pretty severe time; the wounds proved to be bad ones. But he retains a good heart, and is at present on the gain. (It is not uncommon for the men to remain on the field this way, one, two, or even four or five days.)

Hospital Scenes and Persons

Letter Writing.—When eligible, I encourage the men to write, and myself, when called upon, write all sorts of letters for them (including love letters, very tender ones.) Almost as I reel off these memoranda, I write

---

1 *Secesh*: A secessionist, or someone who supported the Confederacy during the American Civil War.

for a new patient to his wife. M. de F., of the 17th Connecticut, company H, has just come up (February 17th) from Windmill point, and is received in ward H, Armory-square. He is an intelligent looking man, has a foreign accent, black-eyed and hair'd, a Hebraic appearance. Wants a telegraphic message sent to his wife, New Canaan, Conn. I agree to send the message—but to make things sure I also sit down and write the wife a letter, and dispatch it to the post-office immediately, as he fears she will come on, and he does not wish her to, as he will surely get well.

Saturday, January 30th.—Afternoon, visited Campbell hospital. Scene of cleaning up the ward, and giving the men all clean clothes—through the ward (6) the patients dressing or being dress'd—the naked upper half of the bodies—the good-humor and fun—the shirts, drawers, sheets of beds, &c., and the general fixing up for Sunday. Gave J. L. 50 cents.

Wednesday, February 4th.—Visited Armory-square hospital, went pretty thoroughly through wards E and D. Supplied paper and envelopes to all who wish'd—as usual, found plenty of men who needed those articles. Wrote letters. Saw and talk'd with two or three members of the Brooklyn 14th regt. A poor fellow in ward D, with a fearful wound in a fearful condition, was having some loose splinters of bone taken from the neighborhood of the wound. The operation was long, and one of great pain yet, after it was well commenced, the soldier bore it in silence. He sat up, propp'd—was much wasted—had lain a long time quiet in one position (not for days only but weeks,) a bloodless, brown-skinn'd face, with eyes full of determination—belong'd to a New York regiment. There was an unusual cluster of surgeons, medical cadets, nurses, &c., around his bed—I thought the whole thing was done with tenderness, and done well. In one case, the wife sat by the side of her husband, his sickness typhoid fever, pretty bad. In another, by the side of her son, a mother—she told me she had seven children, and this was the youngest. (A fine, kind, healthy, gentle mother, good-looking, not very old, with a cap on her head, and dress'd like home—what a charm it gave to the whole ward.) I liked the woman nurse in ward E—I noticed how she sat a long time by a poor fellow who just had, that morning, in addition to his other sickness, bad hemorrhage—she gently assisted him, reliev'd him of the blood, holding a cloth to his mouth, as he coughed it up—he was so weak he could only just turn his head over on the pillow.

One young New York man, with a bright, handsome face, had been lying several months from a most disagreeable wound, receiv'd at Bull Run. A bullet had shot him right through the bladder, hitting him front, low in the belly, and coming out back. He had suffer'd much—the water[2] came out of the wound, by slow but steady quantities, for many weeks—so that he lay almost constantly in a sort of puddle—and there were other disagreeable circumstances. He was of good heart, however. At present comparatively comfortable, had a bad throat, was delighted with a stick of horehound candy I gave him, with one or two other trifles.

The Wounded from Chancellorsville

May '63.—As I write this, the wounded have begun to arrive from Hooker's command from bloody Chancellorsville. I was down among the first arrivals. The men in charge told me the bad cases were yet to come. If that is so I pity them, for these are bad enough. You ought to see the scene of the wounded arriving at the landing here at the foot of Sixth street, at night. Two boat loads came about half-past seven last night. A little after eight it rain'd a long and violent shower. The pale, helpless soldiers had been debark'd, and lay around on the wharf and neighborhood anywhere. The rain was, probably, grateful to them; at any rate they were exposed to it. The few torches light up the spectacle. All around—on the wharf, on the ground, out on side places—the men are lying on blankets, old quilts, &c., with bloody rags bound round heads, arms, and legs. The attendants are few, and at night few outsiders also—only a few hard-work'd transportation men and drivers. (The wounded are getting to be common, and people grow callous.) The men, whatever their condition, lie there, and patiently wait till their turn comes to be taken up. Near by, the ambulances are now arriving in clusters, and one after another is call'd to back up and take its load. Extreme cases are sent off on stretchers. The men generally make little or no ado, whatever their sufferings. A few groans that cannot be suppress'd, and occasionally a scream of pain as they lift a man into the ambulance.

---

2   *Water*: Urine.

To-day, as I write, hundreds more are expected, and to-morrow and the next day more, and so on for many days. Quite often they arrive at the rate of 1000 a day.

Some Specimen Cases

June 18th.—In one of the hospitals I find Thomas Haley, company M, 4th New York cavalry—a regular Irish boy, a fine specimen of youthful physical manliness—shot through the lungs—inevitably dying—came over to this country from Ireland to enlist—has not a single friend or acquaintance here—is sleeping soundly at this moment, (but it is the sleep of death)—has a bullet-hole straight through the lung. I saw Tom when first brought here, three days since, and didn't suppose he could live twelve hours—(yet he looks well enough in the face to a casual observer.) He lies there with his frame exposed above the waist, all naked, for coolness, a fine built man, the tan not yet bleach'd from his cheeks and neck. It is useless to talk to him, as with his sad hurt, and the stimulants they give him, and the utter strangeness of every object, face, furniture, &c., the poor fellow, even when awake, is like some frighten'd, shy animal. Much of the time he sleeps, or half sleeps. (Sometimes I thought he knew more than he show'd.) I often come and sit by him in perfect silence; he will breathe for ten minutes as softly and evenly as a young babe asleep. Poor youth, so handsome, athletic, with profuse beautiful shining hair. One time as I sat looking at him while he lay asleep, he suddenly, without the least start, awaken'd, open'd his eyes, gave me a long steady look, turning his face very slightly to gaze easier—one long, clear, silent look—a slight sigh—then turn'd back and went into his doze again. Little he knew, poor death-stricken boy, the heart of the stranger that hover'd near.

W.H.E., Co. F, 2nd N.Y.—His disease is pneumonia. He lay sick at the wretched hospital below Aquia creek, for seven or eight days before brought here. He was detail'd from his regiment to go there and help as nurse, but was soon taken down himself. Is an elderly, sallow-faced, rather gaunt, gray-hair'd man, a widower, with children. He express'd a great desire for good, strong green tea. An excellent lady, Mrs. W., of Washington, soon sent him a package; also a small sum of money. The doctor said give him the tea at pleasure; it lay on the table by his side, and he used it every day. He slept a great deal; could not talk much, as he grew deaf. Occupied bed 15, ward I, Armory. (The same lady above, Mrs. W., sent the men a large package of tobacco.)

J. G. lies in bed 52, ward I; is of company B, 7th Pennsylvania. I gave him a small sum of money, some tobacco, and envelopes. To a man adjoining also gave twenty-five cents; he flush'd in the face when I offer'd it—refused at first, but as I found he had not a cent, and was very fond of having the daily papers to read, I pressed it on him. He was evidently very grateful, but said little.

J.T.L., of company F, 9th New Hampshire, lies in bed 37, ward I. Is very fond of tobacco. I furnish him some; also with a little money. Has gangrene of the feet; a pretty bad case; will surely have to lose three toes. Is a regular specimen of an old-fashion'd, rude, hearty, New England countryman, impressing me with his likeness to that celebrated singed cat, who was better than she look'd.[3]

Bed 3, ward E, Armory, has a great hankering for pickles, something pungent. After consulting the doctor, I gave him a small bottle of horse-radish; also some apples; also a book. Some of the nurses are excellent. The woman-nurse in this ward I like very much. (Mrs. Wright—a year afterwards I found her in Mansion house hospital, Alexandria—she is a perfect nurse.)

In one bed a young man, Marcus Small, company K, 7th Maine—sick with dysentery and typhoid fever—pretty critical case—I talk with him often—he thinks he will die—looks like it indeed. I write a letter for him home to East Livermore, Maine—I let him talk to me a little, but not much, advise him to keep very quiet—do most of the talking myself—stay quite a while with him, as he holds on to my hand—talk to him in a cheering, but slow, low and measured manner—talk about his furlough, and going home as soon as he is able to travel.

Thomas Lindly, 1st Pennsylvania cavalry, shot very badly through the foot—poor young man, he suffers horribly, has to be constantly dosed with morphine, his face ashy and glazed, bright young eyes—I give him

---

3 *That celebrated singed cat*: The phrase "singed cat" was a relatively common idiom referring to a person who looks worse than they actually are.

a large handsome apple, lay it in sight, tell him to have it roasted in the morning, as he generally feels easier then, and can eat a little breakfast. I write two letters for him.

Opposite, an old Quaker lady sits by the side of her son, Amer Moore, 2d U. S. artillery—shot in the head two weeks since, very low, quite rational—from hips down paralyzed—he will surely die. I speak a very few words to him every day and evening—he answers pleasantly—wants nothing—(he told me soon after he came about his home affairs, his mother had been an invalid, and he fear'd to let her know his condition.) He died soon after she came.

My Preparations for Visits

In my visits to the hospitals I found it was in the simple matter of personal presence, and emanating ordinary cheer and magnetism, that I succeeded and help'd more than by medical nursing, or delicacies, or gifts of money, or anything else. During the war I possess'd the perfection of physical health. My habit, when practicable, was to prepare for starting out on one of those daily or nightly tours of from a couple to four or five hours, by fortifying myself with previous rest, the bath, clean clothes, a good meal, and as cheerful an appearance as possible.

A New York Soldier

This afternoon, July 22d, I have spent a long time with Oscar F. Wilber, company G, 154th New York, low with chronic diarrhea, and a bad wound also. He asked me to read him a chapter in the New Testament. I complied, and ask'd him what I should read. He said, "Make your own choice." I open'd at the close of one of the first books of the evangelists,[4] and read the chapters describing the latter hours of Christ, and the scenes at the crucifixion. The poor, wasted young man ask'd me to read

---

4   *First books of the evangelists*: The accounts by Matthew, Mark, Luke, and John in the New Testament of the Christian Bible.

the following chapter also, how Christ rose again. I read very slowly, for Oscar was feeble. It pleased him very much, yet the tears were in his eyes. He ask'd me if I enjoy'd religion. I said, "Perhaps not, my dear, in the way you mean, and yet, may-be, it is the same thing." He said, "It is my chief reliance." He talk'd of death, and said he did not fear it. I said, "Why, Oscar, don't you think you will get well?" He said, "I may, but it is not probable." He spoke calmly of his condition. The wound was very bad, it discharg'd much. Then the diarrhea had prostrated him, and I felt that he was even then the same as dying. He behaved very manly and affectionate. The kiss I gave him as I was about leaving he return'd fourfold. He gave me his mother's address, Mrs. Sally D. Wilber, Alleghany pest-office, Cattaraugus county, N. Y. I had several such interviews with him. He died a few days after the one just described.

Hospital Scenes—Incidents

It is Sunday afternoon, middle of summer, hot and oppressive, and very silent through the ward. I am taking care of a critical case, now lying in a half lethargy. Near where I sit is a suffering rebel, from the 8th Louisiana; his name is Irving. He has been here a long time, badly wounded, and lately had his leg amputated; it is not doing very well. Right opposite me is a sick soldier-boy, laid down with his clothes on, sleeping, looking much wasted, his pallid face on his arm. I see by the yellow trimming on his jacket that he is a cavalry boy. I step softly over and find by his card that he is named William Cone, of the 1st Maine cavalry, and his folks live in Skowhegan.

Ice Cream Treat.—One hot day toward the middle of June, I gave the inmates of Carver hospital a general ice cream treat, purchasing a large quantity, and, under convoy of the doctor or head nurse, going around personally through the wards to see to its distribution. *An Incident.*—In one of the rights before Atlanta, a rebel soldier, of large size, evidently a young man, was mortally wounded top of the head, so that the brains partially exuded. He lived three days, lying on his back on the spot where he first dropped. He dug with his heel in the ground during that time a hole big enough to put in a couple of ordinary knapsacks. He just lay there in the open air, and with little intermission kept his heel going night and day. Some of our soldiers then moved him to a house, but he died in a few minutes.

Another.—After the battles at Columbia, Tennessee, where we repuls'd about a score of vehement rebel charges, they left a great many wounded on the ground, mostly within our range. Whenever any of these wounded attempted to move away by any means, generally by crawling off, our men without exception brought them down by a bullet. They let none crawl away, no matter what his condition.

Wounds and Diseases

The war is over, but the hospitals are fuller than ever, from former and current cases. A large majority of the wounds are in the arms and legs. But there is every kind of wound, in every part of the body. I should say of the sick, from my observation, that the prevailing maladies are typhoid fever and the camp fevers generally, diarrhea, catarrhal affections and bronchitis, rheumatism and pneumonia. These forms of sickness lead; all the rest follow. There are twice as many sick as there are wounded. The deaths range from seven to ten per cent, of those under treatment.[5]

Hospitals Closing

October 3.—There are two army hospitals now remaining. I went to the largest of these (Douglas) and spent the afternoon and evening. There are many sad cases, old wounds, incurable sickness, and some of the wounded from the March and April battles before Richmond. Few realize how sharp and bloody those closing battles were. Our men exposed themselves more than usual; press'd ahead without urging. Then the

---

5 [Whitman's note: In the U. S. Surgeon-General's office since, there is a formal record and treatment of 153,142 cases of wounds by government surgeons. What must have been the number unofficial, indirect—to say nothing of the Southern armies?]

southerners fought with extra desperation. Both sides knew that with the successful chasing of the rebel cabal from Richmond, and the occupation of that city by the national troops, the game was up. The dead and wounded were unusually many. Of the wounded the last lingering driblets have been brought to hospital here. I find many rebel wounded here, and have been extra busy to-day 'tending to the worst cases of them with the rest.

Oct., Nov. and Dec., '65—Sundays—Every Sunday of these months visited Harewood hospital out in the woods, pleasant and recluse, some two and a half or three miles north of the capitol. The situation is healthy, with broken ground, grassy slopes and patches of oak woods, the trees large and fine. It was one of the most extensive of the hospitals, now reduced to four or five partially occupied wards, the numerous others being vacant. In November, this became the last military hospital kept up by the government, all the others being closed. Cases of the worst and most incurable wounds, obstinate illness, and of poor fellows who have no homes to go to, are found here.

Dec. 10—Sunday—Again spending a good part of the day at Harewood. I write this about an hour before sundown. I have walk'd out for a few minutes to the edge of the woods to soothe myself with the hour and scene. It is a glorious, warm, golden-sunny, still afternoon. The only noise is from a crowd of cawing crows, on some trees three hundred yards distant. Clusters of gnats swimming and dancing in the air in all directions. The oak leaves are thick under the bare trees, and give a strong and delicious perfume. Inside the wards everything is gloomy. Death is there. As I enter'd, I was confronted by it the first thing; a corpse of a poor soldier, just dead, of typhoid fever. The attendants had just straighten'd the limbs, put coppers on the eyes, and were laying it out.

The roads—A great recreation, the past three years, has been in taking long walks out from Washington, five, seven, perhaps ten miles and back; generally with my friend Peter Doyle, who is as fond of it as I am. Fine moonlight nights, over the perfect military roads, hard and smooth—or Sundays—we had these delightful walks, never to be forgotten. The roads connecting Washington and the numerous forts around the city, made one useful result, at any rate, out of the war.

Notes from Sick Rooms[*]

JULIA STEPHEN
(English, 1846–1895)

Julia Stephen, mother of English author Virginia Woolf, is perhaps best known for having been an artist's model for Romantic-era painting and photography. However, she was also an advocate for the poor and the sick, and worked as a volunteer nurse. It was this experience that led her to write *Notes from Sick Rooms* in 1883. She prefaces the work by noting that her advice is drawn from "actual observation" of practices that help and hinder patient comfort and recovery. She also highlights the importance of practical experience, reminding readers that useful instruction in nursing doesn't come exclusively from formal training. The excerpt comes from the opening section of the work, which emphasizes this practical approach. As you read, consider her characterization of nursing and the relationship nurses have with patients and their families.

---

[*] Reprinted from Julia Stephen, *Notes from Sick Rooms* (London: Smith, Elder, and Co., 1883), 1–7, Google Books.

[On Nurses and Patients]

I have often wondered why it is considered a proof of virtue in anyone to become a nurse. The ordinary relations between the sick and the well are far easier and pleasanter than between the well and the well.

There are no doubt people to whom the sight of physical suffering is so distasteful as to turn a sick room into a real Chamber of Horrors for them. That such unlucky persons should ever have authority in a sick room ought to be an impossibility; but if by some unlucky chance they ever have, we should surely reserve our pity for the unfortunate invalids in their charge.

Illness has, or ought to have, much of the leveling power of death. We forget, or at all events cease to dwell on, the unfavorable sides to a character when death has claimed its owner, and in illness we can afford to ignore the details which in health make familiar intercourse difficult.

The ways in which our friends dress, bring up their children, or spend their money, are apt to cause disagreement more or less marked between us when there is no thought of suffering or loss; but the moment we are threatened by either, how slight such matters seem! We can contemplate without irritation the vivid fringe of hair when the head which it disfigures is aching and fevered; and we feel equal to allowing the spoiled children to put their feet in the 'crystal butter-boat,' like the never-to-be-forgotten little boy of our childhood, if it will give any pleasure to the over indulgent mother who is racked with pain.

A nurse's life is certainly not a dull one, and the more skillful the nurse the less dull she will be. The more she cultivates that *art* of nursing, the more enjoyment she will get, and the same may be said of the patient. The art of being ill is no easy one to learn, but it is practiced to perfection by many of the greatest sufferers.

The greatest sufferer is by no means the worst patient, and to give relief, even if it be only temporary, to such patients is perhaps a greater pleasure than can be found in the performance of any other duty.

It ought to be quite immaterial to a nurse whom she is nursing. I have often heard it urged against trained nurses that they look upon their patients as *cases*. If to look on patients as a case is to feel indifference towards them, then the charge is indeed a reproof; but assuming that the nurse is not indifferent, how should she look on her patient but as a case; and further, why should she?

The genuine love of her 'case' and not of the individual patient seems to me the sign of the true nursing instinct.

It would be hard if those who were specially charming, or those whose antecedents interested, were alone to be tenderly nursed. Every nurse, whether trained or amateur, should look on her patient as a 'case,' nursing with the same undeviating tenderness and watchful care the entire stranger, the unsympathetic friend, or the one who is nearest and dearest.

In most cases of illness nursed at home, even if there be a trained nurse, there is generally some member of the family watching and helping—more often hindering the work of the sick room.

Much may be done by helpers to make the lives of both patient and nurse easier and brighter; but unless such outsiders help with skill and tact, as well as with zeal, their presence in the sick room is to be dreaded instead of desired.

To avoid confusion I have used the word 'nurse,' but many of the little hints which I have noted down are for such watchers. One imperative duty of all those in attendance on the sick is that they should be cheerful; not an elaborate, forced cheerfulness, but a quiet brightness which makes their presence a cheer and not an oppression. It may seem difficult to follow this advice, but it is not. Cheerfulness is a habit, and no one should venture to attend the sick who wears a gloomy face. The atmosphere of the sick room should be cheerful and peaceful. Domestic disturbances, money matters, worries, and discussions of all kinds should be kept away.

There can be no half dealing in such matters; hints and whispers are worse than the whole truth. There is no limit to a sick person's imagination, and this is a fact which is too often ignored, even by the tenderest friends. The answers, "O, it is nothing," "Don't worry yourself," when suspicion is once aroused, are enough to fret the unfortunate patient into a fever. She will torture herself with suspicion of every possible calamity, and at last, when she has nerved herself to insist on being told, her unconscious tormentor discloses the fact that one of the pipes has burst!

If trouble should come, and it is important that the invalid should be kept in ignorance, her watchers must make peace with their consciences as best they can; and if questions are asked, they must 'lie freely.'

Among the number of small evils which haunt illness, the greatest, in the misery which it can cause, though smallest in size, is crumbs. The origin of most things has been decided on, but the origin of crumbs in bed has never excited sufficient attention among the scientific world, though it is a problem which has tormented many a sufferer. I will forbear to give my own explanation, which would be neither scientific nor orthodox, and will merely beg that their evil existence may be recognized and, as far as human nature allows, guarded against. The torment of crumbs should be stamped out of the sick bed as if it were the Colorado beetle in a potato field.[1] Anyone who has been ill will at once take her precautions, feeble though they will prove. She will have a napkin under her chin, stretch her neck out of bed, eat in the most uncomfortable way, and watch that no crumbs get into the folds of her night-dress or jacket. When she lies back in bed, in the vain hope that she may have baffled the enemy, he is before her: a sharp crumb is buried in her back, and grains of sand seem sticking to her toes. If the patient is able to get up and have her bed made, when she returns she will find the crumbs are waiting for her. The housemaid will protest that the sheets were shaken, and the nurse that she swept out the crumbs, but there they are, and there they will remain unless the nurse determines to conquer them. To do this she must first believe in them, and there are few assertions that are met with such incredulity as the one—I have crumbs in my bed. After every meal the nurse should put her hand into the bed and feel for the crumbs. When the bed is made, the nurse and housemaid must not content themselves with shaking or sweeping. They tiny crumbs stick in the sheets, and the nurse must patiently take each crumb out; if there are many very small ones, she must even wet her fingers, and get the crumbs to stick to them. The patient's night-clothes must be searched; crumbs lurk in each tiny fold or frill. They go up the sleeve of the night-gown, and if the patient is in bed when the search is going on, her arms should hang out of bed, so that the crumbs which are certain to be there

---

1 Stephen likens the irritation of crumbs to a common North American garden pest.

may be induced to fall down. When crumbs are banished—that is to say, temporarily, for with each meal they return, and for this the nurse must make up her mind—she must see that there are no rucks in the bed-sheets. A very good way of avoiding these is to pin the lower sheet firmly down on the mattress with nursery pins, first stretching the sheet smoothly and straightly over the mattress. Many people are not aware of the importance of putting on a sheet *straight*, but if it is not, it will certainly drag, and if pinned it will probably tear.

A Book of Medical Discourses: In Two Parts*

REBECCA LEE CRUMPLER
American (1831–1895)

During a time when it was rare for Black men and women to have access to higher education, let alone study medicine, Rebecca Lee Crumpler gained admission to medical school and became the only Black woman to graduate from the New England Female Medical College, which later merged with Boston University. Crumpler was the first African American woman to earn a Doctorate in Medicine in 1864, a year before the end of the Civil War. After the war, she moved to Richmond, Virginia, to work with the Freedmen's Bureau, a government organization founded in 1865 to help the formerly enslaved and poor in southern states. She returned to practice in Boston around 1869 and stayed in Massachusetts for the rest of her life. In 1883, Crumpler published *A Book of Medical Discourses: In Two Parts*, which focused on the medical care of women and children. As you read, consider the practical medical advice she offers for new mothers and her approach to some medical folk wisdom of the time.

---

* Reprinted from Rebecca Lee Crumpler, *A Book of Medical Discourses: in Two Parts* (Boston: Cashman, Keating, 1883), chaps. 2, 7, U.S. National Library of Medicine, National Institutes for Health.

Washing and Dressing the New-Born

Usually, as soon as the birth of a child is announced, a basin or tub of hot water is ordered. The washing begins with a "wee bit of rag" and a great cake of perfumed soap purchased long, long before, for the occasion. Then follows wiping with a great linen towel, during which time the creature gets well aired, being indirectly exhibited to as many as have courage to look on and admire "the cunning little thing."

"The water must be hot, to get off the grease,"[1] said an old nurse. Aye, but with ignorant help would it be surprising if a little of the skin came off first? In more favored circles a nice bath tub is prepared, the water of an equal temperature with the room. Some fine soap is put in to make a suds, which is applied after the surface of the body is oiled. Some cold water adherents persist in using ice-cold water upon a new-born babe, depending on "rubbing it to get up a circulation." I once knew a divine (divines have rules sometimes) whose customs led him to have his only child washed in this way, and believing in the adage of "the hair of the dog curing the bite," he continued to doctor it himself for eighteen months, from its birth to its death, with cold water. The babe received a severe cold, stopping up its nostrils and air tubes, and rendering its little life wholly miserable. To the cause of all this suffering they gave the technical name, Catarrh.

The methods of washing infants just described are more common even in this, enlightened age of humanity than is generally known. The excuse for cold baths may exist in the mode of life of the erratic tribes, or among uncivilized nations whose minds are dark upon the construction and office of a nervous system. The several sad results that I myself have witnessed at times, and places, that it was not deemed my business to speak, have led me to adopt what seemed a more humane course. With the use of cold water some judgment is required, as many infants, when born, are weak, and ready to yield up life upon the application of the slightest sedative. The skin being so largely supplied with nerves which transmit all sensations to the internal organs, as telegraph wires

---

1 *The grease*: The vernix caseosa (Latin for "cheesy varnish"), a waxy, greasy coating often found on the skin of newborns.

do the electric current. Thus cold water may send a chill to some vital part, the result of which no effort in the power of man can counteract. It is next to impossible to keep a babe as warm as it should be going through with the customary routine. Indeed it is not at all uncommon for a babe to be laid beside its mother (if not alone in a crib) lips purple and cold as a lump of clay. I once looked upon a babe who from this cause had for three days resisted all attempts to get it warm. Thus, I fear, many come and go. Does any desire to preserve the vitality of a new being? Then it will not suffice to be too self-assured or too oriental to seek to improve in the matter.

I deeply regret to have to state that I have heard many apparently intelligent persons express opposition to the continuation of the human species. But let me ask, What devastating visitations may we not expect if we seek to diminish God's images by any selfish or misguided motives?

There are many kinds of soap in use for the purpose of washing clothes, cleansing paint, etc. Then there are not a few advertised as superior for washing the skin. But the fact that water into which soap is rubbed turns white, or becomes sudsy, is sufficient evidence that it contains an alkali, or something having the nature of potash. To use it on the tender skin of infants is but to experiment for the benefit of the dealer, at the expense of the babe. Again, soap is irritating to the more tender surfaces, as the lips and eyelids. If the suds is sucked by the child while the sponge is passed over the face, severe purging may occur. Then if soap gets in the eyes, it is liable to cause sore or inflamed eyes, perhaps for life. I truly believe that more children are afflicted with sore eyes, ears, noses, and heads, whose friends took the precaution to have them washed with "pure baby soap," than could be counted in a hundred years. The germs of bronchitis, which means cold settled in the air-tubes leading to the lungs, pneumonia, which means lung fever, indigestion, each or all, can be inducted into the system in the first washing. The male physician, unlike the woman physician, does not always remain long enough to see this important duty properly performed. This may be owing to the fact that, among the poorer classes, two or three women are present who are expected to be experts in baby-washing. But, as a fact, many old women sit around on such occasions who have almost as little knowledge what and how to do, as the babe whose expected advent has called them together. Therefore we cannot too strongly protest against the practice of many physicians, that of leaving a woman in the hands of an inexperienced person as soon as the navel cord is severed. For it is not at all reasonable to conclude, that because a woman is the mother of many children, she is an expert in the matter of washing and dressing the newborn, or of relieving the various ailments incident upon child-bearing.

The Uselessness of "Baby Medicines"

Probably the greatest amount of mischief arising from the administration of "baby teas,"[2] lies in the fact that they are not given with the least certainty as to their effect upon the system of the child, whether to nourish the blood or physic the bowels. Let us take catnip: this is an herb described in some books as being a mild laxative, good to work off cold on the chest and bowels of infants; a sweat-promoter. About a dozen years ago a neighbor of one of my patients, thinking it for the best, gave catnip tea to her three-days'-old son. I was hastily summoned, and on arriving in the room where everything a few hours before was so tranquil, I suspected that catnip tea had been around. Of course no one would own up until, after I had staid by the little victim fifteen hours without sleep, finally succeeding in checking[3] the frequent green discharges and thus saving the child's life, shame, caused the disclosure of the cause of the mischief. The tea had not been given for food, as the mother had a full supply; but as the babe was moving about, it was thought that a little catnip tea would make it sleep. A lady told me with great dignity that her children ate homeopathic pills[4] when they wished. "Why," said she, "my children fatten on them."

---

2   *Baby-teas*: Teas made from catnip and fennel are still sometimes used for the relief of colic in infants.
3   *Checking*: Stopping.
4   Homeopathy, which follows the doctrine that something that causes symptoms in a healthy person can cure that symptom in a sick person when introduced in minuscule amounts ("like cures like"), became increasingly popular in the nineteenth century. By 1835, the U.S. had established its first school of homeopathy, with 22 such schools by 1900.

I saw that she did not know the secret of the "fattening." Another said, "Why, my James eats castor-oil on bread." Now we are aware that there are very many articles used as food that can be prepared and combined so as to act in place of medicine in certain cases; but as a general thing medicine will not answer to nourish the body in place of food. According to the mechanism of man, there are three stages in his life for which due preparation is made, before he comes into existence, to wit: the breasts' milk for infancy, the teeth, with which to eat solid food, and medicine, to heal when sick. As to catnip producing sleep, I cannot agree with old ladies in general; but I do know of a truth that if a child is dosed with it in early infancy, the effect is to loosen the bowels; the fatigue from this over-distension of the stomach causes sleep. Babes should move about if they have life enough in them; they should, by no means, be stupefied. The first milk from the breast is the only medicine needed; when other mixtures are poured into the child's stomach, as teas sweetened with sugar, honey, molasses, either of which is laxative, the danger is greatly augmented, especially if given before the bowels have moved at all. The custom of old-fashioned people, as they style themselves, of giving new-born babes castor-oil and molasses, or soot tea (for that irrepressible belly-ache), and urine and molasses, to clean them out, is, though with reluctance, fast dying out. It would be well to notice that children who are dosed during infancy for every supposed ill are seldom robust. They become physically stunted, and their peevish habits exact for them all sorts of over-indulgence. More food for the blood, and less medicine, should be the motto. Let us follow the tide of progression.

There are no uniform rules by which infants are to have a discharge at birth, either from the bowels or bladder. Therefore, no efforts to induce such should be used until necessity demands it. It is no uncommon thing for infants to pass large quantities from the bowels, just as they are entering the world; a circumstance not likely to be noticed by those unaccustomed to all the incidents of childbirth. It is always safe to await the action of the first food, whether from the breast or artificial; and if it be but a few drops well digested, there need be no fear but that the napkins will be soiled as fast as desired. If such result does not follow, after waiting two or three days, a flannel cloth folded, and wrung out of hot water, laid first on your cheek, then on the child's belly, and that covered with dry flannel, will, with perseverance, bring about the desired result. Sometimes an infant passes large quantities of the dark matter immediately after the fatigue of washing and dressing (old style); then it may pass no more for two or three days, or until time has been given for matter to accumulate. If the organs of the child are all right, all will be well. But should doubts arise as to the best course to take, surely medical advice only needs the seeking. It was formerly the custom, and is now to a great extent with old nurses, to give later in the month certainly before their month was up, as all teas and charms had to be given before they left saffron tea. I have seen them sit by a hot stove and feed infants with saffron tea more patiently than they would like it given to them. I once asked a high-priced nurse why she gave saffron tea. I was kindly, though decidedly, informed that it was to "push the gums." I was none the wiser by asking. I afterward learned from the child's older sister that the doctor said the baby had the jaundice. Well it might have the jaundice, kept in a room with a temperature of 80 degrees, with two adult persons night and day, and fed on saffron tea. Now the crocus, or saffron, sometimes grown in our gardens, is described as possessing sweating properties, being good to promote eruptions of the skin in fevers, and good in fits. Yet thousands of infants, no doubt, have been forced to swallow saffron tea, who have not given the slightest evidence of any unnatural complaint. No paregoric, laudanum, or other preparations containing opium, should ever be given to an infant for the purpose of quieting or making it sleep. Sleep-producers serve only to bind the bowels and stupefy the senses. Carminatives (medicines that expel wind) such as caraway, fennel, anise, cardamon, mints and the like, should never be given unless prescribed by those competent to vouch for their effect.

It is becoming a widespread custom to send a little girl or boy to a druggist's to purchase some advertised baby medicine or food. The patent cough syrups, or those kept on hand in shops, I deem unsafe in the hands of the inexperienced. Most, if not all of them, contain some sleep-producing ingredient, whereby they may check a cough by paralyzing, as it were, the little nerves of sensation in the air tubes; thus giving opportunity for the phlegm to collect in great quantities, with no possible way of escape. Doubtless in this way suffocation is frequently induced, in whooping-cough, bronchitis, or croup.

Several years ago, in the city of Boston, a mother returned from work, and found her baby, which she had left alone, a corpse. Her explanation, as it appeared in the daily papers, was to the effect that she had given the child the rinsings of the vial that contained laudanum, to keep it quiet.

People are getting much wiser nowadays; laudanum and paregoric cannot be easily obtained without a recipe. But they can yet buy and give large doses of "Patent Soothing Syrups."[5]

In all cases of difficult breathing or signs of croup, with or without hot skin, a soft flannel cloth should be wrung out of hot water, and laid over the entire chest, close up under the chin and ears; and if the bowels are bound, it may extend to the belly, the whole being covered with a dry, warm flannel. By this means the force of a cold can be broken, the breathing relieved, and in a majority of cases it is all that is required to be done. Even in severe cases of lung fever, warm water applications are invaluable; acting as an absorbent through the medium of the pores of the skin. If a paste of flax-seed meal is used, it should be applied in the same way. If the applications are to be warm, they should be kept warm, and if they are to be cold, should be kept cold, until relief is obtained.

I may have digressed somewhat, as pneumonia seldom develops in the first month of infancy. At all events, external applications are in place till medical aid is secured. I do not wish to be understood as usurping the power of other physicians; each has his or her own method of procedure.

I merely wish to impress the domestic and common sense means, to be used in cases of emergency.

The old custom of giving infants "a little weak toddy" to "bring up the wind and make them sleep," should henceforth and forever be removed

---

5   *Patent soothing syrups*: Any one of a number of proprietary medicines supposedly patented for use in soothing babies suffering from dysentery, colic, or teething pain. One of the most famous of these was Mrs. Winslow's Soothing Syrup, which contained large quantities of morphine and alcohol (one fluid ounce of the syrup contained up to 65 mg of morphine—an adult dose in an oral solution is now recommended to be 15–30 mg).

from the midst of a more enlightened people. If it is given weak the effect is to intoxicate at first, and then produce sleep; which may be followed by a fearful attack of purging. If given strong, it may induce constipation and dry colic, the very thing it is intended to relieve. Such a course may also have inculcated a desire for tippling in many of our weak-minded youth. Castor-oil is a well-known sickening purgative, and it does seem to be a wonderful interposition of Providence alone, that so many thousand infants have survived the compulsory dosing with this drug. But a few years ago a lady, aged about sixty-five, came to her end from severe diarrhea, brought on, as she testified, by taking a "store-bottle of castor-oil at a dose."

Mothers and nurses should strive to become familiar with all articles of diet; also with the properties and medical uses of all drugs and minerals, and their action upon the animal economy.

Neurasthenia*

AGNES MARY FRANCES ROBINSON
(English, 1857–1944)

English poet Agnes Mary Frances Robinson, fluent in in multiple languages and trained in Greek literature, was the author of several well-regarded books of poetry, and she had many lively connections in society circles. She grew up around writers and artists, and as an adult had a salon, a space for social gatherings dedicated to intellectual and political discussion where she connected with other writers. Later in her life, her social circle grew to include scientists because her second husband was a microbiologist (and successor to Louis Pasteur). Her works often take up philosophical themes, including mortality, and topics related to mental health. The poem included here was first published under the title "In Affliction" in 1888, but was republished in her 1902 collection *The Collected Poems, Lyrical and Narrative, of Mary Robinson (Madame Duclaux)* under the revised title "Neurasthenia," which refers to the ill-defined nervous condition commonly diagnosed in the period (see George Miller Beard, pp. 258–261). As you read, consider the narrator's description of the "affliction" of the title.

---

* Reprinted from Agnes Mary Frances Robinson, *Songs, Ballads, and a Garden Play* (London: T. Fisher Unwin, 1888), 33, Google Books.

In Affliction

I watch the happier people of the house
Come in and out and talk and go their ways;
I sit and gaze at them; I cannot rouse
My heavy mind to share their busy days.

I watch them glide like skaters on a stream [5]
Across the brilliant surface of the world;
But I am underneath; they do not dream
How deep below the eddying flood is whirl'd.

They cannot come to me, nor I to them;
But, if a mightier arm could reach and save, [10]
Should I forget the time I had to stem?
Should I, like these, ignore the abysmal wave?
Yes! In the radiant air how could I know
How black it is, how fast it is, below?

The Yellow Wallpaper*

CHARLOTTE PERKINS GILMAN
(American, 1860–1935)

Known as a social reformer and feminist in her own day, Charlotte Perkins Gilman wrote widely: from the lauded feminist manifesto *Women and Economics* (1898) to a range of novels, short stories, and poems. Among these works, *The Yellow Wallpaper*, published in 1892, is her most famous today. Gilman's short story is widely regarded as a literary classic. In it, the narrator recounts her increasingly surreal experience over the course of a summer stay at an estate in the country, taken in large part to help cure her of a "nervous depression," a kind of neurasthenia (see George Miller Beard, pp. 258–261). The short story offers a picture of some of the dynamics around the status of women and around female health issues in late nineteenth-century society. As you read, consider the approach taken by the narrator's doctor (who is also her husband) in treating her condition and the narrator's own description of her experience.

---

* Reprinted from Charlotte Perkins Stetson [Gilman], *The Yellow Wallpaper* (Boston: Small, Maynard, 1899; Project Gutenberg, 2021).

The Yellow Wallpaper

It is very seldom that mere ordinary people like John and myself secure ancestral halls for the summer.

A colonial mansion, a hereditary estate, I would say a haunted house, and reach the height of romantic felicity—but that would be asking too much of fate!

Still I will proudly declare that there is something queer about it.

Else, why should it be let so cheaply? And why have stood so long untenanted?

John laughs at me, of course, but one expects that in marriage.

John is practical in the extreme. He has no patience with faith, an intense horror of superstition, and he scoffs openly at any talk of things not to be felt and seen and put down in figures.

John is a physician, and *perhaps*—(I would not say it to a living soul, of course, but this is dead paper and a great relief to my mind)—*perhaps* that is one reason I do not get well faster.

You see, he does not believe I am sick!

And what can one do?

If a physician of high standing, and one's own husband, assures friends and relatives that there is really nothing the matter with one but temporary nervous depression—a slight hysterical tendency—what is one to do?

My brother is also a physician, and also of high standing, and he says the same thing.

So I take phosphates or phosphites[1]—whichever it is, and tonics, and journeys, and air, and exercise, and am absolutely forbidden to "work" until I am well again.[2]

---

1 *Phosphates and phosphites*: Salts of phosphoric and phosphorous acids, respectively. Both were considered useful for the treatment of neurasthenia (though drugs were not the primary method of treatment). Phosphorus deficiency can result in anxiety, fatigue and pain, weakness, numbness, and irritability.

2 The narrator has been prescribed the "Rest Cure," devised by Silas Weir Mitchell to treat neurasthenia in women. This treatment restricted exertion and "brain work" like writing, studying, or other creative intellectual activity. It also involved long periods of bed rest and, sometimes, electrotherapy. The treatment for neurasthenia

Personally, I disagree with their ideas.

Personally, I believe that congenial work, with excitement and change, would do me good.

But what is one to do?

I did write for a while in spite of them; but it *does* exhaust me a good deal—having to be so sly about it, or else meet with heavy opposition.

I sometimes fancy that in my condition if I had less opposition and more society and stimulus—but John says the very worst thing I can do is to think about my condition, and I confess it always makes me feel bad.

So I will let it alone and talk about the house.

The most beautiful place! It is quite alone, standing well back from the road, quite three miles from the village. It makes me think of English places that you read about, for there are hedges and walls and gates that lock, and lots of separate little houses for the gardeners and people.

There is a *delicious* garden! I never saw such a garden—large and shady, full of box-bordered paths, and lined with long grape-covered arbors with seats under them.

There were greenhouses, too, but they are all broken now.

There was some legal trouble, I believe, something about the heirs and co-heirs; anyhow, the place has been empty for years.

That spoils my ghostliness, I am afraid; but I don't care—there is something strange about the house—I can feel it.

I even said so to John one moonlight evening, but he said what I felt was a *draught*, and shut the window.

I get unreasonably angry with John sometimes. I'm sure I never used to be so sensitive. I think it is due to this nervous condition.

But John says if I feel so I shall neglect proper self-control; so I take pains to control myself,—before him, at least,—and that makes me very tired.

I don't like our room a bit. I wanted one downstairs that opened on the piazza and had roses all over the window, and such pretty old-fashioned chintz hangings! but John would not hear of it.

---

in men was quite different: they were required to travel to the western U.S. to hike, enjoy nature, and then write about their experience.

He said there was only one window and not room for two beds, and no near room for him if he took another.

He is very careful and loving, and hardly lets me stir without special direction.

I have a scheduled prescription for each hour in the day; he takes all care from me, and so I feel basely ungrateful not to value it more.

He said we came here solely on my account, that I was to have perfect rest and all the air I could get. "Your exercise depends on your strength, my dear," said he, "and your food somewhat on your appetite; but air you can absorb all the time." So we took the nursery, at the top of the house.

It is a big, airy room, the whole floor nearly, with windows that look all ways, and air and sunshine galore. It was nursery first and then playground and gymnasium, I should judge; for the windows are barred for little children, and there are rings and things in the walls.

The paint and paper look as if a boys' school had used it. It is stripped off—the paper—in great patches all around the head of my bed, about as far as I can reach, and in a great place on the other side of the room low down. I never saw a worse paper in my life.

One of those sprawling flamboyant patterns committing every artistic sin.

It is dull enough to confuse the eye in following, pronounced enough to constantly irritate, and provoke study, and when you follow the lame, uncertain curves for a little distance they suddenly commit suicide—plunge off at outrageous angles, destroy themselves in unheard-of contradictions.

The color is repellent, almost revolting; a smoldering, unclean yellow, strangely faded by the slow-turning sunlight.

It is a dull yet lurid orange in some places, a sickly sulphur tint in others.

No wonder the children hated it! I should hate it myself if I had to live in this room long.

There comes John, and I must put this away,—he hates to have me write a word.

*

We have been here two weeks, and I haven't felt like writing before, since that first day.

I am sitting by the window now, up in this atrocious nursery, and there is nothing to hinder my writing as much as I please, save lack of strength.

John is away all day, and even some nights when his cases are serious.

I am glad my case is not serious!

But these nervous troubles are dreadfully depressing.

John does not know how much I really suffer. He knows there is no *reason* to suffer, and that satisfies him.

Of course it is only nervousness. It does weigh on me so not to do my duty in any way!

I meant to be such a help to John, such a real rest and comfort, and here I am a comparative burden already!

Nobody would believe what an effort it is to do what little I am able—to dress and entertain, and order things.

It is fortunate Mary is so good with the baby. Such a dear baby!

And yet I *cannot* be with him, it makes me so nervous.

I suppose John never was nervous in his life. He laughs at me so about this wallpaper!

At first he meant to repaper the room, but afterwards he said that I was letting it get the better of me, and that nothing was worse for a nervous patient than to give way to such fancies.

He said that after the wallpaper was changed it would be the heavy bedstead, and then the barred windows, and then that gate at the head of the stairs, and so on.

"You know the place is doing you good," he said, "and really, dear, I don't care to renovate the house just for a three months' rental."

"Then do let us go downstairs," I said, "there are such pretty rooms there."

Then he took me in his arms and called me a blessed little goose, and said he would go down cellar if I wished, and have it whitewashed into the bargain.

But he is right enough about the beds and windows and things.

It is as airy and comfortable a room as any one need wish, and, of course, I would not be so silly as to make him uncomfortable just for a whim.

I'm really getting quite fond of the big room, all but that horrid paper.

Out of one window I can see the garden, those mysterious deep-shaded arbors, the riotous old-fashioned flowers, and bushes and gnarly trees.

Out of another I get a lovely view of the bay and a little private wharf belonging to the estate. There is a beautiful shaded lane that runs down there from the house. I always fancy I see people walking in these numerous paths and arbors, but John has cautioned me not to give way to fancy in the least. He says that with my imaginative power and habit of story-making a nervous weakness like mine is sure to lead to all manner of excited fancies, and that I ought to use my will and good sense to check the tendency. So I try.

I think sometimes that if I were only well enough to write a little it would relieve the press of ideas and rest me.

But I find I get pretty tired when I try.

It is so discouraging not to have any advice and companionship about my work. When I get really well John says we will ask Cousin Henry and Julia down for a long visit; but he says he would as soon put fire-works in my pillow-case as to let me have those stimulating people about now.

I wish I could get well faster.

But I must not think about that. This paper looks to me as if it *knew* what a vicious influence it had!

There is a recurrent spot where the pattern lolls like a broken neck and two bulbous eyes stare at you upside-down.

I get positively angry with the impertinence of it and the everlastingness. Up and down and sideways they crawl, and those absurd, unblinking eyes are everywhere. There is one place where two breadths didn't match, and the eyes go all up and down the line, one a little higher than the other.

I never saw so much expression in an inanimate thing before, and we all know how much expression they have! I used to lie awake as a child and get more entertainment and terror out of blank walls and plain furniture than most children could find in a toy-store.

I remember what a kindly wink the knobs of our big old bureau used to have, and there was one chair that always seemed like a strong friend.

I used to feel that if any of the other things looked too fierce I could always hop into that chair and be safe.

The furniture in this room is no worse than inharmonious, however, for we had to bring it all from downstairs. I suppose when this was used as a playroom they had to take the nursery things out, and no wonder! I never saw such ravages as the children have made here.

The wallpaper, as I said before, is torn off in spots, and it sticketh closer than a brother—they must have had perseverance as well as hatred.

Then the floor is scratched and gouged and splintered, the plaster itself is dug out here and there, and this great heavy bed, which is all we found in the room, looks as if it had been through the wars.

But I don't mind it a bit—only the paper.

There comes John's sister. Such a dear girl as she is, and so careful of me! I must not let her find me writing.

She is a perfect, and enthusiastic housekeeper, and hopes for no better profession. I verily believe she thinks it is the writing which made me sick!

But I can write when she is out, and see her a long way off from these windows.

There is one that commands the road, a lovely, shaded, winding road, and one that just looks off over the country. A lovely country, too, full of great elms and velvet meadows.

This wallpaper has a kind of sub-pattern in a different shade, a particularly irritating one, for you can only see it in certain lights, and not clearly then.

But in the places where it isn't faded, and where the sun is just so, I can see a strange, provoking, formless sort of figure, that seems to sulk about behind that silly and conspicuous front design.

There's sister on the stairs!

*

Well, the Fourth of July is over! The people are gone and I am tired out. John thought it might do me good to see a little company, so we just had mother and Nellie and the children down for a week.

Of course I didn't do a thing. Jennie sees to everything now.

But it tired me all the same.

John says if I don't pick up faster he shall send me to Weir Mitchell[3] in the fall.

But I don't want to go there at all. I had a friend who was in his hands once, and she says he is just like John and my brother, only more so!

Besides, it is such an undertaking to go so far.

I don't feel as if it was worth while to turn my hand over for anything, and I'm getting dreadfully fretful and querulous.

I cry at nothing, and cry most of the time.

Of course I don't when John is here, or anybody else, but when I am alone.

And I am alone a good deal just now. John is kept in town very often by serious cases, and Jennie is good and lets me alone when I want her to.

So I walk a little in the garden or down that lovely lane, sit on the porch under the roses, and lie down up here a good deal.

I'm getting really fond of the room in spite of the wallpaper. Perhaps *because* of the wallpaper.

It dwells in my mind so!

I lie here on this great immovable bed—it is nailed down, I believe—and follow that pattern about by the hour. It is as good as gymnastics, I assure you. I start, we'll say, at the bottom, down in the corner over there where it has not been touched, and I determine for the thousandth time that I *will* follow that pointless pattern to some sort of a conclusion.

I know a little of the principle of design, and I know this thing was not arranged on any laws of radiation, or alternation, or repetition, or symmetry, or anything else that I ever heard of.

It is repeated, of course, by the breadths, but not otherwise.

---

3 *Weir Mitchell*: Silas Weir Mitchell (1824–1914), the physician who developed the Rest Cure. He spent much of his career working on nervous conditions and neuroscience.

Looked at in one way each breadth stands alone, the bloated curves and flourishes—a kind of "debased Romanesque" with *delirium tremens*—go waddling up and down in isolated columns of fatuity.

But, on the other hand, they connect diagonally, and the sprawling outlines run off in great slanting waves of optic horror, like a lot of wallowing seaweeds in full chase.

The whole thing goes horizontally, too, at least it seems so, and I exhaust myself in trying to distinguish the order of its going in that direction.

They have used a horizontal breadth for a frieze, and that adds wonderfully to the confusion.

There is one end of the room where it is almost intact, and there, when the cross-lights fade and the low sun shines directly upon it, I can almost fancy radiation after all,—the interminable grotesques seem to form around a common center and rush off in headlong plunges of equal distraction.

It makes me tired to follow it. I will take a nap, I guess.

*

I don't know why I should write this.

I don't want to.

I don't feel able.

And I know John would think it absurd. But I *must* say what I feel and think in some way—it is such a relief!

But the effort is getting to be greater than the relief.

Half the time now I am awfully lazy, and lie down ever so much.

John says I mustn't lose my strength, and has me take cod-liver oil and lots of tonics and things, to say nothing of ale and wine and rare meat.[4]

Dear John! He loves me very dearly, and hates to have me sick. I tried to have a real earnest reasonable talk with him the other day, and tell him how I wish he would let me go and make a visit to Cousin Henry and Julia.

---

4 A rich diet, including red meat, was also part of the Rest Cure.

But he said I wasn't able to go, nor able to stand it after I got there; and I did not make out a very good case for myself, for I was crying before I had finished.

It is getting to be a great effort for me to think straight. Just this nervous weakness, I suppose.

And dear John gathered me up in his arms, and just carried me upstairs and laid me on the bed, and sat by me and read to me till it tired my head.

He said I was his darling and his comfort and all he had, and that I must take care of myself for his sake, and keep well.

He says no one but myself can help me out of it, that I must use my will and self-control and not let any silly fancies run away with me.

There's one comfort, the baby is well and happy, and does not have to occupy this nursery with the horrid wallpaper.

If we had not used it that blessed child would have! What a fortunate escape! Why, I wouldn't have a child of mine, an impressionable little thing, live in such a room for worlds.

I never thought of it before, but it is lucky that John kept me here after all. I can stand it so much easier than a baby, you see.

Of course I never mention it to them any more,—I am too wise,—but I keep watch of it all the same.

There are things in that paper that nobody knows but me, or ever will.

Behind that outside pattern the dim shapes get clearer every day.

It is always the same shape, only very numerous.

And it is like a woman stooping down and creeping about behind that pattern. I don't like it a bit. I wonder—I begin to think—I wish John would take me away from here!

*

It is so hard to talk with John about my case, because he is so wise, and because he loves me so.

But I tried it last night.

It was moonlight. The moon shines in all around, just as the sun does.

I hate to see it sometimes, it creeps so slowly, and always comes in by one window or another.

John was asleep and I hated to waken him, so I kept still and watched the moonlight on that undulating wallpaper till I felt creepy.

The faint figure behind seemed to shake the pattern, just as if she wanted to get out.

I got up softly and went to feel and see if the paper *did* move, and when I came back John was awake.

"What is it, little girl?" he said. "Don't go walking about like that—you'll get cold."

I thought it was a good time to talk, so I told him that I really was not gaining here, and that I wished he would take me away.

"Why darling!" said he, "our lease will be up in three weeks, and I can't see how to leave before.

"The repairs are not done at home, and I cannot possibly leave town just now. Of course if you were in any danger I could and would, but you really are better, dear, whether you can see it or not. I am a doctor, dear, and I know. You are gaining flesh and color, your appetite is better. I feel really much easier about you."

"I don't weigh a bit more," said I, "nor as much; and my appetite may be better in the evening, when you are here, but it is worse in the morning when you are away."

"Bless her little heart!" said he with a big hug; "she shall be as sick as she pleases! But now let's improve the shining hours by going to sleep, and talk about it in the morning!"

"And you won't go away?" I asked gloomily.

"Why, how can I, dear? It is only three weeks more and then we will take a nice little trip of a few days while Jennie is getting the house ready. Really, dear, you are better!"

"Better in body perhaps"—I began, and stopped short, for he sat up straight and looked at me with such a stern, reproachful look that I could not say another word.

"My darling," said he, "I beg of you, for my sake and for our child's sake, as well as for your own, that you will never for one instant let that idea enter your mind! There is nothing so dangerous, so fascinating, to a temperament like yours. It is a false and foolish fancy. Can you not trust me as a physician when I tell you so?"

So of course I said no more on that score, and we went to sleep before long. He thought I was asleep first, but I wasn't,—I lay there for hours trying to decide whether that front pattern and the back pattern really did move together or separately.

On a pattern like this, by daylight, there is a lack of sequence, a defiance of law, that is a constant irritant to a normal mind.

The color is hideous enough, and unreliable enough, and infuriating enough, but the pattern is torturing.

You think you have mastered it, but just as you get well under way in following, it turns a back somersault and there you are. It slaps you in the face, knocks you down, and tramples upon you. It is like a bad dream.

The outside pattern is a florid arabesque, reminding one of a fungus. If you can imagine a toadstool in joints, an interminable string of toadstools, budding and sprouting in endless convolutions,—why, that is something like it.

That is, sometimes!

There is one marked peculiarity about this paper, a thing nobody seems to notice but myself, and that is that it changes as the light changes.

When the sun shoots in through the east window—I always watch for that first long, straight ray—it changes so quickly that I never can quite believe it.

That is why I watch it always.

By moonlight—the moon shines in all night when there is a moon—I wouldn't know it was the same paper.

At night in any kind of light, in twilight, candlelight, lamplight, and worst of all by moonlight, it becomes bars! The outside pattern I mean, and the woman behind it is as plain as can be.

I didn't realize for a long time what the thing was that showed behind,—that dim sub-pattern,—but now I am quite sure it is a woman.

By daylight she is subdued, quiet. I fancy it is the pattern that keeps her so still. It is so puzzling. It keeps me quiet by the hour.

I lie down ever so much now. John says it is good for me, and to sleep all I can.

Indeed, he started the habit by making me lie down for an hour after each meal.

It is a very bad habit, I am convinced, for, you see, I don't sleep.

And that cultivates deceit, for I don't tell them I'm awake,—oh, no!

The fact is, I am getting a little afraid of John.

He seems very queer sometimes, and even Jennie has an inexplicable look.

It strikes me occasionally, just as a scientific hypothesis, that perhaps it is the paper!

I have watched John when he did not know I was looking, and come into the room suddenly on the most innocent excuses, and I've caught him several times *looking at the paper!* And Jennie too. I caught Jennie with her hand on it once.

She didn't know I was in the room, and when I asked her in a quiet, a very quiet voice, with the most restrained manner possible, what she was doing with the paper she turned around as if she had been caught stealing, and looked quite angry—asked me why I should frighten her so!

Then she said that the paper stained everything it touched, that she had found yellow smooches[5] on all my clothes and John's, and she wished we would be more careful!

Did not that sound innocent? But I know she was studying that pattern, and I am determined that nobody shall find it out but myself!

*

Life is very much more exciting now than it used to be. You see I have something more to expect, to look forward to, to watch. I really do eat better, and am more quiet than I was.

John is so pleased to see me improve! He laughed a little the other day, and said I seemed to be flourishing in spite of my wallpaper.

I turned it off with a laugh. I had no intention of telling him it was *because* of the wallpaper—he would make fun of me. He might even want to take me away.

I don't want to leave now until I have found it out. There is a week more, and I think that will be enough.

---

5 *Smooches*: Smudges.

*

I'm feeling ever so much better! I don't sleep much at night, for it is so interesting to watch developments; but I sleep a good deal in the daytime.

In the daytime it is tiresome and perplexing.

There are always new shoots on the fungus, and new shades of yellow all over it. I cannot keep count of them, though I have tried conscientiously.

It is the strangest yellow, that wallpaper! It makes me think of all the yellow things I ever saw—not beautiful ones like buttercups, but old foul, bad yellow things.

But there is something else about that paper—the smell! I noticed it the moment we came into the room, but with so much air and sun it was not bad. Now we have had a week of fog and rain, and whether the windows are open or not, the smell is here.

It creeps all over the house.

I find it hovering in the dining-room, skulking in the parlor, hiding in the hall, lying in wait for me on the stairs.

It gets into my hair.

Even when I go to ride, if I turn my head suddenly and surprise it—there is that smell!

Such a peculiar odor, too! I have spent hours in trying to analyze it, to find what it smelled like.

It is not bad—at first, and very gentle, but quite the subtlest, most enduring odor I ever met.

In this damp weather it is awful. I wake up in the night and find it hanging over me.

It used to disturb me at first. I thought seriously of burning the house—to reach the smell.

But now I am used to it. The only thing I can think of that it is like is the *color* of the paper! A yellow smell.

There is a very funny mark on this wall, low down, near the mopboard.[6] A streak that runs round the room. It goes behind every piece of

---

6 *Mopboard*: Baseboard trim.

furniture, except the bed, a long, straight, even *smooch*, as if it had been rubbed over and over.

I wonder how it was done and who did it, and what they did it for. Round and round and round—round and round and round—it makes me dizzy!

*

I really have discovered something at last.

Through watching so much at night, when it changes so, I have finally found out.

The front pattern *does* move—and no wonder! The woman behind shakes it!

Sometimes I think there are a great many women behind, and sometimes only one, and she crawls around fast, and her crawling shakes it all over.

Then in the very bright spots she keeps still, and in the very shady spots she just takes hold of the bars and shakes them hard.

And she is all the time trying to climb through. But nobody could climb through that pattern—it strangles so; I think that is why it has so many heads.

They get through, and then the pattern strangles them off and turns them upside-down, and makes their eyes white!

If those heads were covered or taken off it would not be half so bad.

*

I think that woman gets out in the daytime!

And I'll tell you why—privately—I've seen her!

I can see her out of every one of my windows!

It is the same woman, I know, for she is always creeping, and most women do not creep by daylight.

I see her on that long shaded lane, creeping up and down. I see her in those dark grape arbors, creeping all around the garden.

I see her on that long road under the trees, creeping along, and when a carriage comes she hides under the blackberry vines.

I don't blame her a bit. It must be very humiliating to be caught creeping by daylight!

I always lock the door when I creep by daylight. I can't do it at night, for I know John would suspect something at once.

And John is so queer now, that I don't want to irritate him. I wish he would take another room! Besides, I don't want anybody to get that woman out at night but myself.

I often wonder if I could see her out of all the windows at once.

But, turn as fast as I can, I can only see out of one at one time.

And though I always see her she *may* be able to creep faster than I can turn!

I have watched her sometimes away off in the open country, creeping as fast as a cloud shadow in a high wind.

*

If only that top pattern could be gotten off from the under one! I mean to try it, little by little.

I have found out another funny thing, but I shan't tell it this time! It does not do to trust people too much.

There are only two more days to get this paper off, and I believe John is beginning to notice. I don't like the look in his eyes.

And I heard him ask Jennie a lot of professional questions about me. She had a very good report to give.

She said I slept a good deal in the daytime.

John knows I don't sleep very well at night, for all I'm so quiet!

He asked me all sorts of questions, too, and pretended to be very loving and kind.

As if I couldn't see through him!

Still, I don't wonder he acts so, sleeping under this paper for three months.

It only interests me, but I feel sure John and Jennie are secretly affected by it.

*

Hurrah! This is the last day, but it is enough. John is to stay in town over night, and won't be out until this evening.

Jennie wanted to sleep with me—the sly thing! but I told her I should undoubtedly rest better for a night all alone.

That was clever, for really I wasn't alone a bit! As soon as it was moonlight, and that poor thing began to crawl and shake the pattern, I got up and ran to help her.

I pulled and she shook, I shook and she pulled, and before morning we had peeled off yards of that paper.

A strip about as high as my head and half around the room.

And then when the sun came and that awful pattern began to laugh at me I declared I would finish it to-day!

We go away to-morrow, and they are moving all my furniture down again to leave things as they were before.

Jennie looked at the wall in amazement, but I told her merrily that I did it out of pure spite at the vicious thing.

She laughed and said she wouldn't mind doing it herself, but I must not get tired.

How she betrayed herself that time!

But I am here, and no person touches this paper but me—not *alive*!

She tried to get me out of the room—it was too patent! But I said it was so quiet and empty and clean now that I believed I would lie down again and sleep all I could; and not to wake me even for dinner—I would call when I woke.

So now she is gone, and the servants are gone, and the things are gone, and there is nothing left but that great bedstead nailed down, with the canvas mattress we found on it.

We shall sleep downstairs to-night, and take the boat home to-morrow.

I quite enjoy the room, now it is bare again.

How those children did tear about here!

This bedstead is fairly gnawed!

But I must get to work.

I have locked the door and thrown the key down into the front path.

I don't want to go out, and I don't want to have anybody come in, till John comes.

I want to astonish him.

I've got a rope up here that even Jennie did not find. If that woman does get out, and tries to get away, I can tie her!

But I forgot I could not reach far without anything to stand on!

This bed will *not* move!

I tried to lift and push it until I was lame, and then I got so angry I bit off a little piece at one corner—but it hurt my teeth.

Then I peeled off all the paper I could reach standing on the floor. It sticks horribly and the pattern just enjoys it! All those strangled heads and bulbous eyes and waddling fungus growths just shriek with derision!

I am getting angry enough to do something desperate. To jump out of the window would be admirable exercise, but the bars are too strong even to try.

Besides I wouldn't do it. Of course not. I know well enough that a step like that is improper and might be misconstrued.

I don't like to *look* out of the windows even—there are so many of those creeping women, and they creep so fast.

I wonder if they all come out of that wallpaper as I did?

But I am securely fastened now by my well-hidden rope—you don't get *me* out in the road there!

I suppose I shall have to get back behind the pattern when it comes night, and that is hard!

It is so pleasant to be out in this great room and creep around as I please!

I don't want to go outside. I won't, even if Jennie asks me to.

For outside you have to creep on the ground, and everything is green instead of yellow.

But here I can creep smoothly on the floor, and my shoulder just fits in that long smooch around the wall, so I cannot lose my way.

Why, there's John at the door!

It is no use, young man, you can't open it!

How he does call and pound!

Now he's crying for an axe.

It would be a shame to break down that beautiful door!

"John dear!" said I in the gentlest voice, "the key is down by the front steps, under a plantain leaf!"

That silenced him for a few moments.

Then he said—very quietly indeed, "Open the door, my darling!"

"I can't," said I. "The key is down by the front door under a plantain leaf!"

And then I said it again, several times, very gently and slowly, and said it so often that he had to go and see, and he got it, of course, and came in. He stopped short by the door.

"What is the matter?" he cried. "For God's sake, what are you doing!"

I kept on creeping just the same, but I looked at him over my shoulder.

"I've got out at last," said I, "in spite of you and Jane! And I've pulled off most of the paper, so you can't put me back!"

Now why should that man have fainted? But he did, and right across my path by the wall, so that I had to creep over him every time!

Books and Men*

WILLIAM OSLER
(Canadian, 1849–1919)

One of the founding faculty members of Johns Hopkins Hospital and the creator of the first formal residency program for medical students, physician William Osler is also often referred to as "the father of modern medicine." In addition to revolutionizing medical education, he was a renowned physician and wrote prolifically; his *Principles and Practice of Medicine* (1892) quickly became the standard textbook for clinical medicine. The work included here is a lecture originally given at the Boston Medical Library in 1901. As you read, consider his advocacy for the importance not just of scientific and practical training for practitioners but also of deep reading (that is, of the need for and value of books and libraries for physicians).

---

* Reprinted from William Osler, *Aequanimitas, with other Addresses to Medical Students, Nurses, and Practitioners of Medicine* (Philadelphia: P. Blakiston's Son, 1905), 219–225, Google Books.

Books and Men

Those of us from other cities who bring congratulations this evening can hardly escape the tinglings of envy when we see this noble treasure house; but in my own case the bitter waters of jealousy which rise in my soul are at once diverted by two strong sensations. In the first place I have a feeling of lively gratitude towards this library. In 1876 as a youngster interested in certain clinical subjects to which I could find no reference in our library at McGill, I came to Boston, and I here found what I wanted, and I found moreover a cordial welcome and many friends. It was a small matter I had in hand but I wished to make it as complete as possible, and I have always felt that this library helped me to a good start. It has been such a pleasure in recurring visits to the library to find Dr. Brigham in charge, with the same kindly interest in visitors that he showed a quarter of a century ago. But the feeling which absorbs all others is one of deep satisfaction that our friend, Dr. Chadwick, has at last seen fulfilled the desire of his eyes. To few is given the tenacity of will which enables a man to pursue a cherished purpose through a quarter of a century—"*Ohne Hast, aber ohne Rast*"[1] ('tis his favorite quotation); to fewer still is the fruition granted. Too often the reaper is not the sower. Too often the fate of those who labor at some object for the public good is to see their work pass into other hands, and to have others get the credit for enterprises which they have initiated and made possible. It has not been so with our friend, and it intensifies a thousandfold the pleasure of this occasion to feel the fitness, in every way, of the felicitations which have been offered to him.

It is hard for me to speak of the value of libraries in terms which would not seem exaggerated. Books have been my delight these thirty years, and from them I have received incalculable benefits. To study the phenomena of disease without books is to sail an uncharted sea, while to study books without patients is not to go to sea at all. Only a maker of books can appreciate the labors of others at their true value. Those of us who have brought forth fat volumes should offer hecatombs at these

---

1   *Ohne Hast, aber ohne Rast*: Without haste, but without rest.

shrines of Minerva Medica.² What exsuccous, attenuated offspring they would have been but for the pabulum furnished through the placental circulation of a library.³ How often can it be said of us with truth, "*Das beste was er ist verdankt er Andern!*"⁴

For the teacher and the worker a great library such as this is indispensable. They must know the world's best work and know it at once. They mint and make current coin the ore so widely scattered in journals, transactions and monographs. The splendid collections which now exist in five or six of our cities and the unique opportunities of the Surgeon-General's Library have done much to give to American medicine a thoroughly eclectic character.

But when one considers the unending making of books, who does not sigh for the happy days of that thrice happy Sir William Browne⁵ whose pocket library sufficed for his life's needs; drawing from a Greek testament his divinity, from the aphorisms of Hippocrates his medicine, and from an Elzevir Horace⁶ his good sense and vivacity. There should be in connection with every library a corps of instructors in the art of reading, who would, as a labor of love, teach the young idea how to read. An old writer says that there are four sorts of readers: "Sponges which attract all without distinguishing; Howre-glasses which receive and powre out as fast; Bagges which only retain the dregges of the spices and let the wine escape, and Sives which retaine the best onely."⁷ A man wastes

---

2 I.e., authors should offer honor and sacrifice to libraries, which are like temples of Minerva, the Roman goddess of medicine (and wisdom, justice, music, arts and crafts, and defense).

3 I.e., how dry and useless these works would be if their authors hadn't been nourished by libraries.

4 *Das beste was er ist verdankt er Andern*: Whatever is best in oneself is due to others.

5 [Osler's note, regarding English physician William Browne (1692–1774): "In one of the Annual Orations at the Royal College of Physicians he said: 'Behold an instance of human ambition! not to be satisfied but by the conquest, as it were, of three worlds, lucre in the country, honour in the college, pleasure in the medicinal springs.'"]

6 *Elzevir Horace*: The Elzevir printing family in Paris published a well-regarded edition of the ancient Roman poet Horace's works in 1676.

7 The "old writer" here is the English poet and clergy member John Donne (see pp. 109–124); this quote is from the preface of *Biathanatos*, Donne's defense of "self-homicide" (or suicide) on logical and theological grounds. For his part, Donne

a great many years before he reaches the "sieve" stage: For the general practitioner a well-used library is one of the few correctives of the premature senility which is so apt to overtake him. Self-centered, self-taught, he leads a solitary life, and unless his every-day experience is controlled by careful reading or by the attrition of a medical society it soon ceases to be of the slightest value and becomes a mere accretion of isolated facts, without correlation. It is astonishing with how little reading a doctor can practice medicine, but it is not astonishing how badly he may do it. Not three months ago a physician living within an hour's ride of the Surgeon-General's Library brought to me his little girl, aged twelve. The diagnosis of infantile myxedema[8] required only a half glance. In placid contentment he had been practicing twenty years in "Sleepy Hollow" and not even when his own flesh and blood was touched did he rouse from an apathy deep as Rip Van Winkle's sleep. In reply to questions: No, he had never seen anything in the journals about the thyroid gland; he had seen no pictures of cretinism[9] or myxedema; in fact his mind was a blank on the whole subject. He had not been a reader, he said, but he was a practical man with very little time. I could not help thinking of John Bunyan's remarks on the elements of success in the practice of medicine. "Physicians," he says, "get neither name nor fame by the pricking of wheals or the picking out thistles, or by laying of plaisters to the scratch of a pin; every old woman can do this. But if they would have a name and a fame, if they will have it quickly, they must do some great and desperate cures. Let them fetch one to life that was dead, let them recover one to his wits that was mad, let them make one that was born blind to see, or let them give ripe wits to a fool—these are notable cures, and he that can do thus, if he dost thus first, he shall have the name and fame he deserves; he may lie abed till noon."[10] Had my doctor friend been a reader

---

attributes the idea itself to the Jewish historian Josephus Flavius (also known as Joseph ben Gorion and Gorionides).

8   *Myxedema*: Advanced hypothyroidism.
9   *Cretinism*: A condition caused by a congenital thyroid deficiency.
10 English Puritan John Bunyan (1628–1688) was both a preacher and an author, most famous for the 1678 Christian allegorical work *The Pilgrim's Progress* (sometimes referred to as the first English-language novel). This quotation comes from *The Jerusalem Sinner Saved*, a work on forgiveness first published the year Bunyan died.

he might have done a great and notable cure and even have given ripe wits to a fool! It is in utilizing the fresh knowledge of the journals that the young physician may attain quickly to the name and fame he desires.

There is a third class of men in the profession to whom books are dearer than to teachers or practitioners—a small, a silent band, but in reality the leaven[11] of the whole lump. The profane call them bibliomaniacs, and in truth they are at times irresponsible and do not always know the difference between *meum* and *tuum*.[12] In the presence of Dr. Billings or of Dr. Chadwick I dare not further characterize them. Loving books partly for their contents, partly for the sake of the authors, they not alone keep alive the sentiment of historical continuity in the profession, but they are the men who make possible such gatherings as the one we are enjoying this evening. We need more men of their class, particularly in this country, where every one carries in his pocket the tape-measure of utility. Along two lines their work is valuable. By the historical method alone can many problems in medicine be approached profitably. For example, the student who dates his knowledge of tuberculosis from Koch[13] may have a very correct, but he has a very incomplete, appreciation of the subject. Within a quarter of a century our libraries will have certain alcoves devoted to the historical consideration of the great diseases, which will give to the student that mental perspective which is so valuable an equipment in life. The past is a good nurse, as Lowell remarks,[14] particularly for the weanlings of the fold.

'Tis man's worst deed
To let the things that have been, run to waste
And in the unmeaning Present sink the Past.[15]

---

11 *Leaven*: The leavening agent (like yeast) that causes transformation or change.
12 *Meum and tuum*: Latin for "mine" and "yours."
13 German physician and microbiologist Robert Koch (1843–1910) discovered the bacterial origin of tuberculosis in 1882, which radically changed approaches to treatment for the better.
14 From American poet James Russell Lowell's anti-slavery satirical work *The Biglow Papers*, No. V: "The Debate in the Sennit, Sot to a Nusry Rhyme," written in what Lowell called "Yankee dialect."
15 From English author Charles Lamb's (1775–1834) sonnet IX, "To John Lamb, Esq., of the South-Sea-House," lines 9–11.

But in a more excellent way these *laudatores temporis acti*[16] render a royal service. For each one of us to-day, as in Plato's time, there is a higher as well as a lower education. The very marrow and fitness of books may not suffice to save a man from becoming a poor, mean-spirited devil, without a spark of fine professional feeling, and without a thought above the sordid issues of the day. The men I speak of keep alive in us an interest in the great men of the past and not alone in their works, which they cherish, but in their lives, which they emulate. They would remind us continually that in the records of no other profession is there to be found so large a number of men who have combined intellectual pre-eminence with nobility of character. This higher education so much needed to-day is not given in the school, is not to be bought in the market place, but it has to be wrought out in each one of us for himself; it is the silent influence of character on character and in no way more potently than in the contemplation of the lives of the great and good of the past, in no way more than in "the touch divine of noble natures gone."[17]

I should like to see in each library a select company of the Immortals set apart for special adoration. Each country might have its representatives in a sort of alcove of Fame, in which the great medical classics were gathered Not necessarily books, more often the epoch-making contributions to be found in ephemeral journals. It is too early, perhaps, to make a selection of American medical classics, but it might be worth while to gather suffrages in regard to the contributions which ought to be placed upon our Roll of Honor. A few years ago I made out a list of those I thought the most worthy which I carried down to 1850, and it has a certain interest for us this evening. The native modesty of the Boston physician is well known, but in certain circles there has been associated with it a curious psychical phenomenon, a conviction of the utter worthlessness of the *status præsens*[18] in New England, as compared with conditions existing elsewhere. There is a variety to-day of the Back

---

16 *Laudatores temporis acti*: People who praise the past (the phrase comes from the Horace's *Ars poetica*).
17 From James Russell Lowell's poem "Memorie Positum," lines 19–20.
18 *Status praesens*: Present state of affairs.

Bay Brahmin[19] who delights in cherishing the belief that medically things are everywhere better than in Boston, and who is always ready to predict "an Asiatic removal of candlesticks," to borrow a phrase from Cotton Mather.[20] Strange indeed would it have been had not such a plastic profession as ours felt the influences which molded New England into the intellectual center of the New World. In reality, nowhere in the country has the profession been adorned more plentifully with men of culture and of character—not voluminous writers or exploiters of the products of other men's brains—and they manage to get a full share on the Roll of Fame which I have suggested. To 1850, I have counted some twenty contributions of the first rank, contributions which for one reason or another deserve to be called American medical classics. New England takes ten. But in medicine the men she has given to the other parts of the country have been better than books. Men like Nathan R. Smith, Austin Flint, Willard Parker, Alonzo Clark, Elisha Bartlett, John C. Dalton,[21] and others carried away from their New England homes a love of truth, a love of learning and above all a proper estimate of the personal character of the physician.

Dr. Johnson shrewdly remarked that ambition was usually proportionate to capacity,[22] which is as true of a profession as it is of a man. What we have seen to-night reflects credit not less on your ambition than on your capacity. A library after all is a great catalyser, accelerating the nutrition and rate of progress in a profession, and I am sure you will find yourselves the better for the sacrifice you have made in securing this home for your books, this workshop for your members.

---

19 *Back Bay Brahmin*: Also known as the "Boston Brahmins," members of Boston's influential upper class.
20 I.e., ready to predict the isolation and abandonment of New England. Puritan minister Cotton Mather (who influenced the adoption of smallpox inoculation methods in America; see pp. 167–171) uses this phrase—an apparent reference to the biblical book of Revelation—in *The Wonders of the Invisible World* (1693), in which he defends his part in the Salem Witch Trials and argues that witchcraft is an evil tool of Satan.
21 Notable physicians and medical practitioners of nineteenth-century America.
22 English literary figure Samuel Johnson (1709–1784), known especially for his essays, biographies, and dictionary, includes this idea in his biography of the Dutch botanist, chemist, and physician Herman Boerhaave (1668–1738), published in 1739.

On Psychosexual Development*

SIGMUND FREUD
(Austrian, 1856–1939)

There may be no more famous name associated with psychology than that of the Austrian founder of psychoanalysis Sigmund Freud. Psychoanalysis holds that human development and behavior are significantly impacted by unconscious drives and material. Freud's work in psychology began with the nervous disorders, including neurasthenia (see George Miller Beard, pp. 258–261) and so-called hysteria, that had become such prevalent diagnoses during the nineteenth century. With his Viennese colleague Josef Breuer, he developed a theory of the unconscious mind that would inform much of his psychoanalytic work. Among his contributions (many of which, while important, are now contested) is a detailed theory of psychosexual development beginning in infancy. In these excerpts, first published in 1899 and 1905, consider Freud's treatment of the now-famous Oedipus complex and the concept of penis envy.

---

* Reprinted from Sigmund Freud, *The Interpretation of Dreams*, 3rd ed., trans. A. A. Brill (New York: Macmillan, 1913; Bartleby.com, 2010), 182–7; Reprinted from Sigmund Freud, *Three Contributions to the Theory of Sex*, 2nd ed., trans. A. A. Brill (New York: Nervous and Mental Disease Publishing, 1920; Project Gutenberg, 2005), 56.

The Interpretation of Dreams

The Material and Sources of Dreams

According to my experience, which is now large, parents play a leading part in the infantile psychology of all later neurotics, and falling in love with one member of the parental couple and hatred of the other help to make up that fateful sum of material furnished by the psychic impulses, which has been formed during the infantile period, and which is of such great importance for the symptoms appearing in the later neurosis. But I do not think that psychoneurotics are here sharply distinguished from normal human beings, in that they are capable of creating something absolutely new and peculiar to themselves. It is far more probable, as is shown also by occasional observation upon normal children, that in their loving or hostile wishes towards their parents psychoneurotics only show in exaggerated form feelings which are present less distinctly and less intensely in the minds of most children. Antiquity has furnished us with legendary material to confirm this fact, and the deep and universal effectiveness of these legends can only be explained by granting a similar universal applicability to the above-mentioned assumption in infantile psychology.

I refer to the legend of King Oedipus and the drama of the same name by Sophocles. Oedipus, the son of Laius, king of Thebes, and of Jocasta, is exposed while a suckling, because an oracle has informed the father that his son, who is still unborn, will be his murderer. He is rescued, and grows up as the king's son at a foreign court, until, being uncertain about his origin, he also consults the oracle, and is advised to avoid his native place, for he is destined to become the murderer of his father and the husband of his mother. On the road leading away from his supposed home he meets King Laius and strikes him dead in a sudden quarrel. Then he comes to the gates of Thebes, where he solves the riddle of the Sphinx who is barring the way, and he is elected king by the Thebans in gratitude, and is presented with the hand of Jocasta. He reigns in peace and honor for a long time, and begets two sons and two daughters upon his unknown mother, until at last a plague breaks out which causes the Thebans to consult the oracle anew. Here Sophocles' tragedy begins. The messengers bring the advice that the plague will stop as soon as the murderer of Laius is driven from the country. But where is he hidden? "Where are they to be found? How shall we trace the perpetrators of so old a crime where no conjecture leads to discovery?" (Act I Sc. 2)

The action of the play now consists merely in a revelation, which is gradually completed and artfully delayed—resembling the work of a psychoanalysis—of the fact that Oedipus himself is the murderer of Laius, and the son of the dead man and of Jocasta. Oedipus, profoundly shocked at the monstrosities which he has unknowingly committed, blinds himself and leaves his native place. The oracle has been fulfilled.

The *Oedipus Tyrannus* is a so-called tragedy of fate; its tragic effect is said to be found in the opposition between the powerful will of the gods and the vain resistance of the human beings who are threatened with destruction; resignation to the will of God and confession of one's own helplessness is the lesson which the deeply-moved spectator is to learn from the tragedy. Consequently modern authors have tried to obtain a similar tragic effect by embodying the same opposition in a story of their own invention. But spectators have sat unmoved while a curse or an oracular sentence has been fulfilled on blameless human beings in spite of all their struggles; later tragedies of fate have all remained without effect.

If the *Oedipus Tyrannus* is capable of moving modern men no less than it moved the contemporary Greeks, the explanation of this fact cannot lie merely in the assumption that the effect of the Greek tragedy is based upon the opposition between fate and human will, but is to be sought in the peculiar nature of the material by which the opposition is shown. There must be a voice within us which is prepared to recognize the compelling power of fate in *Oedipus*, while we justly condemn the situations occurring in *Die Ahnfrau*[1] or in other tragedies of later date as arbitrary inventions. And there must be a factor corresponding to this inner voice in the story of King Oedipus. His fate moves us only for

---

1 *Die Ahnfrau*: A five-act tragedy by Austrian dramatist Franz Grillparzer (1791–1872), which, like *Oedipus*, investigates the relationship between fate and the consequence of one's own actions.

the reason that it might have been ours, for the oracle has put the same curse upon us before our birth as upon him. Perhaps we are all destined to direct our first sexual impulses towards our mothers, and our first hatred and violent wishes towards our fathers; our dreams convince us of it. King Oedipus, who has struck his father Laius dead and has married his mother Jocasta, is nothing but the realized wish of our childhood. But more fortunate than he, we have since succeeded, unless we have become psychoneurotics, in withdrawing our sexual impulses from our mothers and in forgetting our jealousy of our fathers. We recoil from the person for whom this primitive wish has been fulfilled with all the force of the repression which these wishes have suffered within us. By his analysis, showing us the guilt of Oedipus, the poet urges us to recognize our own inner self, in which these impulses, even if suppressed, are still present. The comparison with which the chorus leaves us—

"…Behold! this Oedipus, who unravelled the famous riddle and who was a man of eminent virtue; a man who trusted neither to popularity nor to the fortune of his citizens; see how great a storm of adversity hath at last overtaken him" (Act v. sc. 4).

This warning applies to ourselves and to our pride, to us, who have grown so wise and so powerful in our own estimation since the years of our childhood. Like Oedipus, we live in ignorance of the wishes that offend morality, wishes which nature has forced upon us, and after the revelation of which we want to avert every glance from the scenes of our childhood.

Three Contributions to the Theory of Sex

The Infantile Sexual Investigation

The Riddle of the Sphinx.—It is not theoretical but practical interests which start the work of the investigation activity in the child. The threat to the conditions of his existence through the actual or expected arrival of a new child, the fear of the loss in care and love which is connected with this event, cause the child to become thoughtful and sagacious. Corresponding with the history of this awakening, the first problem with which it occupies itself is not the question as to the difference between the sexes, but the riddle: from where do children come? In a distorted form, which can easily be unraveled, this is the same riddle which was given by the Theban Sphinx. The fact of the two sexes is usually first accepted by the child without struggle and hesitation. It is quite natural for the male child to presuppose in all persons it knows a genital like his own, and to find it impossible to harmonize the lack of it with his conception of others.

The Castration Complex.—This conviction is energetically adhered to by the boy and tenaciously defended against the contradictions which soon result, and are only given up after severe internal struggles (castration complex). The substitutive formations of this lost penis of the woman play a great part in the formation of many perversions.

The assumption of the same (male) genital in all persons is the first of the remarkable and consequential infantile sexual theories. It is of little help to the child when biological science agrees with his preconceptions and recognizes the feminine clitoris as the real substitute for the penis. The little girl does not react with similar refusals when she sees the differently formed genital of the boy. She is immediately prepared to recognize it, and soon becomes envious of the penis; this envy reaches its highest point in the consequentially important wish that she also should be a boy.

Selected Works*

OHIYESA/CHARLES ALEXANDER EASTMAN
(Santee Sioux, 1858–1939)

Ohiyesa ("The Winner" in Dakota, the language of the Sioux tribe) was raised by his grandmother, a respected midwife. His mother died shortly after giving birth to him, and his father was thought to have been killed in an uprising against white colonizers. Years later, Ohiyesa learned that his father was alive and had been imprisoned and converted to Christianity. Under the Christian name of Jacob Eastman, Ohiyesa's father returned home. Ohiyesa, taking the name Charles Alexander Eastman, was sent to a mission school, one of hundreds of government-run boarding schools tasked with converting Native children to Christianity and enforcing Euro-American culture. Later, Ohiyesa graduated from Dartmouth College in 1887 and, in 1890, was one of the first Native Americans to graduate medical school.[1] As a government physician for the Pine Ridge Agency on the Pine Ridge Reservation, Ohiyesa cared for members of the Oglala Sioux tribe. While there, he tended the wounded at the Wounded Knee Massacre in 1890. Later, he served with the Bureau of Indian Affairs, helped found the first Native American rights organization, and cofounded the Boy Scouts of America. He wrote a great deal about Indigenous culture, including several autobiographical works. The works excerpted here were published in 1911 and 1902. As you read, consider Ohiyesa's depiction of his culture's medicine and beliefs and of his own early life.

1 Ohiyesa's predecessors included Waowawanaonk, later Peter Wilson (Cayuga), an 1844 graduate of Geneva Medical College in New York; Susan La Flesche Picotte (Omaha), an 1889 graduate of Woman's Medical College of Pennsylvania; Wassaja, later Carlos Montezuma (Yavapai), an 1889 graduate of Chicago Medical College.

The Soul of the Indian: An Interpretation[2]

Ceremonial and Symbolic Worship

Perhaps the most remarkable organization ever known among American Indians, that of the "Grand Medicine Lodge," was apparently an indirect result of the labors of the early Jesuit missionaries. In it Caucasian ideas are easily recognizable, and it seems reasonable to suppose that its founders desired to establish an order that would successfully resist the encroachments of the "Black Robes." However that may be, it is an unquestionable fact that the only religious leaders of any note who have arisen among the native tribes since the advent of the white man, the "Shawnee Prophet" in 1762,[3] and the half-breed prophet of the "Ghost Dance" in 1890,[4] both founded their claims or prophecies upon the Gospel story. Thus in each case an Indian religious revival or craze, though more or less threatening to the invader, was of distinctively alien origin.

---

2   The term *Indian* was "commonly used to describe the hundreds of distinct nations of Indigenous Peoples through North, Central, and South America and the Caribbean" (56). Today, the use of this term as a marker of identity is discouraged unless embraced by a particular Nation, Tribe, or individual. Gregory Younging, *Elements of Indigenous Style* (Edmonton, AB: Brush Education, 2018), 56–57.

3   *Shawnee prophet*: Tenskatwawa (1775–1836), a younger brother of Tecumseh, chief of the Shawnee in the central United States. Tenskatwawa became known as a prophet after falling into a trance in which the Master of Life visited him and told him that Native Americans must reject all of the customs of the white colonizers in the country. The date 1762 appears to be a mistake, as Tenskatwawa was not yet born. However, in 1762, another spiritual prophet of the Lenni Lanape people named Neolin, referred to as the "Delaware Prophet," was active in the same area and had similar visions in which he met with the Master of Life.

4   Wovoka (ca. 1856–1932), also known as Jack Wilson, was a spiritual leader of the Paiute people and founded the Ghost Dance, a new religious movement aimed at stopping the westward expansion of white colonizers and promoting peace among Native American communities.

---

*   Reprinted from Ohiyesa [Charles A. Eastman], *The Soul of the Indian: An Interpretation* (London: Constable & Co., 1911; Project Gutenberg, 2016), chap. 3; Reprinted from Ohiyesa, *Indian Boyhood* (New York: McClure, Phillips, & Co., 1902; Project Gutenberg, 2016), part 1 (Earliest Recollections), chaps. 1, 3.

The Medicine Lodge originated among the Algonquin tribe, and extended gradually throughout its branches, finally affecting the Sioux of the Mississippi Valley, and forming a strong bulwark against the work of the pioneer missionaries, who secured, indeed, scarcely any converts until after the outbreak of 1862, when subjection, starvation, and imprisonment turned our broken-hearted people to accept Christianity, which seemed to offer them the only gleam of kindness or hope.

The order was a secret one, and in some respects not unlike the Free Masons, being a union or affiliation of a number of lodges, each with its distinctive songs and medicines. Leadership was in order of seniority in degrees, which could only be obtained by merit, and women were admitted to membership upon equal terms, with the possibility of attaining to the highest honors. No person might become a member unless his moral standing was excellent, all candidates remained on probation for one or two years, and murderers and adulterers were expelled. The commandments promulgated by this order were essentially the same as the Mosaic Ten,[5] so that it exerted a distinct moral influence, in addition to its ostensible object, which was instruction in the secrets of legitimate medicine.

In this society the uses of all curative roots and herbs known to us were taught exhaustively and practiced mainly by the old, the younger members being in training to fill the places of those who passed away. My grandmother was a well-known and successful practitioner, and both my mother and father were members, but did not practice.

A medicine or "mystery feast" was not a public affair, as members only were eligible, and upon these occasions all the "medicine bags" and totems of the various lodges were displayed and their peculiar "medicine songs" were sung. The food was only partaken of by invited guests, and not by the hosts, or lodge making the feast. The "Grand Medicine Dance" was given on the occasion of initiating those candidates who had finished their probation, a sufficient number of whom were designated to take the places of those who had died since the last meeting. Invitations were sent out in the form of small bundles of tobacco. Two

---

5 *Mosaic Ten*: The Ten Commandments of Moses, described in the books of Exodus and Deuteronomy in the Hebrew Torah and Christian Old Testament.

very large teepees were pitched facing one another, a hundred feet apart, half open, and connected by a roofless hall or colonnade of fresh-cut boughs. One of these lodges was for the society giving the dance and the novices, the other was occupied by the "soldiers," whose duty it was to distribute the refreshments, and to keep order among the spectators. They were selected from among the best and bravest warriors of the tribe.

The preparations being complete, and the members of each lodge garbed and painted according to their rituals, they entered the hall separately, in single file, led by their oldest man or "Great Chief." Standing before the "Soldiers' Lodge," facing the setting sun, their chief addressed the "Great Mystery" directly in a few words, after which all extending the right arm horizontally from the shoulder with open palm, sang a short invocation in unison, ending with a deep: "E-ho-ho-ho!" This performance, which was really impressive, was repeated in front of the headquarters lodge, facing the rising sun, after which each lodge took its assigned place, and the songs and dances followed in regular order.

The closing ceremony, which was intensely dramatic in its character, was the initiation of the novices, who had received their final preparation on the night before. They were now led out in front of the headquarters lodge and placed in a kneeling position upon a carpet of rich robes and furs, the men upon the right hand, stripped and painted black, with a round spot of red just over the heart, while the women, dressed in their best, were arranged upon the left. Both sexes wore the hair loose, as if in mourning or expectation of death. An equal number of grand medicine-men, each of whom was especially appointed to one of the novices, faced them at a distance of half the length of the hall, or perhaps fifty feet.

After silent prayer, each medicine-man in turn addressed himself to his charge, exhorting him to observe all the rules of the order under the eye of the Mysterious One, and instructing him in his duty toward his fellow-man and toward the Ruler of Life. All then assumed an attitude of superb power and dignity, crouching slightly as if about to spring forward in a foot-race, and grasping their medicine bags firmly in both hands. Swinging their arms forward at the same moment, they uttered their guttural "Yo-ho-ho-ho!" in perfect unison and with startling effect.

In the midst of a breathless silence, they took a step forward, then another and another, ending a rod or so from the row of kneeling victims, with a mighty swing of the sacred bags that would seem to project all their mystic power into the bodies of the initiates. Instantly they all fell forward, apparently lifeless.

With this thrilling climax, the drums were vigorously pounded and the dance began again with energy. After a few turns had been taken about the prostrate bodies of the new members, covering them with fine robes and other garments which were later to be distributed as gifts, they were permitted to come to life and to join in the final dance. The whole performance was clearly symbolic of death and resurrection.

While I cannot suppose that this elaborate ritual, with its use of public and audible prayer, of public exhortation or sermon, and other Caucasian features, was practiced before comparatively modern times, there is no doubt that it was conscientiously believed in by its members, and for a time regarded with reverence by the people. But at a later period it became still further demoralized and fell under suspicion of witchcraft.

There is no doubt that the Indian held medicine close to spiritual things, but in this also he has been much misunderstood; in fact everything that he held sacred is indiscriminately called "medicine," in the sense of mystery or magic. As a doctor he was originally very adroit and often successful. He employed only healing bark, roots, and leaves with whose properties he was familiar, using them in the form of a distillation or tea and always singly. The stomach or internal bath was a valuable discovery of his, and the vapor or Turkish bath was in general use. He could set a broken bone with fair success, but never practiced surgery in any form. In addition to all this, the medicine-man possessed much personal magnetism and authority, and in his treatment often sought to reestablish the equilibrium of the patient through mental or spiritual influences—a sort of primitive psychotherapy.

The Sioux word for the healing art is "wah-pee-yah," which literally means readjusting or making anew. "Pay-jee-hoo-tah," literally root, means medicine, and "wakan" signifies spirit or mystery. Thus the three ideas, while sometimes associated, were carefully distinguished.

It is important to remember that in the old days the "medicine-man" received no payment for his services, which were of the nature of an honorable function or office. When the idea of payment and barter was introduced among us, and valuable presents or fees began to be demanded for treating the sick, the ensuing greed and rivalry led to many demoralizing practices, and in time to the rise of the modern "conjurer," who is generally a fraud and trickster of the grossest kind. It is fortunate that his day is practically over.

Ever seeking to establish spiritual comradeship with the animal creation, the Indian adopted this or that animal as his "totem," the emblematic device of his society, family, or clan. It is probable that the creature chosen was the traditional ancestress, as we are told that the First Man had many wives among the animal people. The sacred beast, bird, or reptile, represented by its stuffed skin, or by a rude painting, was treated with reverence and carried into battle to insure the guardianship of the spirits. The symbolic attribute of beaver, bear, or tortoise, such as wisdom, cunning, courage, and the like, was supposed to be mysteriously conferred upon the wearer of the badge. The totem or charm used in medicine was ordinarily that of the medicine lodge to which the practitioner belonged, though there were some great men who boasted a special revelation.

There are two ceremonial usages which, so far as I have been able to ascertain, were universal among American Indians, and apparently fundamental. These have already been referred to as the "eneepee," or vapor-bath, and the "chan-du-hu-pah-yu-za-pee," or ceremonial of the pipe. In our Siouan legends and traditions these two are preeminent, as handed down from the most ancient time and persisting to the last.

In our Creation myth or story of the First Man, the vapor-bath was the magic used by The-one-who-was-First-Created, to give life to the dead bones of his younger brother, who had been slain by the monsters of the deep. Upon the shore of the Great Water he dug two round holes, over one of which he built a low enclosure of fragrant cedar boughs, and here he gathered together the bones of his brother. In the other pit he made a fire and heated four round stones, which he rolled one by one into the lodge of boughs. Having closed every aperture save one, he sang a mystic chant while he thrust in his arm and sprinkled water upon the stones with a bunch of sage. Immediately steam arose, and as the legend says, "there was an appearance of life." A second time he sprinkled water, and the dry bones rattled together. The third time he seemed to hear soft singing from within the lodge; and the fourth time a voice exclaimed: "Brother, let me out!" (It should be noted that the number four is the magic or sacred number of the Indian.)

This story gives the traditional origin of the "eneepee," which has ever since been deemed essential to the Indian's effort to purify and recreate his spirit. It is used both by the doctor and by his patient. Every man must enter the cleansing bath and take the cold plunge which follows, when preparing for any spiritual crisis, for possible death, or imminent danger.

Not only the "eneepee" itself, but everything used in connection with the mysterious event, the aromatic cedar and sage, the water, and especially the water-worn boulders, are regarded as sacred, or at the least adapted to a spiritual use. For the rock we have a special reverent name—"Tunkan," a contraction of the Sioux word for Grandfather.

The natural boulder enters into many of our solemn ceremonials, such as the "Rain Dance," and the "Feast of Virgins." The lone hunter and warrior reverently holds up his filled pipe to "Tunkan," in solitary commemoration of a miracle which to him is as authentic and holy as the raising of Lazarus to the devout Christian.

There is a legend that the First Man fell sick, and was taught by his Elder Brother the ceremonial use of the pipe, in a prayer to the spirits for ease and relief. This simple ceremony is the commonest daily expression of thanks or "grace," as well as an oath of loyalty and good faith when the warrior goes forth upon some perilous enterprise, and it enters even into his "hambeday," or solitary prayer, ascending as a rising vapor or incense to the Father of Spirits.

In all the war ceremonies and in medicine a special pipe is used, but at home or on the hunt the warrior employs his own. The pulverized weed is mixed with aromatic bark of the red willow, and pressed lightly into the bowl of the long stone pipe. The worshiper lights it gravely and takes a whiff or two; then, standing erect, he holds it silently toward the Sun, our father, and toward the earth, our mother. There are modern variations, as holding the pipe to the Four Winds, the Fire, Water, Rock, and other elements or objects of reverence.

Indian Boyhood

Hadakah, "The Pitiful Last"

…Of course I myself do not remember when I first saw the day, but my brothers have often recalled the event with much mirth; for it was a custom of the Sioux that when a boy was born his brother must plunge into the water, or roll in the snow naked if it was winter time; and if he was not big enough to do either of these himself, water was thrown on him. If the new-born had a sister, she must be immersed. The idea was that a warrior had come to camp, and the other children must display some act of hardihood.

I was so unfortunate as to be the youngest of five children who, soon after I was born, were left motherless. I had to bear the humiliating name "Hakadah," meaning "the pitiful last," until I should earn a more dignified and appropriate name. I was regarded as little more than a plaything by the rest of the children.

My mother, who was known as the handsomest woman of all the Spirit Lake and Leaf Dweller Sioux, was dangerously ill, and one of the medicine men who attended her said: "Another medicine man has come into existence, but the mother must die. Therefore let him bear the name 'Mysterious Medicine.'" But one of the bystanders hastily interfered, saying that an uncle of the child already bore that name, so, for the time, I was only "Hakadah."

My beautiful mother, sometimes called the "Demi-Goddess" of the Sioux, who tradition says had every feature of a Caucasian descent with the exception of her luxuriant black hair and deep black eyes, held me tightly to her bosom upon her death-bed, while she whispered a few words to her mother-in-law. She said: "I give you this boy for your own. I cannot trust my own mother with him; she will neglect him and he will surely die."

The woman to whom these words were spoken was below the average in stature, remarkably active for her age (she was then fully sixty), and possessed of as much goodness as intelligence. My mother's judgment concerning her own mother was well founded, for soon after her death that old lady appeared, and declared that Hakadah was too young to live without a mother. She offered to keep me until I died, and then she would put me in my mother's grave. Of course my other grandmother denounced the suggestion as a very wicked one, and refused to give me up.

My Indian Grandmother

As a motherless child, I always regarded my good grandmother as the wisest of guides and the best of protectors. It was not long before I began to realize her superiority to most of her contemporaries. This idea was not gained entirely from my own observation, but also from a knowledge of the high regard in which she was held by other women. Aside from her native talent and ingenuity, she was endowed with a truly wonderful memory. No other midwife in her day and tribe could compete with her in skill and judgment. Her observations in practice were all preserved in her mind for reference, as systematically as if they had been written upon the pages of a note-book.

I distinctly recall one occasion when she took me with her into the woods in search of certain medicinal roots. "Why do you not use all kinds of roots for medicines?" said I.

"Because," she replied, in her quick, characteristic manner, the Great Mystery does not will us to find things too easily. In that case everybody would be a medicine-giver, and Ohiyesa must learn that there are many secrets which the Great Mystery will disclose only to the most worthy. Only those who seek him fasting and in solitude will receive his signs." With this and many similar explanations she wrought in my soul wonderful and lively conceptions of the "Great Mystery" and of the effects of prayer and solitude. I continued my childish questioning.

"But why did you not dig those plants that we saw in the woods, of the same kind that you are digging now?"

"For the same reason that we do not like the berries we find in the shadow of deep woods as well as the ones which grow in sunny places. The latter have more sweetness and flavor. Those herbs which have medicinal virtues should be sought in a place that is neither too wet nor too dry, and where they have a generous amount of sunshine to maintain their vigor.

"Some day Ohiyesa will be old enough to know the secrets of medicine; then I will tell him all. But if you should grow up to be a bad man, I must withhold these treasures from you and give them to your brother, for a medicine man must be a good and wise man. I hope Ohiyesa will be a great medicine man when he grows up. To be a great warrior is a noble ambition; but to be a mighty medicine man is a nobler!" She said these things so thoughtfully and impressively that I cannot but feel and remember them even to this day.

Our native women gathered all the wild rice, roots, berries and fruits which formed an important part of our food. This was distinctively a woman's work. Uncheedah (grandmother) understood these matters perfectly, and it became a kind of instinct with her to know just where to look for each edible variety and at what season of the year. This sort of labor gave the Indian women every opportunity to observe and study Nature after their fashion; and in this Uncheedah was more acute than most of the men. The abilities of her boys were not all inherited from their father; indeed, the stronger family traits came obviously from her. She was a leader among the native women, and they came to her, not only for medical aid, but for advice in all their affairs.

"Out, Out—"

ROBERT FROST
(American, 1874–1963)

Perhaps one of the most iconic of American poets and certainly one of the most lauded, with four Pulitzer Prizes and a Congressional Gold medal both recognizing his poetry, Robert Frost often wrote poems invoking the rural and rustic as they explore their (often dark or ironic) themes. The most famous of these include "The Road Not Taken" (1915) and "Stopping by the Woods on a Snowy Evening" (1923). "Out, Out—" (1916), the poem included here, also fits into this mold. It is a narrative poem describing the aftermath of an accident involving a young boy and a buzzsaw, which includes the use of ether as an anesthetic (see Crawford Williamson Long, pp. 232–234). As you read, consider the tone of the poem and the actions of those who have come to his aid.

---

* Reprinted from Robert Frost, *Mountain Interval*, 2nd ed. (New York: Henry Holt, 1921; Project Gutenberg, 2009), 50–51.

"Out, Out—"

The buzz-saw snarled and rattled in the yard
And made dust and dropped stove-length sticks of wood,
Sweet-scented stuff when the breeze drew across it.
And from there those that lifted eyes could count
Five mountain ranges one behind the other [5]
Under the sunset far into Vermont.
And the saw snarled and rattled, snarled and rattled,
As it ran light, or had to bear a load.
And nothing happened: day was all but done.
Call it a day, I wish they might have said [10]
To please the boy by giving him the half hour
That a boy counts so much when saved from work.
His sister stood beside them in her apron
To tell them "Supper." At the word, the saw,
As if to prove saws knew what supper meant, [15]
Leaped out at the boy's hand, or seemed to leap—
He must have given the hand. However it was,
Neither refused the meeting. But the hand!
The boy's first outcry was a rueful laugh,
As he swung toward them holding up the hand [20]
Half in appeal, but half as if to keep
The life from spilling. Then the boy saw all—
Since he was old enough to know, big boy
Doing a man's work, though a child at heart—
He saw all spoiled. "Don't let him cut my hand off— [25]
The doctor, when he comes. Don't let him, sister!"
So. But the hand was gone already.
The doctor put him in the dark of ether.
He lay and puffed his lips out with his breath.
And then—the watcher at his pulse took fright. [30]
No one believed. They listened at his heart.
Little—less—nothing!—and that ended it.
No more to build on there. And they, since they
Were not the one dead, turned to their affairs.

On the Asylum Road*

CHARLOTTE MARY MEW
(English, 1869–1928)

Poet Charlotte Mary Mew grew up in a large family that experienced a great deal of sadness. As the oldest of seven children, Mew lost three siblings to death and two to psychiatric institutions. She and her sister Anne remained close throughout their lives, and neither married (scholars have also convincingly suggested that Mew was attracted to women, but that all her pursuits went unrequited). In adulthood, Mew began to publish short stories and poems, and became active in literary circles. Her sister died of cancer in 1927, and Mew was so stricken with the loss that she committed suicide less than a year later. Her work, which often took up themes of death, loneliness, and mental illness, gained praise both from critics and other poets, including Siegfried Sassoon (see pp. 344–346) and Virginia Woolf. The poem included here was first published in the 1916 volume *The Farmer's Bride*. As you read, consider the poem's perspective, which features a narrator on the outside of an asylum considering the patients within.

---

* Reprinted from Charlotte Mary Mew, *Saturday Market* (New York: Macmillan, 1921), 36, Google Books.

On the Asylum Road

Theirs is the house whose windows—every pane—
Are made of darkly stained or clouded glass:
Sometimes you come upon them in the lane,
The saddest crowd that you will ever pass.

But still we merry town or village folk [5]
Throw to their scattered stare a kindly grin,
And think no shame to stop and crack a joke
With the incarnate wages of man's sin.

None but ourselves in our long gallery we meet,
The moor-hen stepping from her reeds with dainty feet, [10]
    The hare-bell bowing on his stem,
Dance not with us; their pulses beat
To fainter music; nor do we to them
    Make their life sweet.

The gayest crowd that they will ever pass [15]
Are we to brother-shadows in the lane:
Our windows, too, are clouded glass
To them, yes, every pane!

Mental Cases*

WILFRED OWEN
(English, 1893–1918)

In 1915, while working as a teacher in a private household, 22-year-old poet Wilfred Owen decided to enlist in the English military in order to serve in World War I. His wartime experiences greatly influenced his writing. He is now known as one of the greatest poets of the First World War, alongside his close friend Siegfried Sassoon (see pp. 344–346). The poem was written around the time that Owen was being treated for shell shock, a stress reaction to war trauma (see W. H. R. Rivers, pp. 334–343). Shell shock was first named in 1915, as the new military technology of the conflict, including airplanes, tanks, poison gas, machine guns and trench warfare, greatly intensified the psychological dangers of war. Shell shock is now described by the larger category of post-traumatic stress disorder, or PTSD, which started to take shape as a recognizable diagnosis in the 1950s. However, the condition wasn't identified as such officially until the *DSM-III* (American Psychiatric Association's classification manual for mental disorders) was published in 1980. As you read, consider the poem's explicit depiction of war's consequences on mental health.

---

* Reprinted from *Poems by Wilfred Owen, with an Introduction by Siegfried Sassoon* (New York: Viking, 1921), 8, Google Books.

Mental Cases

Who are these? Why sit they here in twilight?
Wherefore rocky they, purgatorial shadows,
Drooping tongues from jaws that slob their relish,
Baring teeth that leer like skulls' tongues wicked?
Stroke on stroke of pain,—but what slow panic,   [5]
Gouged these chasms round their fretted sockets?
Ever from their hair and through their hand palms
Misery swelters. Surely we have perished
Sleeping, and walk hell; but who these hellish?

—These are men whose minds the Dead have ravished.   [10]
Memory fingers in their hair of murders,
Multitudinous murders they once witnessed.
Wading sloughs of flesh these helpless wander,
Treading blood from lungs that had loved laughter.
Always they must see these things and hear them,   [15]
Batter of guns and shatter of flying muscles,
Carnage incomparable and human squander
Rucked too thick for these men's extrication.

Therefore still their eyeballs shrink tormented
Back into their brains, because on their sense   [20]
Sunlight seems a bloodsmear; night comes blood-black;
Dawn breaks open like a wound that bleeds afresh
—Thus their heads wear this hilarious, hideous,
Awful falseness of set-smiling corpses.
—Thus their hands are plucking at each other;   [25]
Picking at the rope-knouts of their scourging;
Snatching after us who smote them, brother,
Pawing us who dealt them war and madness.

The Repression of War Experience*

W. H. R. RIVERS

(English, 1894–1922)

William H. R. Rivers conducted research on delirium and the nineteenth-century diagnostic categories of neurasthenia and hysteria prior to the outbreak of World War I. That war brought new developments in military technology, such as machine guns, tanks, and poison gas, that made the conflict one of the deadliest in history. It also brought an increase in cases of a traumatic condition then called shell shock or war neurosis—an early understanding of post-traumatic stress disorder. Sufferers of shell shock were often viewed as unpredictable and weak, even cowardly, and treatments (when soldiers received them) could be harsh; favored methods included the use of anesthetics and electroshock therapy. Rivers's approach was more humane. He used the "talking cure," a guided confrontation of trauma through discussion. One of his patients included Siegfried Sassoon, whose poem in this volume (see pp. 344–346) shares the name of Rivers's work excerpted here (and published in 1918). As you read, consider his approach to treatment and his description of its use for some of his patients.

---

* Reprinted from W. H. R. Rivers, "The Repression of War Experience," *Proceedings of the Royal Society of Medicine* 11, Sect. Psych, 1–20, PubMed Central, U.S. National Library of Medicine, National Institutes of Health.

[On War Neurosis and Its Treatment]

Everyone who has had to treat cases of war-neurosis, and especially that form of neurosis dependent on anxiety, must have been faced by the problem what advice to give concerning the attitude the patient should adopt towards his war experience. It is natural to thrust aside painful memories just as it is natural to avoid dangerous or horrible scenes in actuality. This natural tendency to banish the distressing or the horrible is especially pronounced in those whose powers of resistance have been lowered by the long-continued strains of trench life, the shock of shell explosion, or other catastrophe of warfare. Even if patients were left to themselves, most would naturally strive to forget distressing memories and thoughts. They are, however, very far from being left to themselves, the natural tendency to repress being in my experience almost universally fostered by their relatives and friends, as well as by their medical advisers. Even when patients have themselves realized the impossibility of forgetting their war experiences and have recognized the hopeless and enervating character of the treatment by repression, they are often induced to attempt the task in obedience to medical orders. The advice which has usually been given to my patients in other hospitals is that they should endeavor to banish all thoughts of war from their minds. In some cases all conversation between patients, or with visitors, about the war is strictly forbidden, and the patients are instructed to lead their thoughts to other topics, to beautiful scenery and other pleasant aspects of experience.

To a certain extent this policy is perfectly sound. Nothing annoys a nervous patient more than the continual inquiries of his relatives and friends about his experiences of the Front, not only because it awakens painful memories, but also because of the obvious futility of most of the questions and the hopelessness of bringing the realities home to his hearers. Moreover, the assemblage together in a hospital of a number of men with little in common except their war experiences, naturally leads their conversation far too frequently to this topic, and even among those whose memories are not especially distressing it tends to enhance the state for which the term "fed up" seems to be the universal designation.

It is, however, one thing that those who are suffering from the shocks and strains of warfare should dwell continually on their war experience or be subjected to importunate inquiries; it is quite another matter to attempt to banish such experience from their minds altogether. The cases I am about to record illustrate the evil influence of this latter course of action and the good effects which follow its cessation.

The first case is that of a young officer who was sent home from France on account of a wound received just as he was extricating himself from a mass of earth in which he had been buried. When he reached hospital in England he was nervous and suffered from disturbed sleep and loss of appetite. When his wound had healed he was sent home on leave, where his nervous symptoms became more pronounced so that at his next board[1] his leave was extended. He was for a time an out-patient at a London hospital and was then sent to a convalescent home in the country. Here he continued to sleep badly, with disturbing dreams of warfare, and became very anxious about himself and his prospects of recovery. Thinking he might improve if he rejoined his battalion, he made so light of this condition at his next medical board that he was on the point of being returned to duty when special inquiries about his sleep led to his being sent to Craiglockhart War Hospital for further observation and treatment. On admission he reported that it always took him long to get to sleep at night and that when he succeeded he had vivid dreams of warfare. He could not sleep without a light in his room, because in the dark his attention was attracted by every sound. He had been advised by everyone he had consulted, whether medical or lay, that he ought to banish all unpleasant and disturbing thoughts from his mind. He had been occupying himself for every hour of the day in order to follow this advice and had succeeded in restraining his memories and anxieties during the day, but as soon as he went to bed they would crowd upon him and race through his mind hour after hour, so that every night he dreaded to go to bed.

When he had recounted his symptoms and told me about his method of dealing with his disturbing thoughts, I asked him to tell me candidly his own opinion concerning the possibility of keeping these obtrusive

---

1 *Board*: Military board review.

visitors from his mind. He said at once that it was obvious to him that memories such as those he had brought with him from the war could never be forgotten. Nevertheless, since he had been told by everyone that it was his duty to forget them, he had done his utmost in this. direction. I then told the patient my own views concerning the nature and treatment of his state. I agreed with him that such memories could not be expected to disappear from the mind and advised him no longer to try to banish them, but that he should see whether it was not possible to make them into tolerable, if not even pleasant, companions instead of evil influences which forced themselves upon his mind whenever the silence and inactivity of the night came round. The possibility of such a line of treatment had never previously occurred to him, but my plan seemed reasonable and he promised to give it a trial. We talked about his war experiences and his anxieties, and following this he had the best night he had had for five months. During the following week he had a good deal of difficulty in sleeping, but his sleeplessness no longer had the painful and distressing quality which had been previously given to it by the intrusion of painful thoughts of warfare. In so far as unpleasant thoughts came to him these were concerned with domestic anxieties rather than with the memories of war, and even these no longer gave rise to the dread which had previously troubled him. His general health improved; his power of sleeping gradually increased and he was able after a time to return to duty, not in the hope that this duty might help him to forget, but with some degree of confidence that he was really fit for it.

The case I have just narrated is a straightforward example of anxiety-neurosis which made no real progress as long as the patient tried to keep out of his mind the painful memories and anxieties which had been aroused in his mind by reflection on his past experience, his present state and the chance of his fitness for duty in the future. When in place of running away from these unpleasant thoughts he faced them boldly and allowed his mind to dwell upon them in the day, they no longer raced through his mind at night and disturbed his sleep by terrifying dreams of warfare.

The next case is that of an officer whose burial as the result of a shell explosion had been followed by symptoms pointing to some degree of cerebral concussion. In spite of severe headache, vomiting and disorder of micturition, he remained on duty for more than two months. He then collapsed altogether after a very trying experience in which he had gone out to, seek a fellow officer and had found his body blown into pieces with head and limbs lying separated from the trunk. From that time he had been haunted at night by the vision of his dead and mutilated friend. When he slept he had nightmares in which his friend appeared, sometimes as he had seem him mangled on the field, sometimes in the still more terrifying aspect of one whose limbs and features had been eaten away by leprosy. The mutilated or leprous officer of the dream would come nearer and nearer until the patient suddenly awoke pouring with sweat and in a state of the utmost terror. He dreaded to go to sleep, and spent each day looking forward in painful anticipation of the night. He had been advised to keep all thoughts of war from his mind, but the experience which recurred so often at night was so insistent that he could not keep it wholly from his thoughts, much as he tried to do so. Nevertheless, there is no question but that he was striving by day to dispel memories only to bring them upon him with redoubled force and horror when he slept.

The problem before me in this case was to find some aspect of the painful experience which would allow the patient to dwell upon it in such a way as to relieve its horrible and terrifying character. The aspect to which I drew his attention was that the mangled state of the body of his friend was conclusive evidence that he had been killed outright, and had been spared the prolonged suffering which is too often the fate of those who sustain mortal wounds. He brightened at once, and said that this aspect of the case had never occurred to him, nor had it been suggested by any of those to whom he had. previously related his story. He saw at once that this was an aspect of his experience upon which he could allow his thoughts to dwell. He said he would no longer attempt to banish thoughts and memories of his friend from his mind, but would think of the pain and suffering he had been spared. For several nights he had no dreams at all, and then came a night in which he dreamt that he went out into No Man's Land to seek his friend, and saw his mangled body just as in other dreams, but without the horror which had always previously been present. He knelt beside his friend to save for the relatives any objects of value which were upon the body, a pious duty he had fulfilled in the actual scene, and as he was taking off the Sam Browne belt he woke, with none of the horror and terror of the past, but weeping gently, feeling only grief for the loss of a friend. Some nights later he had another dream in which he met his friend, still mangled, but no longer terrifying. They talked together, and the patient told the history of his illness and how he was now able to speak to him in comfort and without horror or undue distress. Once only during his stay in hospital did he again experience horror in connection with any dream of his friend. During the few days following his discharge from hospital the dream recurred once or twice with some degree of its former terrifying quality, but in his last report to me he had only had one unpleasant dream with a different content, and was regaining his normal health and strength. ...

In the cases recorded in this paper the patients had been repressing certain painful elements of their mental content. They had been deliberately practicing what we must regard as a definite course of treatment, in nearly every case adopted on medical advice, in which they were either deliberately thrusting certain unpleasant memories or thoughts from their minds or were occupying every moment of the day in some activity in order that these thoughts might not come into the focus of attention. At the same time they were suffering from certain highly distressing symptoms which disappeared or altered in character when the process of repression ceased. Moreover, the symptoms by which they had been troubled were such as receive a natural, if not obvious, explanation as the result of the repression they had been practicing. If a person voluntarily represses unpleasant thoughts during the day, it is natural that they should rise into activity when the control of the waking state is removed by sleep or lessened in the state which precedes or follows sleep or occupies its intervals. If the painful thoughts have been kept from the attention throughout the day by means of occupation, it is again natural that they should come into activity when the silence and isolation of the night make occupation no longer possible. It seems as if the thoughts repressed by day assume a painful quality when they come to the surface at night far more intense than is ever attained if they are allowed to occupy the attention during the day. It is as if the process of repression keeps the painful memories or thoughts under a kind of pressure during the day, accumulating such energy by the time night comes that they race through the mind with abnormal speed and violence when the patient is wakeful, or take the most vivid and painful forms when expressed by the imagery of dreams.

When such distressing, if not terrible, symptoms disappear or alter in character as soon as repression ceases, it is natural to conclude that the two processes stand to one another. in the relation of cause and effect, but so great is the complexity of the conditions with which we are dealing in the medicine of the mind that it is necessary to consider certain alternative explanations.

The disappearance or improvement of symptoms on the cessation of voluntary repression may be regarded as due to the action of one form of the principle of catharsis. This term is generally used for the agency which is operative when a suppressed or dissociated body of experience is brought to the surface so that it again becomes reintegrated with. the ordinary personality. It is no great step from this to the mode of action recorded in this paper, in which experience on its way towards suppression has undergone a similar, though necessarily less extensive, process of reintegration. There is, however, another form of catharsis which may have been operative in some of the cases I have described. It often happens in cases of war-neurosis, as in neurosis in general, that the sufferers do not suppress their painful thoughts, but brood over them constantly until their experience assumes vastly exaggerated and often distorted importance and significance. In such cases the greatest relief is afforded by the mere communication of these troubles to another. This form of catharsis may have been operative in relation to certain kinds of experience in some of my cases, and this complicates our estimation of the therapeutic value of the cessation of repression. I have, however, carefully chosen for record on this occasion cases in which the second form of catharsis, if present at all, formed, an agency altogether subsidiary to that afforded by the cessation of repression.

Another complicating factor which may have entered into the therapeutic process in some of the cases is re-education. This certainly came into play in the case of the patient who had the terrifying dreams of his mangled friend. In his case the cessation of repression was accompanied by the direction of the attention of the patient to an aspect of his painful memories which he had hitherto completely ignored. The process by which his attention was thus directed to a neglected aspect of his experience introduced a factor which must be distinguished from the removal of repression itself. The two processes are intimately associated, for it was largely, if not altogether, the new view of his experience which made it possible for the patient to dwell upon his painful memories. In some of the other cases this factor of re-education undoubtedly played a part, not merely in making possible the cessation of repression, but also in helping the patient to adjust himself to the situation with which he was faced, thus contributing positively to the recovery or improvement which followed the cessation of repression.

A more difficult and more contentious problem arises when we consider how far the success which attended the cessation of repression may have been, wholly or in part, due to faith and suggestion. Here, as in every branch of therapeutics, whether it be treatment by drugs, diet, baths, electricity, persuasion, re-education or psycho-analysis, we come up against the difficulty raised by the pervasive and subtle influence of these agencies working behind the scenes. In the subject before us, as in every other kind of medical treatment, we have to consider whether the changes which occurred may have been due, not to the agency which lay on the surface and was the motive of the treatment, but at any rate, in part, to the influence, so difficult to exclude, of faith and suggestion. In my later, work I have come to believe so thoroughly in the injurious action of repression, and have acquired so lively a faith in the efficacy of my mode of treatment, that this agency cannot be excluded as a factor in any success I may have. In my earlier work, however, I certainly had no such faith, and advised the discontinuance of repression with the utmost diffidence. Faith on the part of the patient may, however, be present even when the physician is diffident. It is of more importance that several of the patients had been under my care for some time without improvement until it was discovered that they were repressing painful experience. It was only when the repression ceased that improvement began.

Definite evidence against the influence of suggestion is provided by the case in which the dream of the mangled friend came to lose its horror, this state being replaced by the far more bearable emotion of grief. The change which followed the cessation of repression in this case could not have been suggested by me, for its possibility had not, so far as I am aware, entered my mind. So far as suggestions, witting or unwitting, were given, these would have had the form that the nightmares would cease altogether, and the change in the affective character of the dream, not having been anticipated by myself, can hardly have been communicated to the patient. It is, of course, possible that my own belief in the improvement which would follow the adoption of my advice acted in a general manner by bringing the agencies of faith and suggestion into action, but these agencies can hardly have produced the specific and definite form which the improvement took. In other of the cases I have recorded, faith and suggestion probably played some part, that of the officer with the sudden and overwhelming attacks of depression being especially open to the possibility of these influences.

Such complicating factors as I have just considered can no more be excluded in this than in any other branch of therapeutics, but I am confident that their part is small beside that due to stopping a course of action whereby patients were striving to carry out an impossible task. In some cases faith and suggestion, re-education and sharing troubles with another, undoubtedly form the chief agents in the removal or amendment of the symptoms of neurosis, but in the cases I have recorded there can be little doubt that they contributed only in a minor degree to the success which attended the giving up of repression. …

Because I advocate the facing of painful memories, and deprecate the ostrich-like policy of attempting to banish them from the mind, it must not be thought that I recommend the concentration of the thoughts on such memories. On the contrary, in my opinion it is just as harmful to dwell persistently upon painful memories or anticipations, and brood upon feelings of regret and shame, as to attempt to banish them wholly from the mind. It is necessary to be explicit on this matter when dealing with patients. In a recent case in which I neglected to do so, the absence of any improvement led me to inquire into the patient's method of following my advice, and I found that, thinking he could not have too much of a good thing, he had substituted for the system of repression he had followed before coming under my care, one in which he spent the whole day talking, reading, and thinking of war. He even spent the interval between dinner and going to bed in reading a book dealing with warfare.

There are also some victims of neurosis, especially the very young, for whom the horrors of warfare seem to have a peculiar fascination, so that when the opportunity presents itself they cannot refrain from talking by the hour about war experiences, although they know quite well that it is bad for them to do so. Here, as in so many other aspects of the treatment of neurosis, we have to steer a middle course. Just as we prescribe moderation in exercise, moderation at work and play, moderation in eating, drinking, and smoking, so is moderation necessary in talking, reading, and thinking about war experience. Moreover, we must not be content merely to advise our patients to give up repression, we must help them by every means in our power to put this advice into practice. We must show them how to overcome the difficulties which are put in their way by enfeebled volition, and by the distortion of their experience due to its having for long been seen exclusively from some one point of view. It is often only by a process of prolonged reeducation that it becomes possible for the patient to give up the practice of repressing war experience.

The Repression of War Experience*

SIEGFRIED SASSOON
(English, 1886–1967)

Both decorated for his courage on the battlefield of World War I and openly critical of its continuation, author Siegfried Sassoon became known as one of the War's greatest poets. After lodging a formal protest against the war effort—one which made it all the way to the halls of Parliament—Sassoon was removed from duty and sent off to be treated for neurasthenia and war neurosis (or shell shock). During his hospitalization, he met fellow poet Wilfred Owen (see pp. 332–333) and was treated for his condition by W. H. R. Rivers (see pp. 334–343). The poem included here shares its title with Rivers's treatise on the nature and treatment of shell shock. As you read, consider how it depicts some of the impacts of attempting to repress war memories.

---

* Reprinted from Siegfried Sassoon, *Counter-Attack and Other Poems* (New York: E. P. Dutton, 1918), 51–53, Google Books.

The Repression of War Experience

Now light the candles; one; two; there's a moth;
What silly beggars they are to blunder in
And scorch their wings with glory, liquid flame—
No, no, not that,—it's bad to think of war,
When thoughts you've gagged all day come back to scare you; [5]
And it's been proved that soldiers don't go mad
Unless they lose control of ugly thoughts
That drive them out to jabber among the trees.

Now light your pipe; look, what a steady hand.
Draw a deep breath; stop thinking; count fifteen, [10]
And you're as right as rain...
                      Why won't it rain?...
I wish there'd be a thunder-storm to-night,
With bucketsful of water to sluice the dark,
And make the roses hang their dripping heads. [15]

Books; what a jolly company they are,
Standing so quiet and patient on their shelves,
Dressed in dim brown, and black, and white, and green,
And every kind of colour. Which will you read?
Come on; O *do* read something; they're so wise. [20]
I tell you all the wisdom of the world
Is waiting for you on those shelves; and yet
You sit and gnaw your nails, and let your pipe out,
And listen to the silence: on the ceiling
There's one big, dizzy moth that bumps and flutters; [25]

And in the breathless air outside the house
The garden waits for something that delays.
There must be crowds of ghosts among the trees,—
Not people killed in battle,—they're in France,—
But horrible shapes in shrouds—old men who died [30]

Slow, natural deaths,—old men with ugly souls,
Who wore their bodies out with nasty sins.

*

You're quiet and peaceful, summering safe at home;
You'd never think there was a bloody war on!...
O yes, you would...why, you can hear the guns. [35]
Hark! Thud, thud, thud,—quite soft.. they never cease—
Those whispering guns—O Christ, I want to go out
And screech at them to stop—I'm going crazy;
I'm going stark, staring mad because of the guns.

A Country Doctor[*]

FRANZ KAFKA
(Bohemian, 1883–1924)

Franz Kafka was born in Prague into an Ashkenazi Jewish family[1] and became well-known for his short stories and novels. His works are often marked by the nightmarish, the peculiar, and the complex—features so pronounced they led to the coining of the word "Kafkaesque" to describe works and scenarios that are disorienting and strange. The short story included here was published in a volume of the same name in 1919, and was written in an era when many patients were treated at home, rather than in clinics, by doctors who would make house calls (often at all hours). As you read, consider the experience of the narrator, an unfortunate doctor tasked with an urgent house call in the middle of a cold winter's night, as he attempts to reach and treat a young patient.

---

1 Ashkenazi Jewish people trace their ancestry to groups who settled along the Rhine River (in Germany and France) in the Middle Ages, then spread throughout Central and Eastern Europe. Prior to World War II (1939–1945), the Ashkenazim are estimated to have represented the majority of Europe's Jewish population (around 57%).

---

[*] Reprinted from Franz Kafka, *A Country Doctor*, trans. Ian Johnston (Rosings Digital Publications, 2003).

A Country Doctor

I was in great difficulty. An urgent journey was facing me. A seriously ill man was waiting for me in a village ten miles distant. A severe snowstorm filled the space between him and me. I had a carriage—a light one, with large wheels, entirely suitable for our country roads. Wrapped up in furs with the bag of instruments in my hand, I was already standing in the courtyard ready for the journey; but the horse was missing—the horse. My own horse had died the previous night, as a result of overexertion in this icy winter. My servant girl was at that very moment running around the village to see if she could borrow a horse, but it was hopeless—I knew that—and I stood there useless, increasingly covered with snow, becoming all the time more immobile. The girl appeared at the gate, alone. She was swinging the lantern. Of course, who is now going to lend her his horse for such a journey? I walked once again across the courtyard. I couldn't see what to do. Distracted and tormented, I kicked my foot against the cracked door of the pig sty which had not been used for years. The door opened and banged to and fro on its hinges. A warmth and smell as if from horses came out. A dim stall lantern on a rope swayed inside. A man huddled down in the stall below showed his open blue-eyed face. "Shall I hitch up?" he asked, crawling out on all fours. I didn't know what to say and bent down to see what was still in the stall. The servant girl stood beside me. "One doesn't know the sorts of things one has stored in one's own house," she said, and we both laughed. "Hey, Brother, hey Sister," the groom cried out, and two horses, powerful animals with strong flanks, shoved their way one behind the other, legs close to the bodies, lowering their well-formed heads like camels, and getting through the door space, which they completely filled, only through the powerful movements of their rumps. But right away they stood up straight, long legged, with thick steaming bodies. "Help him," I said, and the girl obediently hurried to hand the wagon harness to the groom. But as soon as she was beside him, the groom puts his arms around her and pushes his face against hers. She screams out and runs over to me. On the girl's cheek were red marks from two rows of teeth. "You brute," I cry out in fury, "do you want the whip?". But I immediately remember that he is a stranger, that

I don't know where he comes from, and that he's helping me out of his own free will, when everyone else is refusing to. As if he knows what I was thinking, he takes no offense at my threat, but turns around to me once more, still busy with the horses. Then he says, "Climb in," and, in fact, everything is ready. I notice that I have never before traveled with such a beautiful team of horses, and I climb in happily. "But I'll take the reins. You don't know the way," I say. "Of course," he says; "I'm not going with you. I'm staying with Rosa." "No," screams Rosa and runs into the house, with an accurate premonition of the inevitability of her fate. I hear the door chain rattling as she sets it in place. I hear the lock click. I see how in addition she runs down the corridor and through the rooms putting out all the lights in order to make herself impossible to find. "You're coming with me," I say to the groom, "or I'll give up the journey, no matter how urgent it is. It's not my intention to give you the girl as the price of the trip." "Giddy up," he says and claps his hands. The carriage is torn away, like a piece of wood in a current. I still hear how the door of my house is breaking down and splitting apart under the groom's onslaught, and then my eyes and ears are filled with a roaring sound which overwhelms all my senses at once. But only for a moment. Then I am already there, as if the farm yard of my invalid opens up immediately in front of my courtyard gate. The horses stand quietly. The snowfall has stopped, moonlight all around. The sick man's parents rush out of the house, his sister behind them. They almost lift me out of the carriage. I get nothing from their confused talking. In the sick room one can hardly breathe the air. The neglected cooking stove is smoking. I want to push open the window, but first I'll look at the sick man. Thin, without fever, not cold, not warm, with empty eyes, without a shirt, the young man under the stuffed quilt heaves himself up, hangs around my throat, and whispers in my ear, "Doctor, let me die." I look around. No one has heard. The parents stand silently, leaning forward, and wait for my opinion. The sister has brought a stool for my handbag. I open the bag and look among my instruments. The young man constantly gropes at me from the bed to remind me of his request. I take some tweezers, test them in the candle light, and put them back. "Yes," I think blasphemously, "in such cases the gods do help. They send the missing horse, even add a second one because it's urgent, and even throw in a groom as a bonus." Now for the first time I think once more of Rosa. What am I doing? How am I saving her? How do I pull her out from under this groom, ten miles away from her, with uncontrollable horses in the front of my carriage? These horses, who have somehow loosened their straps, are pushing open the window from outside, I don't know how. Each one is sticking its head through a window and, unmoved by the crying of the family, is observing the invalid. "I'll go back right away," I think, as if the horses were ordering me to journey back, but I allow the sister, who thinks I am in a daze because of the heat, to take off my fur coat. A glass of rum is prepared for me. The old man claps me on the shoulder; the sacrifice of his treasure justifies this familiarity. I shake my head. In the narrow circle of the old man's thinking I was not well; that's the only reason I refuse to drink. The mother stands by the bed and entices me over. I follow and, as a horse neighs loudly at the ceiling, lay my head on the young man's chest, which trembles under my wet beard. That confirms what I know: the young man is healthy. His circulation is a little off, saturated with coffee by his caring mother, but he's healthy and best pushed out of bed with a shove. I'm no improver of the world and let him lie there. I am employed by the district and do my duty to the full, right to the point where it's almost too much. Badly paid, but I'm generous and ready to help the poor. I still have to look after Rosa, and then the young man may have his way, and I want to die too. What am I doing here in this endless winter! My horse is dead, and there is no one in the village who'll lend me his. I have to drag my team out of the pig sty. If they hadn't happened to be horses, I'd have had to travel with pigs. That's the way it is. And I nod to the family. They know nothing about it, and if they did know, they wouldn't believe it. Incidentally, it's easy to write prescriptions, but difficult to come to an understanding with people. Now, at this point my visit might have come to an end—they have once more called for my help unnecessarily. I'm used to that. With the help of my night bell[2] the entire region torments me, but that this time I had to sacrifice Rosa as well, this beautiful girl, who lives in my house all year long and whom I scarcely notice—this sacrifice is too great, and

2 *Night bell*: An alarm used to call on physicians after hours, so they can make necessary house calls.

I must somehow in my own head subtly rationalize it away for the moment, in order not to let loose at this family who cannot, even with their best will, give me Rosa back again. But as I am closing up by hand bag and calling for my fur coat, the family is standing together, the father sniffing the glass of rum in his hand, the mother, probably disappointed in me—what more do these people expect?—tearfully biting her lips, and the sister flapping a very bloody hand towel, I am somehow ready, in the circumstances, to concede that the young man is perhaps nonetheless sick. I go to him. He smiles up at me, as if I was bringing him the most nourishing kind of soup—ah, now both horses are whinnying, the noise is probably supposed to come from higher regions in order to illuminate my examination—and now I find out that, yes indeed, the young man is ill. On his right side, in the region of the hip, a wound the size of the palm of one's hand has opened up. Rose colored, in many different shadings, dark in the depths, brighter on the edges, delicately grained, with uneven patches of blood, open to the light like a mine. That's what it looks like from a distance. Close up a complication is apparent. Who can look at that without whistling softly? Worms, as thick and long as my little finger, themselves rose colored and also spattered with blood, are wriggling their white bodies with many limbs from their stronghold in the inner of the wound towards the light. Poor young man, there's no helping you. I have found out your great wound. You are dying from this flower on your side. The family is happy; they see me doing something. The sister says that to the mother, the mother tells the father, the father tells a few guests who are coming in on tip toe through the moonlight of the open door, balancing themselves with outstretched arms. "Will you save me?" whispers the young man, sobbing, quite blinded by the life inside his wound. That's how people are in my region. Always demanding the impossible from the doctor. They have lost the old faith. The priest sits at home and tears his religious robes to pieces, one after the other. But the doctor is supposed to achieve everything with his delicate surgeon's hand. Well, it's what they like to think. I have not offered myself. If they use me for sacred purposes, I let that happen to me as well. What more do I want, an old country doctor, robbed of my servant girl! And they come, the families and the village elders, and take my clothes off. A choir of school children with the teacher at the head stands in front of the house and sings an extremely simple melody with the words Take his clothes off, then he'll heal and if he doesn't cure, then kill him. It's only a doctor; it's only a doctor. Then I am stripped of my clothes and, with my fingers in my beard and my head tilted to one side, I look at the people quietly. I am completely calm and clear about everything and stay that way, too, although it is not helping me at all, for they are now taking me by the head and feet and dragging me into bed. They lay me against the wall on the side of wound. Then they all go out of the room. The door is shut. The singing stops. Clouds move in front of the moon. The bedclothes lie warmly around me. In the open space of the windows the horses' heads sway like shadows. "Do you know," I hear someone saying in my ear, "my confidence in you is very small. You were shaken out from somewhere. You don't come on your own feet. Instead of helping, you give me less room on my deathbed. The best thing would be if I scratch your eyes out." "Right," I say, "it's a disgrace. But now I'm a doctor. What am I supposed to do? Believe me, things are not easy for me either." "Should I be satisfied with this excuse? Alas, I'll probably have to be. I always have to make do. I came into the world with a beautiful wound; that was all I was furnished with." "Young friend," I say, "your mistake is that you have no perspective. I've already been in all the sick rooms, far and wide, and I tell you your wound is not so bad. Made in a tight corner with two blows from an ax. Many people offer their side and hardly hear the ax in the forest, to say nothing of the fact that it's coming closer to them." "Is that really so, or are you deceiving me in my fever?" "It is truly so. Take the word of honor of a medical doctor." He took my word and grew still. But now it was time to think about my escape. The horses were still standing loyally in place. Clothes, fur coat, and bag were quickly snatched up. I didn't want to delay by getting dressed; if the horses rushed as they had on the journey out, I should, in fact, be springing out of that bed into my own, as it were. One horse obediently pulled back from the window. I threw the bundle into the carriage. The fur coat flew too far and was caught on a hook by only one arm. Good enough. I swung myself up onto the horse. The reins dragging loosely, one horse barely harnessed to the other, the carriage swaying behind, last of all the fur coat in the snow. "Giddy up," I said, but there was no giddying up about it. We dragged through the snowy desert like old men; for a long time the fresh but inaccurate singing of the children resounded behind us: Enjoy yourselves, you patients. The doctor's laid in bed with you. I'll never come home at this rate. My flourishing practice is lost. A successor is robbing me, but to no avail, for he cannot replace me. In my house the disgusting groom is wreaking havoc. Rosa is his victim. I will not think it through. Naked, abandoned to the frost of this unhappy age, with an earthly carriage and unearthly horses, I drive around by myself, an old man. My fur coat hangs behind the wagon, but I cannot reach it, and no one from the nimble rabble of patients lifts a finger. Betrayed! Betrayed! Once one responds to a false alarm on the night bell, there's no making it good again—not ever.

Complaint*

WILLIAM CARLOS WILLIAMS
(Puerto-Rican American, 1883–1963)

William Carlos Williams was born in New Jersey and raised in a bilingual, multicultural household by his English father and Puerto Rican mother. Known as one of the leading modernist poets, he won the first National Book Award for poetry during his lifetime and posthumously earned a Pulitzer Prize for his final collection of poems. He was also an accomplished physician. He attended the University of Pennsylvania's Medical School (where William Osler—see pp. 306–312—taught for a time) and graduated with a degree in pediatrics and obstetrics. He practiced in his home state of New Jersey, making countless house calls and eventually working as Chief Pediatrician of Passaic General Hospital. The influence of his profession is felt in much of his writing, including the poem here, which was first published in 1921. As you read, consider the perspective of the narrator, a physician on a house call to visit a woman in labor.

---

* Reprinted from William Carlos Williams, *Sour Grapes: A Book of Poems* (Boston: The Four Seas, 1921), 37, Google Books.

Complaint

They call me and I go
It is a frozen road
past midnight, a dust
of snow caught
in the rigid wheeltracks. [5]
The door opens.
I smile, enter and
shake off the cold.
Here is a great woman
on her side in the bed. [10]
She is sick,
perhaps vomiting,
perhaps laboring
to give birth to
a tenth child. Joy! Joy! [15]
Night is a room
darkened for lovers,
through the jalousies the sun
has sent one gold needle!
I pick the hair from her eyes [20]
and watch her misery
with compassion.

WPA Ex-Slaves Narrative Project[*]

FEDERAL WRITERS PROJECT
American 1936–1938

As part of the tremendous New Deal public works effort known as the Work Progress Administration (WPA), Federal Project Number One worked to promote American arts and culture by providing jobs for tens of thousands of previously unemployed workers during the Great Depression. Among its endeavors was the Federal Writers Project, which undertook a vast effort in oral history known as the Slave Narrative Collection. From 1936 to 1938, more than two thousand interviews were conducted with survivors of the bondage of slavery, spanning seventeen states and leading to over ten thousand pages of first-person accounts. Included here is a selection of these accounts, drawn from the narrative records of several different southern states. As you read, consider the accounts of health and sickness that the formerly enslaved interviewees describe.

---

[*] Reprinted from Works Progress Administration, *Slave Narratives: A Folk History of Slavery in the United States from Interviews with Former Slaves: Volume I, Alabama Narratives, Part 1; Volume II, Arkansas Narratives, Part 1, 3, 4; Volume IV, Georgia Narratives, Part 1, 4* (Washington, DC.: Library of Congress, 1941; Project Gutenberg, 2011).

Alabama Narratives, Volume 1

Interview with William Henry Townes

Levi D. Shelby, Jr., Tuscumbia, Alabama

"Slaves never got sick much, but when dey did dey got de bes'.[1] Dere was always a nurse on de farm, and when a slave got sick dey was righ' dere to give dem treatments. Back in dose days dey used all sorts of roots and yarbs[2] for medicine. Peach tree leaves was one of de mos' of'en. Sassafras was anudder what was used of'en; hit was used mostly in de spring made in tea. Asafetida was anudder what was use to keep you from havin' azma. Hit was wore 'round de neck in a lil bag. Prickler ash was anudder what was tooken in de spring. Hit was 'spose ter clean de blood. Some of de folks would use brass, copper an' dimes wid holes in 'em to keep from havin' their rumertiz.[3]

Arkansas Narratives, Part 1

Name of Interviewer: Beulah Sherwood Hagg

Name of Ex-Slave; Boston Blackwell
  Age: 98
  Residence: 520 Plum, North Little Rock

"When I finally get up I went to farming right here in Pulaski county. Lordy, no, miss, I didn't buy no land. Nothing to buy with. I went share

---

1 The language presented here tends to be an interpretation of dialect and accent markers transcribed by the predominantly White interviewers. Although interviewers were encouraged to be attentive to the idioms more than the accents, they were typically not trained in phonetics or linguistics; much of the language is thus heavily stereotyped.
2 *Yarbs*: Herbs.
3 *Rumertiz*: Rheumatism, any one of a range of painful disorders affecting the joints and connective tissue.

cropping with a white man, Col. Baucum. You asking me what was the shares? Worked on halvers.[4] I done all the work and fed myself. No'um, I wasn't married yit. I took the rheumatiz in my legs, and got short winded. Then I was good for nothing but picking cotton. I kept on with that till my eyes, they got so dim I couldn't see to pick the rows clean. Heap o' times I needed medicine—heap o'times I needed lots of things I never could get. Iffen I could of had some help when I been sick, I mought not be so no account now. My daughter has taked keer of me ever since I not been able to work no more."

Arkansas Narratives, Part 3

Name of Interviewer—S. S. Taylor

Person interviewed—H. B. Holloway (Dad or Pappy)

"My wife was sick, down, couldn't do nothin'. Someone got to telling her about Cain Robertson. Cain Robertson was a hoodoo[5] doctor in Georgia. They there wasn't nothin' Cain couldn't do. She says, 'Go and see Cain and have him come up here.'

"I says, 'There ain't no use to send for Cain. Cain ain't coming up here because they say he is a "two-head" Nigger.'[6] (They called all them hoodoo men 'two-head' Niggers; I don't know why they called them two-head.) 'And you know he knows the white folks will put him in jail if he comes to town.'

"But she says, 'You go and get him.'

---

4   *Halvers*: Sharecroppers who leased home, land, and tools from a landlord, and then did all the work on the property before turning over half (or more) of the crop back to that landlord at the end of the season.
5   *Hoodoo*: A spiritual tradition developed by enslaved people from Africa in the United States, which collected practices and beliefs from a range of traditional African religions and Indigenous botanical knowledge in the U.S.
6   This term and its subsequent uses are retained to preserve the historical record. Its use as a derogatory and offensive variation on the word *Negro* first entered the Merriam-Webster dictionary in 1864.

"So I went.

"I left him at the house and when I came back in, he said, 'I looked at your wife and she had one of then spells while I was there. I'm afraid to tackle this thing because she has been poisoned and it's been goin' on a long time. And if she dies, they'll say I killed her and they already don't like me and lookin' for an excuse to do somethin' to me.'

"My wife overheard him and says, 'You go on, you got to do somethin.''

"So he made me go to town and get a pint of corn whiskey. When I brought it back, he drunk a half of it at one gulp, and I started to knock him down. I'd thought he'd get drunk with my wife lying there sick.

"Then he said, 'I'll have to see your wife's stomach.' Then he scratched it, and put three little horns on the place he scratched. Then he took another drink of whiskey and waited about ten minutes. When he took them off her stomach, they were full of blood. He put them in the basin in some water and sprinkled some powder on them, and in about ten minutes more, he made me get them and they were full of clear water and there was a lot of little things that looked like wiggle tails swimming around in it.

"He told me when my wife got well to walk in a certain direction a certain distance and the woman that caused all the trouble would come to my house and start a fuss with me.

"I said, 'Can't you put this same thing back on her.'

"He said, 'Yes, but it would kill my hand.' He meant that he had a curing hand and that if he made anybody sick or killed them, all his power to cure would go from him.

"I showed the stuff he took out of my wife's stomach to old Doc Matthews and he said, 'You can get anything into a person by putting it in them.' He asked me how I found out about it, and how it was taken out, and who did it.

"I told him all about it, and he said, 'I'm going to see that that Nigger practices anywhere in this town he wants to and nobody bothers him.' And he did."

Arkansas Narratives, Part 4

Interviewer: Watt McKinney

Person interviewed: Tines Kendricks, Trenton, Arkansas
  Age: 104

"Just to show you, Boss, how 'twas with Mars Sam, on' how contrary an' fractious an' wicked dat young white man was, I wants to tell you 'bout de time dat Aunt Hannah's little boy Mose died. Mose, he sick 'bout er week. Aunt Hannah, she try to doctor on him an' git him well an' she tell old mis' dat she think Mose bad off an' orter have de doctor. Old mis', she wouldn't git de doctor. She say Mose ain't sick much, an' bless my Soul, Aunt Hannah she right. In a few days from then Mose is dead. Mars Sam, he come cussin' an' tole Gabe to get some planks an' make de coffin an' sont some of dem to dig de grave over dere on de far side of de place where dey had er buryin'-groun' for de niggers. Us toted de coffin over to where de grave was dug an' gwine bury little Mose dar an' Uncle Billy Jordan, he was dar and begun to sing an' pray an' have a kind of funeral at de buryin'. Every one was moanin' an' singin' an' prayin' and Mars Sam heard 'em all come sailin' over dar on he hoss an' lit right in to cussin' an' rarein' an' say dat if dey don't hurry an' bury dat nigger an' shut up dat singin' an' carryin' on, he gwine lash every one of dem, an' then he went to cussin' worser an' 'busin' Uncle Billy Jordan. He say iffen he ever hear of him doin' any more preachin' or prayin' 'round 'mongst de niggers at de grave-yard or anywheres else, he gwine lash him to death. No suh, Boss, Mars Sam wouldn't even 'low no preachin' or singin' or nothin' like dat. He was wicked. I tell you he was.

"Old mis' she ginrally looked after de niggers when dey sick an' give dem de medicine. An' too, she would get de doctor iffen she thing dey real bad off 'cause like I said, old mis', she mighty stingy an' she never want to lose no nigger by dem dyin'. How-some-ever it was hard some time to get her to believe you sick when you tell her dat you was, an' she would think you just playin' off from work. I have seen niggers what would be mighty near dead before old mis' would believe them sick at all.

Georgia Narratives, Part 1

Julia Brown (Aunt Sally), 710 Griffin Place, N.W. Atlanta, Ga, July 25, 1936; by Geneva Tonsill.

"Doctors wuzn't so plentiful then. They'd go 'round in buggies and on hosses. Them that rode on a hoss had saddle pockets jest filled with little bottles and lots of them. He'd try one medicine and if it didn't do not[7] good he'd try another until it did do good and when the doctor went to see a sick pusson he'd stay rat there until he wuz better. He didn't jest come in and write a 'scription fur somebody to take to a drug store. We used herbs a lots in them days. When a body had dropsy we'd set him in a tepid bath made of mullein leaves. There wuz a jimson weed we'd use fur rheumatism, and fur asthma we'd use tea made of chestnut leaves. We'd git the chestnut leaves, dry them in the sun jest lak tea leaves, and we wouldn't let them leaves git wet fur nothin' in the world while they wuz dryin'. We'd take poke salad roots, boil them and then take sugar and make a syrup. This wuz the best thing fur asthma. It was known to cure it too. Fur colds and sich we used ho'hound; made candy out'n it with brown sugar. We used a lots of rock candy and whiskey fur colds too. They had a remedy that they used fur consumption—take dry cow manure, make a tea of this and flavor it with mint and give it to the sick pusson. We didn't need many doctors then fur we didn't have so much sickness in them days, and nachelly they didn't die so fast; folks lived a long time then. They used a lot of peachtree leaves too for fever, and when the stomach got upsot we'd crush the leaves, pour water over them and wouldn't let them drink any other kind of water 'till they wuz better. Ah still believes in them ole ho'made medicines too and ah don't believe in so many doctors."

---

7 [Transcriber's note: no?]

Georgia Narratives, Part 4

John F. Van Hook, Age 76; Newton Bridge Road, Athens, Georgia

Written by: Mrs. Sadie B. Hornsby, Area 6 Athens
Edited by: Sarah H. Hall (Athens) and John N. Booth (Area Supervisor of Federal Writers' Project—Areas 6 & 7, Augusta, Ga.); Dec. 1, 1938

"We learned to use lots of herbs and other home-made remedies during the war when medicine was scarce at the stores, and some old folks still use these simple teas and poultices. Comfrey was a herb used much for poultices on risings, boils, and the like, and tea made from it is said to be soothing to the nerves. Garlic tea was much used for worms, but it was also counted a good pneumonia remedy, and garlic poultices helped folks to breathe when they had grippe or pneumonia. Boneset tea was for colds. Goldenrod was used leaf, stem, blossom, and all in various ways, chiefly for fever and coughs. Black snake root was a good cure for childbed fever, and it saved the life of my second wife after her last child was born. Slippery ellum[8] was used for poultices to heal burns, bruises, and any abrasions, and we gargled slippery ellum tea to heal sore throats, but red oak bark tea was our best sore throat remedy. For indigestion and shortness of the breath we chewed calamus root or drank tea made from it. In fact, we still think it is mighty useful for those purposes. It was a long time after the war before there were any darkies with enough medical education to practice as doctors. Dr. Doyle in Gainesville was the first colored physician that I ever saw."

---

8   *Slippery ellum*: Slippery Elm.

Themes

Manus Dei
FAITH AND MEDICINE

Although it's now common to think of science and medicine as purely secular and separate from religion, historically medicine has been associated with deities and theology much more often than not. Greek physician Herophilos (335–280 BCE), a pioneer in anatomy and surgery, claimed that the physician is the "hand of God," or *manus Dei*. This connection to the divine finds its way into medical texts and codes of ethics for centuries after. For example, "The Oath" by Hippocrates (ca. fifth–fourth century BCE, pp. 25–26) begins with an invocation of the Greek gods of medicine. And in the sixteenth century, Paracelsus defends his own methods by deferring to the Christian God, who "composed the recipe of Nature" and is Himself both "Physician and the Remedy" (p. 89). Additionally, sickness was (and sometimes still is) seen as a punishment for sin or misbehavior. The word "plague" derives from the Latin word *plaga*, meaning "to strike or hit," and gods were thought to use such plagues to strike down the wicked. This negative connotation remains when modern epidemic outbreaks are labeled as plagues. In this section, we look at a few intersections between sickness and medicine and theological belief.

Sutrasthanam: Sushruta's Compendium*

SUSHRUTA
(Indian, ca. sixth century BCE)

Ayurveda is an ancient Indian medical system that emphasizes balance and moderation and is widely practiced across the Indian subcontinent. Although modern Western science often disregards Ayurveda, along with other alternative medicines, the system's practices are acknowledged by the World Health Organization as an important contribution to health care. *Sushruta's Compendium* (*Sushruta Samhita*) is an ancient Sanskrit Ayurvedic text and a comprehensive collection of medicine and surgery. It was composed by the Indian physician Sushruta (see also pp. 11–17). The Sutrasthanam, which refers to the first part of the text, opens with the legend of the divine origins of medicine.

---

* Reprinted from *An English Translation of* The Sushruta Samhita, *Based on Original Sanskrit Text*, 3 vols. trans. and ed. Kaviraj Kunja Lal Bhishagratna (Calcutta, 1907), 1: 1–2, Internet Archive.

The Origin of the Science of Medicine

Well, we shall now describe the origin of the Science of Medicine, as disclosed by the holy Dhanvantari[1] to his disciple Sushruta.

Once upon a time, when the holy Dhanvantari, the greatest of the mighty celestials, incarnated in the form of Divodása, the king of Kási, was blissfully seated, in his hermitage, surrounded by a concourse of holy Rishis; Aupadhenava, Vaitarana, Aurabhra, Paushkalávata, Karavirya, Gopura-rakshita, Sushruta[2] and others addressed him as follows: "O Sire, it grieves us much to find men, though otherwise well befriended by their kin and relations, falling a prey to diseases, mental, physical, traumatic, or natural, and piteously wailing in agony like utterly friendless creatures on earth; and we supplicate thee, O Lord, to illumine our minds with the truths of the Eternal Ayurveda (Medical Science) so that we may faithfully discharge the duties allotted to us in life, and alleviate the sufferings of humanity at large. Bliss in this life and hereafter, is in the gift of this eternal Ayurveda, and for this, O Lord, we have made bold to approach thee as thy humble disciples." To them, thus replied the holy Dhanvantari: "Welcome to all of you to this blissful hermitage. All of you are worth of the honor of true pupilship or tutelage."

---

1   *Dhanvantari*: Hindu god of medicine.
2   In Vedic traditions, Rishis are enlightened sages; the Rishis listed here are responsible for important medical and surgical Ayurvedic works.

Biblical and Apocryphal Sources*

VARIOUS AUTHORS
(ca. eighth–third century BCE)

The development of the biblical canon has a rich and complex history. Within the many books that have been, at some point, considered for inclusion in Jewish and Christian scripture, several works see divine workings in the practice of medicine. In the selection included here from Isaiah 38, Hezekiah, the thirteenth king of Judah (ca. 739–ca. 687 BCE), was seen as righteous and pious, a model of faith and obedience. This account, possibly authored by the prophet Isaiah in the eighth century BCE, describes Hezekiah's faith and the divine intervention that restored him to health after a serious illness. The second selection is an excerpt from Sirach, or Ecclesiasticus, which is an apocryphal (disputed) book of the Bible. It is canonical in Catholic, Eastern Orthodox, and Oriental Orthodox churches, but is omitted from the canon by Protestant Christian denominations and the Hebrew Tanakh. A Hebrew collection of ethical teachings, it contains the designation of the physician as divinely ordained.

---

* Reprinted from Isa. 38:1–22; Sir. 38:1–15 (World English Bible).

Hezekiah's Divine Recovery: Isaiah 38

[1] In those days Hezekiah was sick and near death.[1] Isaiah the prophet, the son of Amoz, came to him, and said to him, "Yahweh[2] says, 'Set your house in order, for you will die, and not live.'"

[2] Then Hezekiah turned his face to the wall and prayed to Yahweh,

[3] and said, "Remember now, Yahweh, I beg you, how I have walked before you in truth and with a perfect heart, and have done that which is good in your sight." Then Hezekiah wept bitterly.

[4] Then Yahweh's word came to Isaiah, saying,

[5] "Go, and tell Hezekiah, 'Yahweh, the God of David your father, says, "I have heard your prayer. I have seen your tears. Behold, I will add fifteen years to your life.

[6] I will deliver you and this city out of the hand of the king of Assyria, and I will defend this city.

[7] This shall be the sign to you from Yahweh, that Yahweh will do this thing that he has spoken.

[8] Behold, I will cause the shadow on the sundial, which has gone down on the sundial of Ahaz with the sun, to return backward ten steps."'" So the sun returned ten steps on the sundial on which it had gone down.

[9] The writing of Hezekiah king of Judah, when he had been sick, and had recovered of his sickness:

[10] I said, "In the middle of my life I go into the gates of Sheol.[3] I am deprived of the residue of my years."

[11] I said, "I won't see Yah, Yah[4] in the land of the living. I will see man no more with the inhabitants of the world.

[12] My dwelling is removed, and is carried away from me like a shepherd's tent. I have rolled up my life like a weaver. He will cut me off from the loom. From day even to night you will make an end of me.

---

1 Versions of this story also occur in the canonical books 2 Kings and 2 Chron.
2 *Yahweh*: A form of the Hebrew name for God, presented as *yhwh* in Scripture (with uncertain and thus unpronounceable vowels).
3 *Sheol*: The place of the dead.
4 *Yah, Yah*: Short for Yahweh and repeated for emphasis; sometimes translated as "the Lord himself."

[13] I waited patiently until morning. He breaks all my bones like a lion. From day even to night you will make an end of me.

[14] I chattered like a swallow or a crane. I moaned like a dove. My eyes weaken looking upward. Lord, I am oppressed. Be my security."

[15] What will I say? He has both spoken to me, and himself has done it. I will walk carefully all my years because of the anguish of my soul.

[16] Lord, men live by these things; and my spirit finds life in all of them. You restore me, and cause me to live.

[17] Behold, for peace I had great anguish, but you have in love for my soul delivered it from the pit of corruption; for you have cast all my sins behind your back.

[18] For Sheol can't praise you. Death can't celebrate you. Those who go down into the pit can't hope for your truth.

[19] The living, the living, he shall praise you, as I do today. The father shall make known your truth to the children.

[20] Yahweh will save me. Therefore we will sing my songs with stringed instruments all the days of our life in Yahweh's house.

[21] Now Isaiah had said, "Let them take a cake of figs, and lay it for a poultice on the boil, and he shall recover."

[22] Hezekiah also had said, "What is the sign that I will go up to Yahweh's house?"

Medicine and the Manus Dei: Sirach 38

[1] Honor a physician according to your need with the honors due to him, for truly the Lord has created him.

[2] For healing comes from the Most High, and he shall receive a gift from the king.

[3] The skill of the physician will lift up his head. He will be admired in the sight of great men.

[4] The Lord created medicines out of the earth. A prudent man will not despise them.

[5] Wasn't water made sweet with wood, that its power might be known?

[6] He gave men skill that he might be glorified in his marvelous works.

[7] With them he heals and takes away pain.

[8] With these, the pharmacist makes a mixture. God's works won't be brought to an end. From him, peace is upon the face of the earth.

[9] My son, in your sickness don't be negligent, but pray to the Lord, and he will heal you.

[10] Put away wrong doing, and direct your hands in righteousness. Cleanse your heart from all sin.

[11] Give a sweet savor and a memorial of fine flour, and pour oil on your offering, according to your means.

[12] Then give place to the physician, for truly the Lord has created him. Don't let him leave you, for you need him.

[13] There is a time when in recovery is in their hands.

[14] For they also shall ask the Lord to prosper them in diagnosis and in healing for the maintenance of life.

[15] He who sins before his Maker, let him fall into the hands of the physician.

Airmed and the Divine Knowledge of Healing Herbs*

UNKNOWN
(Irish, ca. ninth century)

Cath Maighe Tuireadh (*The Second Battle of Mag Tuired*) is a medieval Irish saga, or a long account in prose of historical or legendary events. In this saga, Airmed, a member of the Celtic pantheon called the Tuatha Dé Danann, carries with her the knowledge of all the healing herbs in the world. The legend included here is likely based on a ninth century version. It recounts a deadly dispute between Airmed's brother Miach and her father Dian-cecht over how to treat deposed king Nuada's amputated arm. After 365 healing herbs grow from Miach's body, Airmed gathers them and catalogs them by their medical use. However, Dian-cecht scatters the herbs so widely that no human could know their properties without Airmed's assistance, ensuring the continued connection between physicians and the divine.

---

* Reprinted from Whitley Stokes, trans., *Revue Celtique* (Paris, 1891), 69, Internet Archive. The work is extant in two manuscripts in the British Library, Harley MS 5280 (early sixteenth century) and Royal Irish Academy, MS 24 p. 9 (1651), but it is thought to have been compiled around the twelfth century based on ninth century materials.

The Second Battle of Mag Tuired

Now Nuada was in his sickness, and Dian-cecht put on him a hand of silver with the motion of every hand therein. That seemed evil to his son Miach. He went to the hand (which had been struck off Dian-cecht), and he said "joint to joint of it and sinew to sinew," and he healed Nuada in thrice three days and nights. The first seventy-two hours he put it over against his side, and it became covered with skin. The second seventy-two hours he put it on his breasts. The third seventy-two hours he would cast white ... of black bulrushes when they were blackened in fire.

That cure seemed evil to Dian-cecht. He flung a sword on the crown of his son's head and cut the skin down to the flesh. The lad healed the wound by means of his skill. Dian-cecht smote him again and cut the flesh till he reached the bone. The lad healed this by the same means. He struck him the third blow and came to the membrane of his brain. The lad healed this also by the same means. Then he struck the fourth blow and cut out the brain, so that Miach died, and Dian-cecht said that the leech himself could not heal him of that blow.

Thereafter Miach was buried by Dian-cecht, and herbs three hundred and sixty-five, according to the number of his joints and sinews, grew through the grave. Then Airmed opened her mantle and separated those herbs according to their properties. But Dian-cecht came to her, and he confused the herbs, so that no one knows their proper cures unless the Holy Spirit should teach them afterwards. And Dian-cecht said "If Miach be not, Airmed shall remain."

Erra, the Plague God*

UNKNOWN
(Assyrian, ca. eighth century BCE)

In Assyrian and Mesopotamian theology, which was practiced circa 3500 BCE through 400 CE in parts of what is now the Middle East, fevers and disease were thought to be caused by powerful spirits. These beliefs are recorded in cuneiform inscriptions from the period. Cuneiform, in which symbols were created by pressing a stylus into clay tablets, is one of the earliest writing systems in the world. Also recorded in cuneiform is evidence that epidemics struck the region during this time. At least one widespread outbreak of a possible strain of influenza hit Mesopotamia in 1200 BCE, before spreading to southern Asia. While there were also healing gods to whom practitioners could appeal for cure, the legend of Erra (also known as Irra or Ura), a god associated with plague, promises to not punish with infection those who worship him directly. The excerpt included here was published in 1903 but originally recorded in Leonard William King's *The First Steps in Assyrian* in 1898, which transliterated the song from original cuneiform tablets housed in the British Museum.

---

* Adapted from Reginald Campbell Thompson, *The Devils and Evil Spirits of Babylonia: Being Babylonian and Assyrian Incantations against the Demons* [...] *which Attack Mankind* (London: Luzac, 1903), XLVII, Internet Archive.

The Song of Erra, the Plague-God

The power of spreading particular diseases was attributed to certain demons such as Erra, the plague-spirit, and Ashakku, the fever spirit. There is a legend about Erra, the plague-spirit, which gives the vainglorious speech he made to Ishum:[1]

Erra was angry, and determined
To ravage the whole world,
But Ishum, his counsellor, appeased him
That he abandoned [his wrath]....
And thus spake the hero Erra: [5]
"Whosoever shall praise this song,
In his shrine may plenty abound....
Whosoever shall magnify my name,
May her rule the four quarters of the world;
Whosoever shall proclaim the glory of my valor, [10]
Shall have none to oppose him;
The singer who chants it shall not die in pestilence,
But unto king and noble his speech shall be well-pleasing;
The scribe who learns it shall escape from the foe....
In the shrine of the peoples where he cries my name continually [15]
His understanding will I increase.
In the house where this tablet is set,
Though I, Erra, be angry or the Imina-bi gods[2] bring havoc,
Yet the dagger of pestilence shall not approach it,
Immunity shall rest upon it." [20]

---

1 *Ishum*: God of fire and advisor to Erra.
2 *Imina-bi gods*: The Divine Heptad, or a group of seven warrior gods associated with the Pleiades constellation.

Pythian Odes III—For Hieron of Syracuse[*]

PINDAR
(Greek, ca. 518–438 BCE)

The Greek god of medicine Asclepius exceeded everyone in the healing arts, including his teacher, the centaur Chiron. He was the son of a Thessalian princess and Apollo, god of health and disease—plague outbreaks were attributed to his vengeful arrows—in addition to being the god of music, poetry, and the sun. Asclepius's skill was so great that he wielded the power of resurrection and was killed by the gods, though accounts of this vary. After his earthly death, Asclepius was allowed to enter the pantheon (or group of deities in a religion) on Olympus as the primary god of medicine. Asclepius was father to the Asclepiades: five daughters and three sons who all became associated with the healing arts. His daughters also reached the status of minor deities, each governing a specific aspect of health: Aegle (vigor and beauty), Aceso (the healing process), Iaso (recuperation from illness), Panacea (universal remedy), and Hygeia (health and hygiene). Asclepius is often depicted carrying a staff with a single snake wrapped around it [See Illustration 6]. This object, the "Rod of Asclepius," is the symbol of medicine and health care [See Illustration 7]. Included here is a mythological account of Asclepius's birth and skill as a healer by the Greek lyric poet Pindar.

---

[*] Reprinted from John Edwin Sandys, trans., *The Odes of Pindar, including the Principal Fragments* (New York: Macmillan, 1915), 185–89, Google Books.

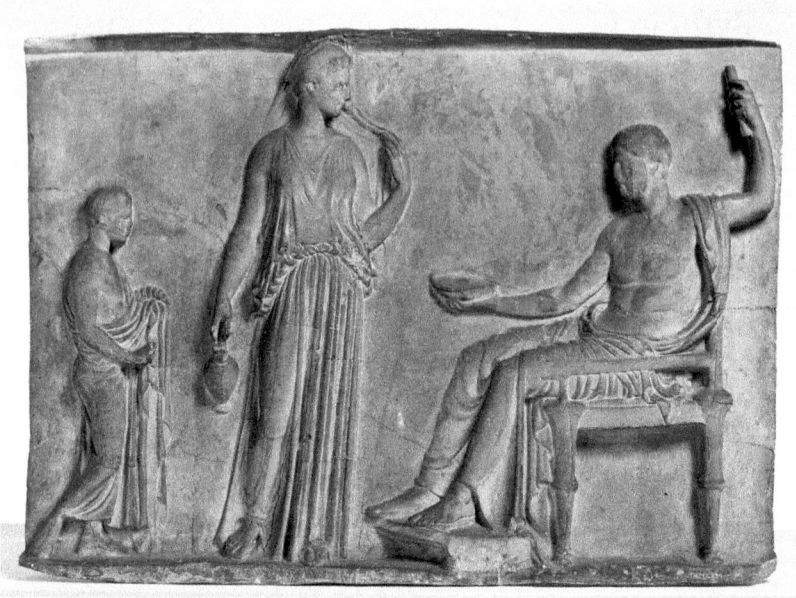

Illustration 6. Greek God of Medicine Asclepius and Hygeia, ca. 400 BCE. Marble relief, 19 × 27.8 in. (48.5 × 70.5 cm). The Gregoriano Etrusco Museum, Hall of the Greek Originals, Vatican.

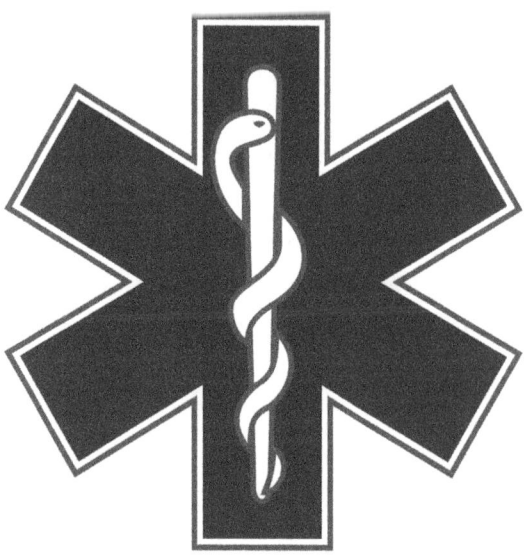

Illustration 7. The Star of Life, a modern medical symbol featuring the Rod of Asclepius.

[Asclepius's Birth]

If the poet's tongue might breathe the prayer that is on the lips of all, I would pray that Chiron, son of Philyra, who is dead and gone, were now alive again—he who once ruled far and wide as the offspring of Cronus, who was the son of Heaven. Would that that rugged monster with spirit kindly unto men, were reigning still in Pelion's glens, even such as when, in olden days, he reared Asclepius, that gentle craftsman who drove pain from the limbs that he healed, that hero who gave aid in all manner of maladies.

Or ever[1] the daughter of Phlegyas could bear him, in the fullness of time, with the aid of Eleithuia, the goddess of child-birth, she was stricken in her chamber by the golden arrows of Artemis, and thus descended to the home of Hades by the counsels of Apollo. Not in vain is the wrath of the sons of Zeus. For she, in the errors of her heart, had lightly regarded that wrath; and, although she had aforetime consorted with Phoebus[2] of the unshorn hair, and bare within her the pure seed of the god, yet without her father's knowledge she consented to be wedded to another. She waited not for the coming of the marriage feast, nor for the music of the full-voiced hymeneal[3] chorus, even the playful strains that maiden-mates love to utter in evening songs. No! she was enamored of an absent love, that passion which many ere now have felt. For among men, there is a foolish company of those who, putting shame on their home, cast their glances afar, and pursue idle dreams in hopes that shall not be fulfilled.

Such was the strong infatuation that the spirit of the fair-robed Coronis had caught. For she slept in the couch of a stranger who came from Arcadia; but she escaped not the ken of the watchful god; for, although he was then at the sacrificial shrine of Pytho, yet Loxias, the king of the temple, perceived it in his mind that knoweth all things, with his thought convinced by an unerring prompter....

---

1 *Or ever*: Before.
2 *Phoebus*: Another name for Apollo.
3 *Hymeneal*: Relating to marriage; named for Hymen, Greek god of marriage (and another son of Apollo's).

But, when the kinsmen had placed the girl in the midst of the wooden walls of the pyre, and the wild flame of the fire-god was playing around it, then spake Apollo: "No longer can I endure in my heart to slay my own child by a death most piteous, at the self-same time as its mother's grievous doom." He stepped forward but once, and anon he found his child, and snatched it from the corpse, while the kindled fire opened for him a path of light; and he bare the babe away, and gave it to the Magnesian Centaur to teach it how to heal mortal men of painful maladies.

And those whosoever came suffering from the sores of nature, or with their limbs wounded either by gray bronze or by far-hurled stone, or with bodies wasting away with summer's heat or winter's cold, he loosed and delivered diverse of them from diverse pains, tending some of them with kindly incantations, giving to others a soothing potion, or, haply, swathing their limbs with simples,[4] or restoring others by the knife.

---

4 *Simples*: Medicines made from a single active ingredient, such as an herb.

Compare & Consider

COMPARE

Examine the explicit connections between medicine and the divine illustrated here with the way belief (either spiritual or secular) is reflected in ethical works (Hippocrates, pp. 26–30; Guy de Chauliac, pp. 67–68; and Thomas Percival, pp. 194–199) or works about disease etiology and treatment (Rhazes, pp. 47–56; Girolamo Fracastoro, pp. 75–83; Paracelsus, pp. 90–95; Zabdiel Boylston, pp. 167–171; and Edward Jenner, pp. 187–193).

CONSIDER

How does thinking of health, sickness, and medicine as a part of spiritual or religious belief help (or impede) medical practice? What, if anything, has taken the place of the "divine" in modern medical science? How do texts change (in approach or in style) when they reflect spiritual versus secular beliefs?

What You See
ASSUMPTION, ANXIETY, AND THE APPEARANCE OF HEALTH

Looks aren't everything, so the saying goes. Yet people are judged based upon their appearances every day. For instance, individuals who appear "monstrous" have historically evoked pity and disgust, regardless of the cause of their appearance. The word "monster" derives from the Latin word *monstrum*, which means sign or portent. In early ancient Greek and Roman accounts, creatures deemed monsters were often seen as frightful, disorderly, and immoral, their existence a sign that something has gone terribly wrong. And "monstrous births" (many of which display features we now recognize as congenital disorders) were understood to be the result of some failing or mistake [See Illustration 8]. They also are often assumed to be immoral or dangerous. In some contexts, the way a person looks has been thought to imply something about their health. Cultural standards for beauty are often tied to ideas of healthfulness, as well, and people who are larger, or smaller, or who have physical differences may all be negatively labeled or ostracized. Additionally, sometimes it's what we can't see that causes problems: someone who "doesn't look sick" may have legitimate concerns regarding pain, disability, or mental health disregarded, and concerns about what happens in the womb (which was long invisible) can prompt intense anxiety. This section provides a glimpse at "monstrosity" as it has sometimes been understood and examines how what we see impacts our assumptions about a person's health.

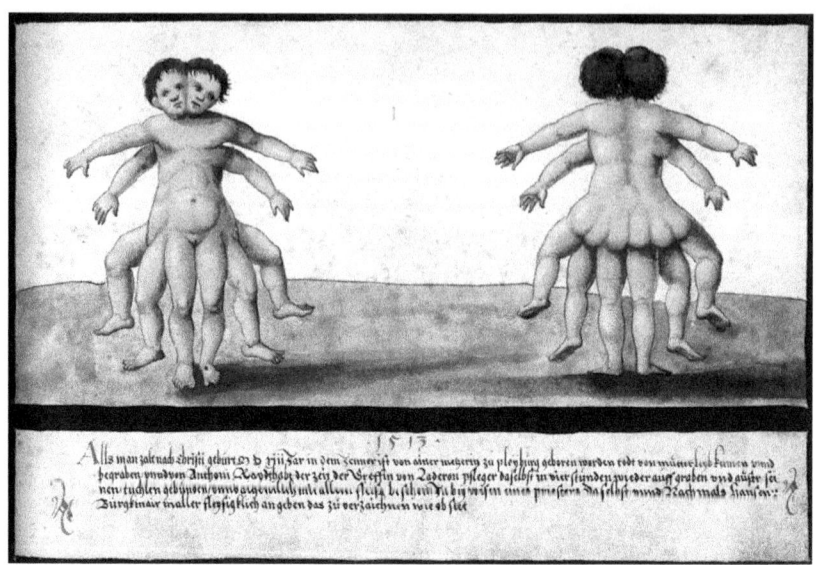

Illustration 8. Depiction of a Monstrous Birth. *Augsburg Book of Miracles*, ca. 1552, folio 93. This illuminated manuscript from Augsburg, Germany, is filled with images depicting events and living beings that were understood as signs of both miracles and warnings. Among them is an illustration of a child born with two heads and extra limbs. Wikimedia Commons.

Of a Monstrous Child*

MICHEL DE MONTAIGNE
(French, 1533–1592)

French philosopher Michel de Montaigne (1533–1592) is known for popularizing the essay as a literary genre. In fact, he was the first to call his short prose works "essays," or *essais* in French, meaning "attempts." In these essays, he often took up issues related to health. He frequently incorporated quotes from ancient Greek philosophers and contemporary writers to underscore his exploration of a topic. Here, he considers monstrous births after encountering a child born with physical deformities, and takes a more sympathetic approach than do many of his contemporaries who take on the issue.

---

* Reprinted from Michel de Montaigne, *Essays of Michel de Montaigne*, vol. 2, trans. Charles Cotton, ed. William Carew Hazlitt (London: Reeves and Turner, 1877; Project Gutenberg, 2016), chap. 30.

Of a Monstrous Child

This story shall go by itself; for I will leave it to physicians to discourse of. Two days ago I saw a child that two men and a nurse, who said they were the father, the uncle, and the aunt of it, carried about to get money by showing it, by reason it was so strange a creature. It was, as to all the rest, of a common form, and could stand upon its feet; could go and gabble much like other children of the same age; it had never as yet taken any other nourishment but from the nurse's breasts, and what, in my presence, they tried to put into the mouth of it, it only chewed a little and spat it out again without swallowing; the cry of it seemed indeed a little odd and particular, and it was just fourteen months old. Under the breast it was joined to another child, but without a head, and which had the spine of the back without motion, the rest entire; for though it had one arm shorter than the other, it had been broken by accident at their birth; they were joined breast to breast, and as if a lesser child sought to throw its arms about the neck of one something bigger. The juncture and thickness of the place where they were conjoined was not above four fingers, or thereabouts, so that if you thrust up the imperfect child you might see the navel of the other below it, and the joining was betwixt the paps and the navel. The navel of the imperfect child could not be seen, but all the rest of the belly, so that all that was not joined of the imperfect one, as arms, buttocks, thighs, and legs, hung dangling upon the other, and might reach to the mid-leg. The nurse, moreover, told us that it urined at both bodies, and that the members of the other were nourished, sensible, and in the same plight with that she gave suck to, excepting that they were shorter and less. This double body and several limbs relating to one head might be interpreted a favorable prognostic to the king—[Henry III.]—of maintaining these various parts of our state under the union of his laws; but lest the event should prove otherwise, 'tis better to let it alone, for in things already past there needs no divination,

> "Ut quum facts sunt, tum ad conjecturam
> aliqui interpretatione revocentur;"

["So as when they are come to pass, they may then by some interpretation be recalled to conjecture"
—Cicero, De Divin., ii. 31.]

as 'tis said of Epimenides, that he always prophesied backward.

I have just seen a herdsman in Medoc, of about thirty years of age, who has no sign of any genital parts; he has three holes by which he incessantly voids his water; he is bearded, has desire, and seeks contact with women.

Those that we call monsters are not so to God, who sees in the immensity of His work the infinite forms that He has comprehended therein; and it is to be believed that this figure which astonishes us has relation to some other figure of the same kind unknown to man. From His all wisdom nothing but good, common; and regular proceeds; but we do not discern the disposition and relation:

"Quod crebro videt, non miratur, etiamsi,
cur fiat, nescit. Quod ante non vidit, id,
si evenerit, ostentum esse censet."

["What he often sees he does not admire, though he be ignorant how
it comes to pass. When a thing happens he never saw before, he thinks that it is a portent."
—Cicero, De Divin., ii. 22.]

Whatever falls out contrary to custom we say is contrary to nature, but nothing, whatever it be, is contrary to her.[1] Let, therefore, this universal and natural reason expel the error and astonishment that novelty brings along with it.

---

1   When something differs from our cultural expectation, we claim that it is unnatural, but nothing made by nature can ever be unnatural.

Of Monsters and Prodigies*

AMBROISE PARÉ
(French, ca. 1510–1590)

French barber-surgeon Ambroise Paré (see pp. 125–132) was a prolific author of works on medicine and surgery. In "Of Monsters and Prodigies," Paré writes of monsters as a sign of God's power and introduces the concept of maternal impression. According to the maternal impression theory—a belief that persisted from antiquity through the nineteenth century—congenital disorders were caused by the thoughts and feelings imprinting themselves on the growing fetus [See Illustration 9]. For example, a pregnant woman frightened by a bear might have a very hirsute child, and a woman experiencing great agitation, anxiety, or depression during pregnancy might transmit those conditions in utero. The following excerpts are drawn from his popular work on monstrosity originally published in French in 1534, and translated into English over a century later.

---

* Reprinted from Ambroise Paré, *The Workes of that Famous Chirurgion Ambrose Parey*, trans. Thomas Johnson (London, 1645), 648, 659, Google Books.

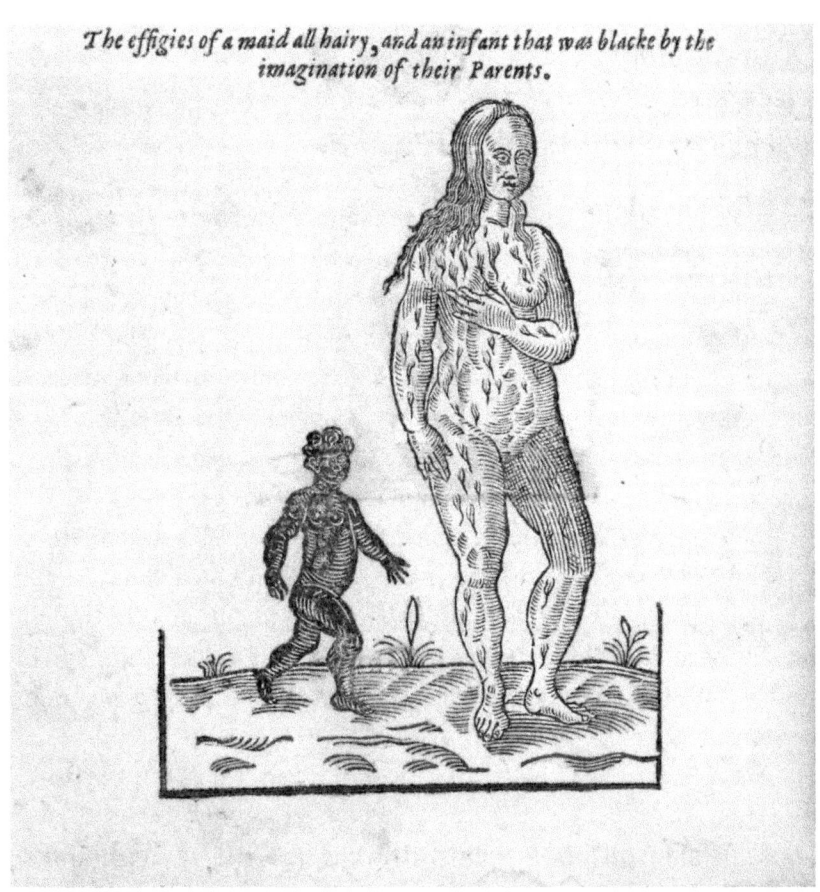

Illustration 9. Effects of Maternal Impression. The text reads, "The effigies of a maid all hairy, and an infant that was blacke by the imagination of their Parents." Woodcut illustration of a woman covered in hair, beside her a small black child. Reprinted from Ambroise Paré, *The Workes of that famous Chirurgion Ambrose Parey Translated out of Latine and Compared with the French*, trans. Thomas Johnson (London: 1634), chap. 7, p. 623. Library of Congress, Rare Book and Special Collections Division.

Of the cause of Monsters; and first of those Monsters which appear for the glory of God, and the punishment of men's wickedness

There are reckoned up many causes of monsters; the first whereof is the glory of God, that his immense power may be manifested to those which are ignorant of it, by the sending of those things which happen contrary to nature: for thus our Savior Christ answered the Disciples (asking whether he or his parents had offended, who, being born blind, received his sight from him) that neither he nor his parents had committed any fault so great, but this to have happened only that the glory and majesty of God should be divulged by that miracle, and such great works.

Another cause is, that God may either punish men's wickedness, or show signs of punishment at hand, because parents sometimes lie and join themselves together without law and measure, or luxuriously and beastly, or at such times as they ought to forbear by the command of God and the Church, such monstrous, horrid and unnatural births do happen.

Of monsters which take their cause and shape by imagination

The ancients having diligently sought into all the secrets of nature, have marked and observed other causes of the generation of monsters: for, understanding the force of imagination to be so powerful in us, as for the most part, it may alter the body of them that imagine, they soon persuaded themselves that the faculty which forms the infant may be led and governed by the firm and strong cogitation of the parents begetting them (often deluded by nocturnal and deceitful apparitions) or by the mother conceiving them, and so that which is strongly conceived in the mind, imprints the force into the infant conceived in the womb: which thing many think to be confirmed by Moses, because he tells[1] that Jacob increased and bettered the part of the sheep granted to him by

---

1   This story appears in Bereshit, or Genesis, the first book of the Hebrew Bible (the Tanakh) and Christian Old Testament—see Gen. 30:25–43.

Laban, his wife's father, by putting rods, having the bark in part pulled off, finely stroked with white and green, in the places where they used to drink, especially at the time they engendered, that the representation apprehended in the conception, should be presently impressed in the young; for the force of imagination hath so much power over the infant, that it sets upon it the notes or characters of the thing conceived.

We have read in Heliodorus[2] that Persinna, Queen of Ethiopia, by her husband Hidustes, being also an Ethiope, had a daughter of a white complexion, because in the embraces of her husband, by which she proved with child, she earnestly fixed her eye and mind upon the picture of the fair Andromeda standing opposite to her. Damascene reports that he saw a maid hairy like a bear, who had that deformity by no other cause or occasion than that her mother earnestly beheld, in the very instant of receiving and conceiving the seed, the image of St. John covered with a camel's skin, hanging upon the posts of the bed.

They say Hippocrates, by this explication of the causes, freed a certain noble woman from suspicion of adultery, who being white her self, and her husband also white, brought forth a child as black as an Ethiopian, because in copulation she strongly and continually had in her mind the picture of the Ethiope.

---

[2] This story appears in Heliodorus of Emesa's *Aethiopica*, an early Greek work rediscovered in the early modern period.

On Reproduction and Generation*

PARACELSUS
(Swiss, ca. 1493–1541)

The works of Paracelsus (see pp. 90–95) include detailed considerations of the nature and process of reproduction, and reflect a great number of concerns about what happens in the then-invisible space of the body during pregnancy. This includes theories of maternal impression and monstrosity, as seen in the writings of Paré and de Montaigne earlier in this section, as well as a theory about bypassing the hidden space of the womb altogether by growing an embryo outside the body.

---

* Reprinted from Arthur Edward Waite, trans., *The Hermetic and Alchemical Writings of Aureolus Philippus Thephrastus Bombast, of Hohenheim, Called Paracelsus the Great*, vol. 1 (London: J. Elliott, 1894), 121–25, Google Books.

On Maternal Impression

Whatever the seed is, such is the herb which springs up from it. From the seed of an onion an onion springs up, not a rose, a nut, or a lettuce. So, too, from corn comes corn; from barley, barley; from oats, oats. Thus it is, too, with all other fruits which have seeds and are sown.

In like manner, it is possible, and not contrary to Nature, that from a woman and a man an irrational animal should be born. Neither on this account should the same judgment be passed on a woman as on a man, that is, she should not on this account be deemed heretical, as if she had acted contrary to Nature; but the result must be assigned to imagination. Imagination is very frequently the cause of this: and the imagination of a pregnant woman is so active that in conceiving seed[1] into her body she can transmute the fetus in different ways: since her interior stars are so strongly directed to the fetus that they produce impression and influence. Wherefore an infant in the mother's womb is, during its formation, as much in the hand and under the will of the mother as clay in the hand of a potter, who from it forms and shapes what he likes and whatever pleases him. So the pregnant mother forms the fruit in her own body according to her imagination, and as her stars are. Thus it often happens that from the seed of a man are begotten cattle or other horrible monsters, as the imagination of the mother was strongly directed towards the embryo.

On Monstrous Births

Monstrous human growths rarely live long. The more wonderful and worthy of regard they are, the sooner death comes upon them; so much so that scarcely any one of them exceeds the third day in the presence of human beings, unless it be at once carried into a secret place and segregated from all men. It should be known, forsooth, that God abhors monsters of this kind. They displease Him, and none of them can be saved when they do not bear the likeness of God. One can only

---

1 *Seed*: Semen.

conjecture that they are shaped by the Devil, and born for the service of the Devil rather than of God; since from no monster was any good work ever derived, but, on the contrary, evil and sin, and all kinds of diabolical craft. For as the executioner marks his sons when he cuts off their ears, gouges out their eyes, brands their cheeks, cuts off their fingers, hands, or head, so the Devil, too, marks his own sons, through the imagination of the mother, which they derive from her evil desires, lusts, and thoughts in conception. All men, therefore, should be avoided who have more or less than the usual numbers of any member, or have any member duplicated. For that is a presage of the Devil, and a certain sign of hidden wickedness and craft.

On the Homunculus

But neither must we by any means forget the generation of homunculi.[2] For there is some truth in this thing, although for a long time it was held in the most occult manner and with secrecy, while there was no little doubt and question among the old Philosophers, whether it was possible to[3] Nature and Art, that a man should be begotten without the female body and the natural womb. I answer hereto, that this is in no way opposed to Spagyric Art and to Nature, nay, that it is perfectly possible.[4] In order to accomplish it, you must proceed thus: Let the semen of a man putrefy by itself in a sealed cucurbite with the highest putrefaction of the *venter equinus*[5] for forty days, or until it begins at last to live, move, and be agitated, which can easily be seen. After this time it will be in some degree like a human being, but, nevertheless, transparent

---

2 One early model of reproductive theory called preformationism asserted that human embryo began as a fully formed but miniscule person (a homunculus, or homunculi in the plural), and that it would grow to its infant size over the course of gestation. This theory was in contrast to epigenesis, in which the embryo developed in parts.
3 *To*: According to.
4 Here Paracelsus tells us that making a homunculus is not impossible—for alchemists.
5 *Venter equinus*: Horse manure, used frequently in alchemy because it emits heat as it decomposes.

and without body. If now, after this, it be every day nourished and fed cautiously and prudently with the arcanum of human blood, and kept for forty weeks in the perpetual and equal heat of a *venter equinus*, it becomes, thenceforth a true and living infant, having all the members of a child that is born from a woman, but much smaller. This we call a homunculus; and it should be afterwards educated with the greatest care and zeal, until it grows up and begins to display intelligence. Now, this is one of the greatest secrets which God has revealed to mortal and fallible man. It is a miracle and marvel of God, an arcanum above all arcana, and deserves to be kept secret until the last times, when there shall be nothing hidden, but all things shall be made manifest. And although up to this time it has not been known to men, it was, nevertheless, known to the wood-sprites and nymphs and giants long ago, because they themselves were sprung from this source; since from such homunculi when they come to manhood are produced giants, pygmies, and other marvelous people, who are the instruments of great things, who get great victories over their enemies, and know all secret and hidden matters.

Mary Toft's Extraordinary Delivery*

NATHANIEL SAINT-ANDRÉ & JOHN HOWARD
(Swiss, 1680–1776) | (English, ca. 1676–1755)

In 1726, young English woman Mary Toft miscarried her third pregnancy. In conversations with curious doctors who flocked to see her, she claimed to have birthed several animal parts during that miscarriage. Among those who attended to Toft were physicians Nathaniel Saint-André and John Howard. Toft explained that she had seen a rabbit while working the fields and determined that the incident had impressed upon the fetus, and thus she had delivered rabbits. Several respected physicians confirmed her reports after being present at the delivery of yet more rabbits, and news of the case spread rapidly. Ultimately, Toft was pressed into confessing: she had fabricated the ordeal in hopes that the renown would improve her economic security. After the hoax was revealed, she and the doctors who believed her were subject to great public ridicule [See Illustration 10]. The following excerpts, published just days before her confession in 1727, tell part of this story.

---

* Reprinted from Nathanial Saint-André and John Howard, *A short narrative of an extraordinary delivery of rabbets, perform'd by Mr John Howard, Surgeon at Guilford* (London, 1727), 4–6, 8–10, Internet Archive.

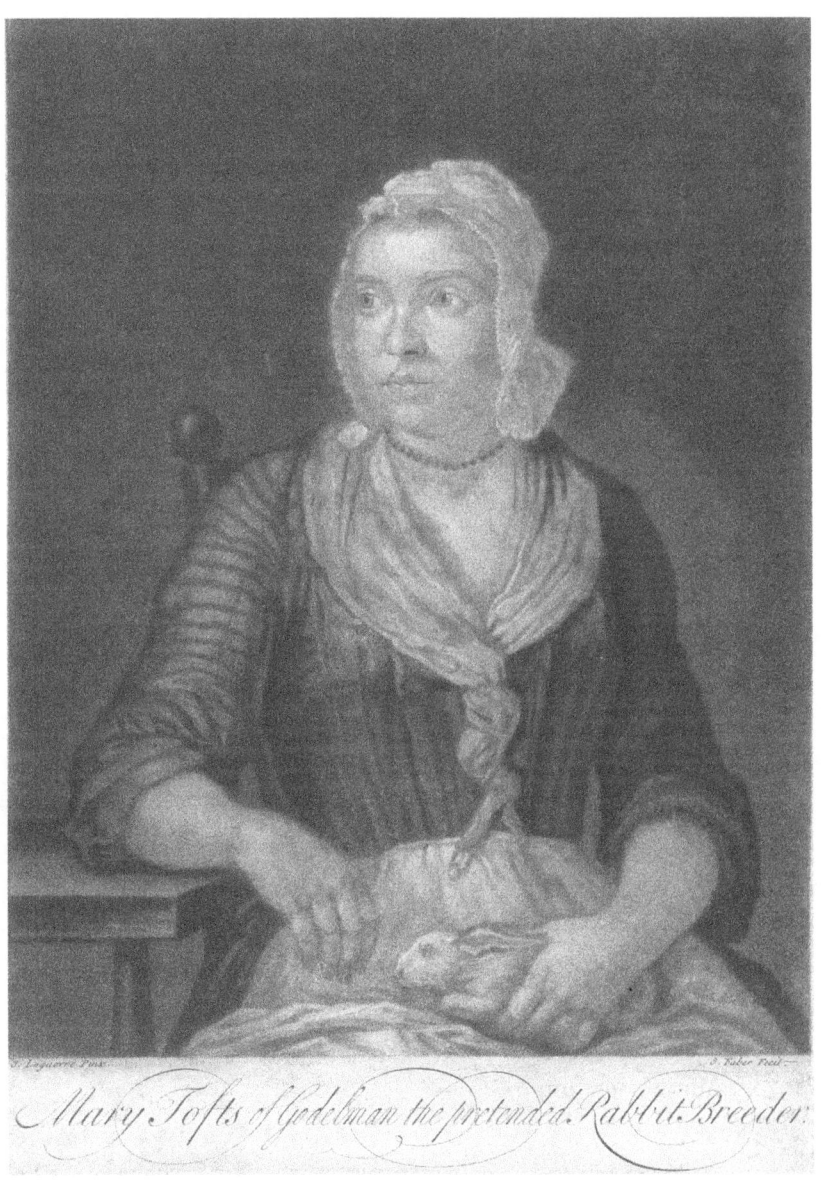

Illustration 10. Portrait of Mary Toft. Lettering reads, "Mary Tofts [sic.] of Godelman the pretended rabbit breeder." Mezzotint by J. Faber, 1726/1727, after J. Laguerre. Wellcome Collection.

A short narrative of an extraordinary delivery of rabbets

The first intelligence I received of this matter, was on the 5th instant, when I saw a very particular account of a woman living at Godlyman lately delivered of five rabbits by Mr. John Howard, surgeon at Guilford in Surrey, a man of known probity, character, and capacity in his profession, who has practiced midwifery for above these thirty years.

This account was again confirmed by two letters from the said Mr. Howard, the first dated Nov. the 6, 4 a clock in the afternoon; the substance of which is, that from the 4th instant to the 6th he had delivered the woman of three more rabbits; that the last of them had leap'd in her belly, for the space of eighteen hours, before it died, and that the moment it was taken away, another was perceived to struggle for birth. The second is dated Nov. the ninth, and is here transcribed verbatim, viz:

Sir,

Since I wrote to you, I have taken or delivered the poor woman of three more rabbits, all three half grown, one of them a dun rabbit; the last leaped twenty three hours in the uterus before it died. As soon as the eleventh rabbit was taken away, up leaped the twelfth rabbit, which is now leaping. If you have any curious person that is pleased to come post, may see another leap in her uterus, and shall take it from her if he pleases; which will be a great satisfaction to the curious: if she had been with child, she has but ten days more to go, so I do not know how many rabbits may be behind; I have brought the woman to Guilford for better convenience.

I am, Sir,
Your humble servant,
John Howard.

*

[Saint-André himself arrives on the scene, to view the curiosity. What follows is his description.]

She was lodged over against Mr. Howard's house, we found her dressed in her stays, sitting on the bed-side with several women near her. I immediately examined her, and, not finding the parts prepared for her labor, I waited for the coming on of fresh pains, which happened in three or four minutes, at which time I delivered her of the entire trunk, stripped of its skin, of a rabbit of about four months growth, in which the heart and lungs were contained with the diaphragm entire....

No person but my self touched her, from the first time I had examined her, to the time of her being delivered by me: her pains were pretty smart,[1] and lasted for some minutes; they went off the moment she was delivered, and she seemed cheerful and easy; walked by herself from the bedside to the Fire, and sat on a chair, where I examined her; and found, that in the course of the Fallopian Tubes, there were some inequalities, but more sensibly on the right side of her belly; which made me conjecture that the rabbits were bred in those tubes, and only came into the uterus, when they gave her those agitations, which, according to the account of Mr Howard, and of several other persons, were sensibly felt many hours before their exclusion.

---

1 *Smart*: Severe.

Phrenology: Topographies of the Skull*

JOHN TAYLOR
(Scottish, nineteenth century)

The notion that a person's character can be judged by their appearance, especially facial features, is an ancient one and common to many cultures. Referred to as physiognomy, the practice of assessing mental or moral qualities in accordance with physical attributes evolved in the late eighteenth century with the theories of German physician named Franz Joseph Gall. He took this idea a step further in developing the field of phrenology: a supposedly scientifically sound study of the shape of the skull and facial features in order to determine a person's character and behavioral traits. Both physiognomy and phrenology are now understood to be pseudoscience. In addition to lacking scientific foundations, tying appearance to beliefs about character and behavior tends to reproduce dangerous ethnic, racial, and cultural stereotypes. Despite this problematic past, phrenology was a fairly popular (if niche) field into the early twentieth century. The first excerpt on phrenology comes from John Taylor, a member of the Edinburgh Phrenological Society and a lecturer on the topic. He wrote *Phrenology Simplified* in 1841 as a guide to the use of a phrenology bust [See Illustration 11].

---

* Reprinted from John Taylor, *Phrenology Simplified*, 2nd ed. (London: Satchwell and Arnold, 1841), iv–v. Wellcome Collection.

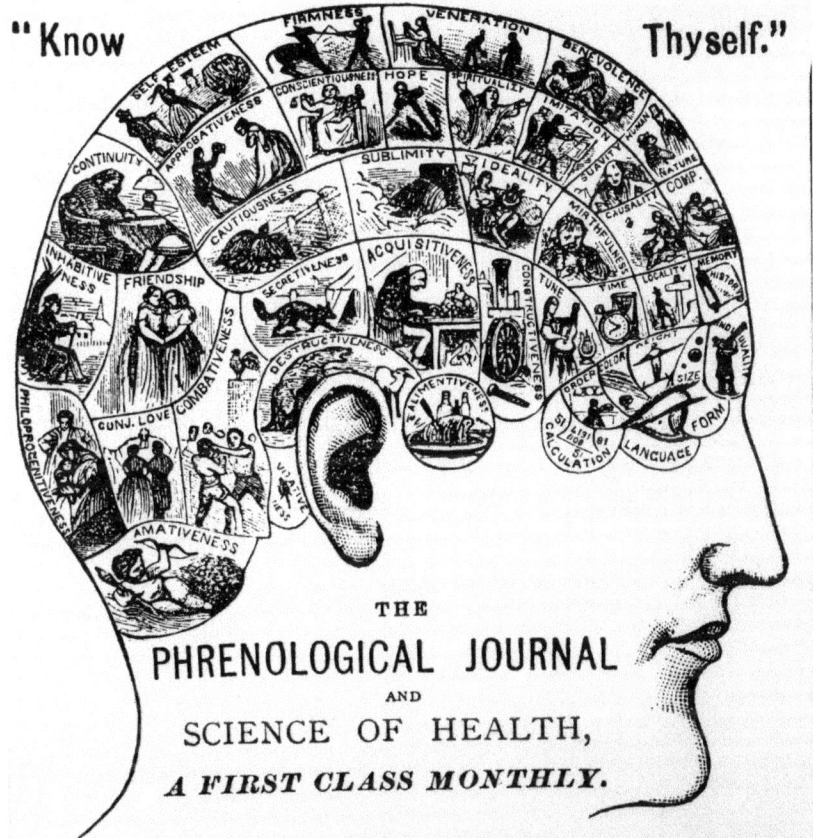

Illustration 11. Know Thyself. Phrenological chart from the *Phrenological Journal* (1881) shows the regions of the skull and the characteristics tied to each. Wellcome Collection.

Phrenology Simplified

With this work and a Phrenological Head,[1] parents, and those having the guardianship of children and youth, will be enabled to discover the capabilities and propensities of those under their charge, and direct their education accordingly....

The author is well satisfied that the Science of Phrenology is only to be properly understood, to be appreciated as one of the most important Sciences that has ever been discovered to the world; bearing as it does on our moral, social, and physical condition—it comes home to every individual, whatever be his conditions, high, low, rich or poor, learned or illiterate, and says to him, "Investigate me and know your capabilities in morals, in intellect, in trade, in science and in art; reject me and for ever remain in doubt and uncertainty, as to those things, yet ever discovering the need of such knowledge."

---

1 *Phrenological head*: A plaster bust of the head with the phrenological regions mapped out on it.

Vaught's Practical Character Reader*

LOUIS ALLEN VAUGHT
(American, 1859–1903)

These illustrations come from the work of American phrenologist Louis Allen Vaught, who sought to guide a general readership in the practical use of phrenological and physiognomic principles in their daily lives. The goal, he asserted, was to "read character," and he believed that "heads, faces, and bodies tell the story." The selections included here present just a few of his ideas about the way character supposedly presents in physical traits. sentimentally [See Illustrations 12, 13, and 14.]

---

* Reprinted from Louis Allen Vaught, *Vaught's Practical Character Reader* (Chicago: L.A. Vaught, 1902), 5, 55–56, Internet Archive.

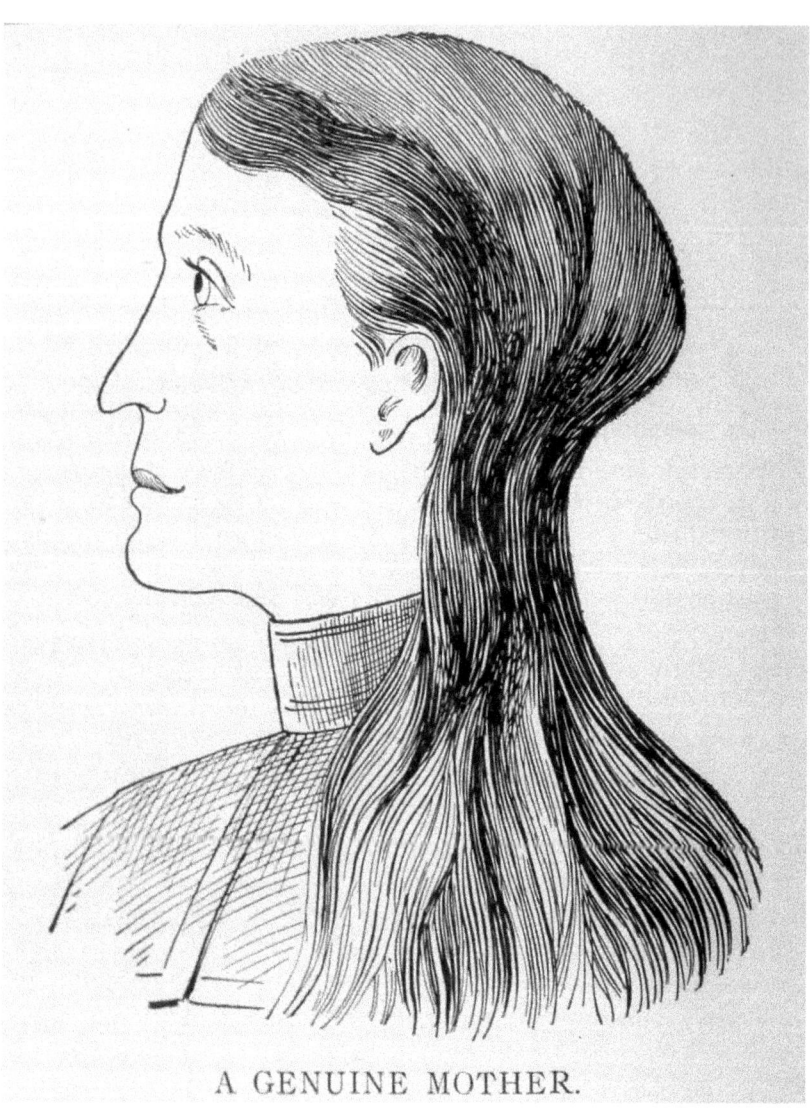

Illustration 12. A Genuine Mother. Accompanying text reads, "We affirm in the most absolute manner that words can be used that mother love is located exactly where this backhead projects most. To be a true, natural mother is to have this faculty highly developed. Young men, fix this picture in your minds." Louis Allen Vaught, *Vaught's Practical Character Reader* (Chicago: L.A. Vaught, 1902), 24, Internet Archive.

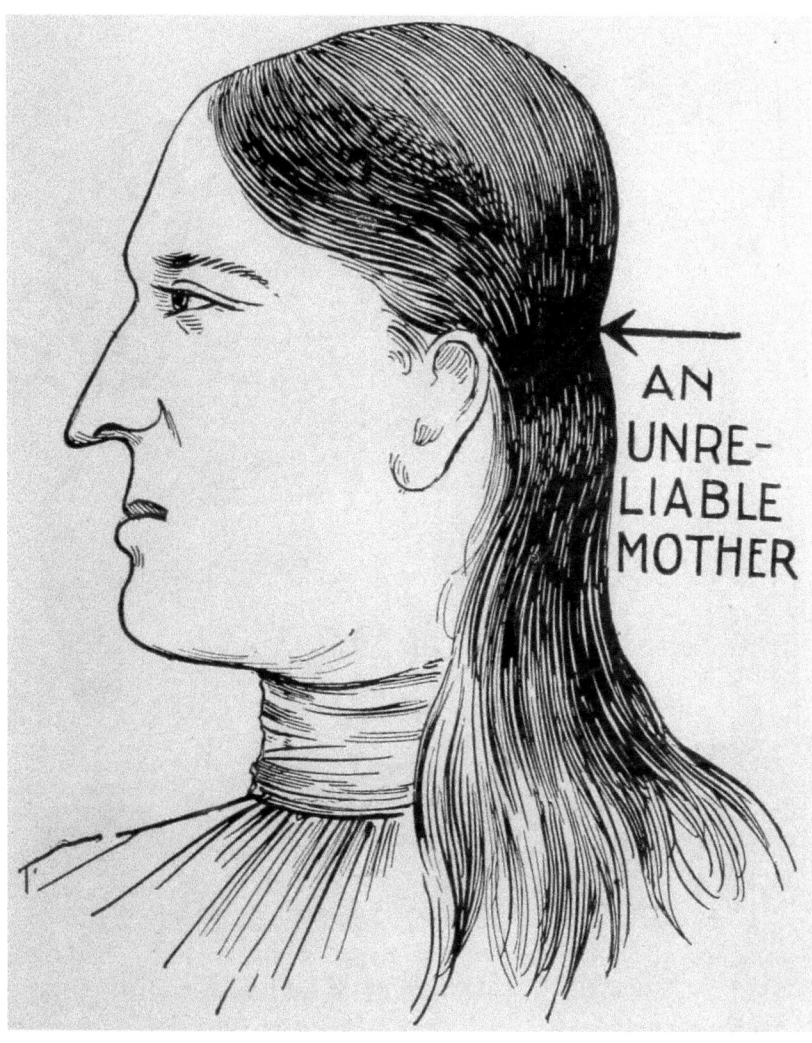

Illustration 13. An Unreliable Mother. Accompanying text reads, "This is a striking illustration. It will pay all to remember this head formation and especially all men who would select wives who will make good mothers." Louis Allen Vaught, *Vaught's Practical Character Reader* (Chicago: L.A. Vaught, 1902), 25, Internet Archive.

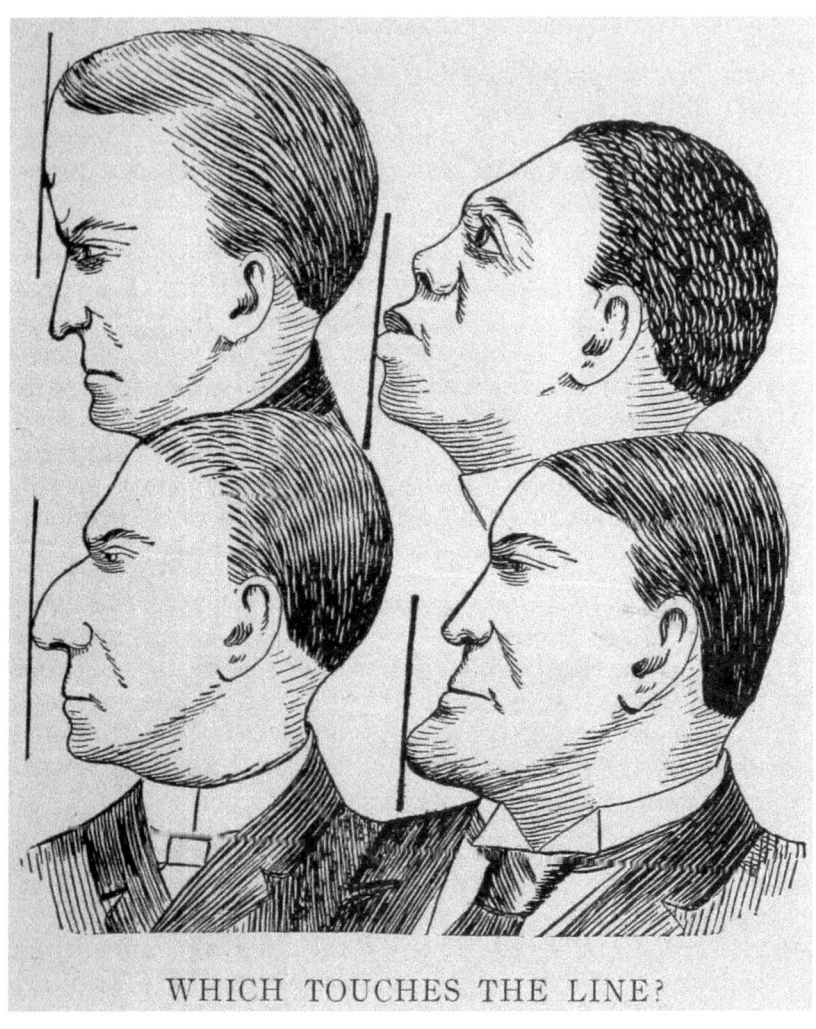

Illustration 14. Which Touches the Line? Louis Allen Vaught, *Vaught's Practical Character Reader* (Chicago: L.A. Vaught, 1902), 55–56, Internet Archive.

Which Touches This Line?

The above illustration is a very instructive one [See Illustration 14]. It will enable our readers to get at the predominant characteristics of anyone at a glance when they fully understand it, and when the individual to be read has one or more of the predominant faculties.

That part of the face or head that projects most forward (if normal) tells what part of the mind is predominant. Special development of parts of head or face means special strength of certain faculties.

When the upper forehead is the most pronounced in development the reasoning or thinking faculties (Causality and Comparison) of the mind are predominant. Such a person will be an abstract, absent-minded thinker. Is very likely to be an ideal theorist. He may be a profound philosopher but not very practical.

When the nose gets to the line first there is a very different character because other faculties are predominant in the mental constitution. In such cases some of the courageous, selfish, forceful faculties predominate. In a word, energetic force is predominant in the individual....

Combativeness and Destructiveness are the two faculties that correspond with the convex anterior projection of the bridge of the nose, while if the nose is thick at the same time, Acquisitiveness and perhaps Secretiveness are also strong. Such people have some kind of active energy, and when the nose is broad, selfish energy.

There is a very different set of faculties predominant when the lips touch the perpendicular line first. Then the appetites and social sentiments predominate. Such are impulsive, sentimental, sensual and often voluptuous. They make emotional speakers and are almost wholly governed by impulse.

When the chin is the most forward feature, tenacity of life is predominant, and if the chin is square and long, persistence is also very strong. Where the chin is not so square and long but thick in muscular coverage, sexual passion is stronger than persistence.

When these four divisions of the face are all strongly developed or when they show a positive convex form, there will be a strong character intellectually, executively, vitally and sentimentally.

The Physiognomy of Insanity*

HUGH WELCH DIAMOND
(British, 1809–1886)

JOHN CONOLLY
(English, 1795–1866)

In 1852, British psychiatrist Dr. Hugh Welch Diamond embarked upon a project that fused photography, phrenology, and psychiatric practice. Diamond believed it was possible to capture, in pictures, the essence of how particular mental illnesses manifest physically in a person's appearance. Diamond's idea was well received in some circles, and in 1858 Dr. John Conolly began to publish a series of articles in the *British Journal of Psychiatry* called "The Physiognomy of Insanity." It was Conolly's hope that the physiognomic study of mental illness could help diagnose and treat sufferers of those conditions. The following images are lithographs based on Diamond's photographs and published in Conolly's articles [See Illustrations 15 and 16]. They offer illustrations of what Conolly considered the "look" of certain forms of mental illness and decline.

---

* Illustrations reprinted from "The Physiognomy of Insanity" in *The Medical Times and Gazette: A Journal of Medical Science, Literature, Criticism, and News*, New Series, vol. 16 (January–February 1858): 14, 144, HathiTrust. Lithographs from photographs by Hugh Diamond and Henry Hering used by John Conolly, Wikimedia Commons.

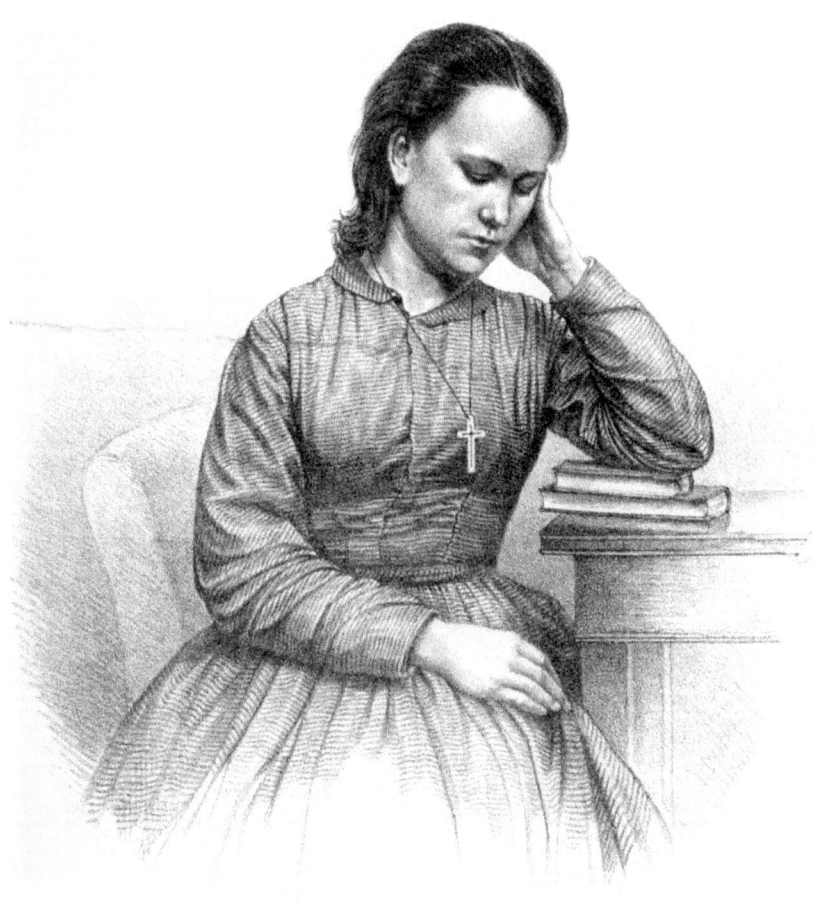

RELIGIOUS MELANCHOLY.

Illustration 15. Religious Melancholy. This condition is described in "The Physiognomy of Insanity" as "a belief of having displeased the Great Creator, and of being hopelessly shut out from mercy and from heaven" (11). Reprinted from "The Physiognomy of Insanity" in *The Medical Times and Gazette: A Journal of Medical Science, Literature, Criticism, and News, New Series*, vol. 16 (January 2, 1858): 14, HathiTrust.

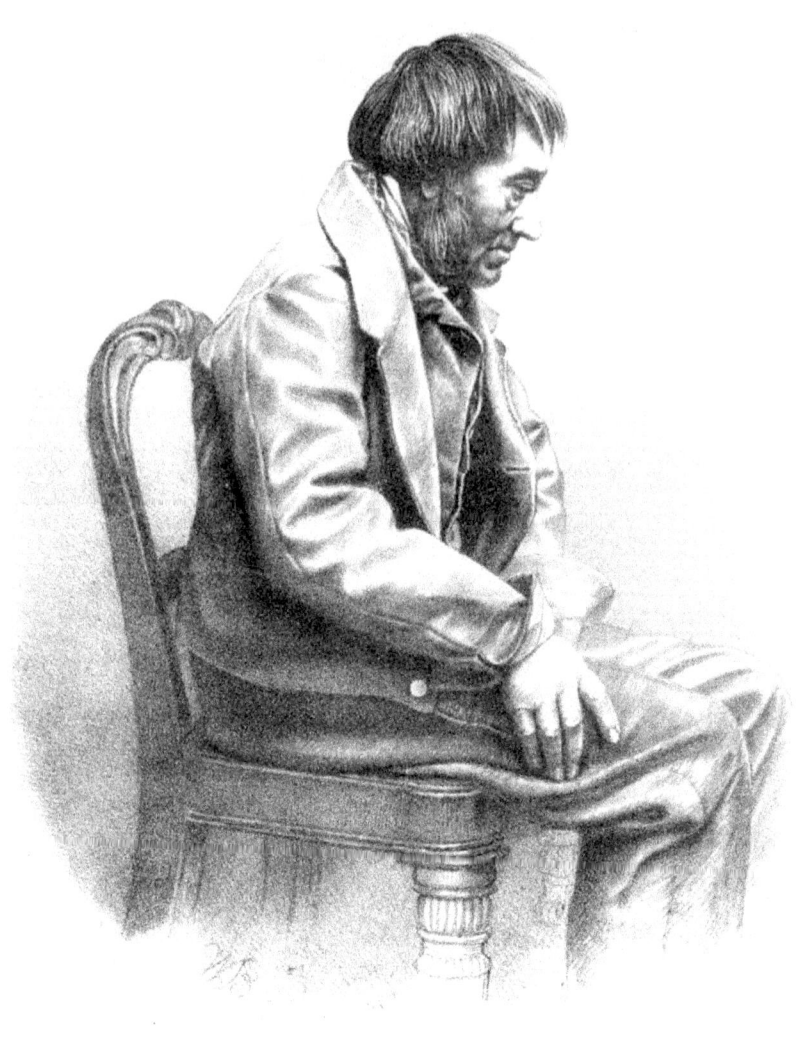

Illustration 16. General Melancholia. Now called melancholic depression, this is a condition in which "the patient has come to a conclusion that insuperable trouble has fallen upon him, and ... the advancing shadow of the dullness of death, rests upon him" (136). Reprinted from "The Physiognomy of Insanity" in *The Medical Times and Gazette: A Journal of Medical Science, Literature, Criticism, and News*, New Series, vol. 16 (February 6, 1858): 144, HathiTrust.

Compare & Consider

COMPARE

Investigate the attitudes towards the health and behavior of individuals deemed physically or mentally "different"—particularly women and people of color—with other works in this volume (Margery Kempe, pp. 69–74; Edward Jorden, pp. 130–108; Jane Sharp, pp. 143–147; William Buchan, pp. 174–177; Mary Prince, pp. 211–221; Emily Dickinson, pp. 246–248; George Miller Beard, pp. 258–261; Agnes Mary Frances Robinson, pp. 285–286; Charlotte Perkins Gilman, pp. 287–305; Charlotte Mary Mew, pp. 330–331; Wilfred Owen, pp. 332–333; W.H.R. Rivers, pp. 334–343; Siegfried Sassoon, pp. 344–346; and the WPA Ex-Slave Narratives, pp. 356–362).

CONSIDER

How does the perspective of a work on mental health (i.e., first person versus third person, or having a personal stake in a topic) impact the audience? How do works that approach complicated, "hidden" issues (like reproduction or mental health and behavior) change—or remain similar—over time and place?

Life in Times of Plague
DEPICTING THE BLACK DEATH

When diseases become epidemics, the impacts are felt in every corner—economics, politics, religion, culture—and at every level, from the individual and the household to the community, country, or even the whole globe. The epidemics that have historically been the most widespread, such as the Black Death, smallpox, cholera, and influenza, have each prompted an outpouring of writing and art beyond the medical works aimed at curbing and curing the diseases. The range of epidemic-related literature and art is enormous. Included here is a very small sampling of works related to the Black Death (bubonic plague, caused by the bacterium *Yersinia pestis*) which came in waves across Asia and Europe from the fourteenth through nineteenth centuries. Also included are two illustrations from pamphlets during the seventeenth century [See Illustrations 17 and 18]. Across three major pandemics, it caused more deaths than any other epidemic in history.

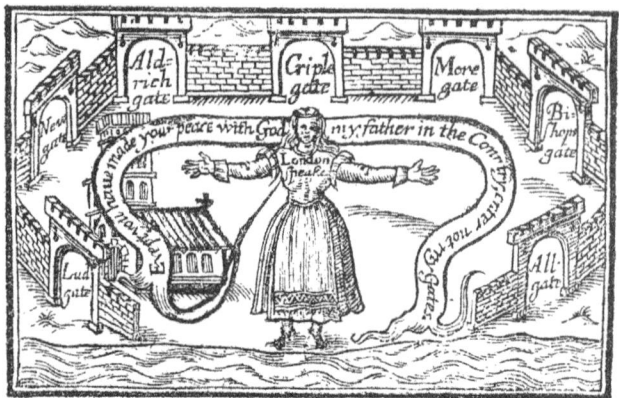

London welcomes home her runaways.

Illustration 17. London Welcomes Home Her Runaways. Woodcut from Henry Petowe's 1625 pamphlet, *The Countrie Ague*. Many city-dwellers who had the means to travel fled the city during outbreaks, and often faced criticism upon returning for abandoning the less fortunate. In this image, a female figure representing the City of London stands with open arms and says to those who fled, "except you have made your peace with God my Father in the country, enter not my gates." Illustration reprinted from Frank P. Wilson, frontispiece to *The Plague in Shakespeare's London* (Oxford: Clarendon Press, 1927), xi. Wikimedia Commons. Attribution 4.0 International (CC BY 4.0).

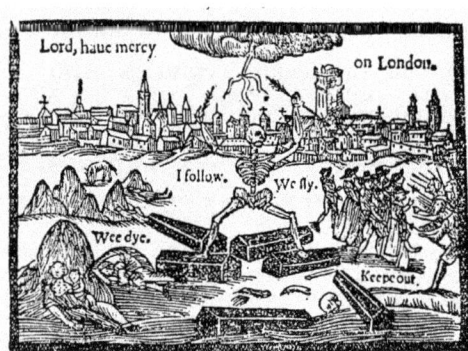

Illustration 18. Lord, Have Mercy on London. Woodcut from Thomas Dekker's 1625 pamphlet, *A Rod for Runaways*. English playwright Thomas Dekker wrote a number of pamphlets detailing the experience of plague in London. This image is featured in one such pamphlet and depicts death (in the form of a skeleton) descending upon the city. Illustration reprinted from Howard W. Haggard, *Devils, Drugs, and Doctors: The Story of the Science of Healing from Medicine-Man to Doctor* (London: William Heinemann, 1953). Wellcome Collection.

The Decameron[*]

GIOVANNI BOCCACCIO
(Italian, 1313–1375)

Boccaccio's sprawling work sets up its one hundred stories as tales told by seven women and ten men isolating themselves outside Florence to avoid the Plague. Though fictional in nature, Boccaccio's work draws from the reality of an outbreak that occurred in 1348, and he incorporates the Plague directly into the introduction to the collection, seen here.

---

[*] Reprinted from Giovanni Boccaccio, *The Decameron*, vol. 1, trans. J. M. Rigg (London, 1903; Project Gutenberg, 2003), Introduction.

Introduction to the first day

...I say, then, that the years of the beatific incarnation of the Son of God had reached the tale of one thousand three hundred and forty-eight when in the illustrious city of Florence, the fairest of all the cities of Italy, there made its appearance that deadly pestilence, which, whether disseminated by the influence of the celestial bodies,[1] or sent upon us mortals by God in His just wrath by way of retribution for our iniquities, had had its origin some years before in the East, whence, after destroying an innumerable multitude of living beings, it had propagated itself without respite from place to place, and so, calamitously, had spread into the West.

In Florence, despite all that human wisdom and forethought could devise to avert it, as the cleansing of the city from many impurities by officials appointed for the purpose, the refusal of entrance to all sick folk, and the adoption of many precautions for the preservation of health; despite also humble supplications addressed to God, and often repeated both in public procession and otherwise, by the devout; towards the beginning of the spring of the said year the doleful effects of the pestilence began to be horribly apparent by symptoms that shewed as if miraculous.

Not such were they as in the East, where an issue of blood from the nose was a manifest sign of inevitable death; but in men and women alike it first betrayed itself by the emergence of certain tumors in the groin or the armpits, some of which grew as large as a common apple, others as an egg, some more, some less, which the common folk called *gavoccioli*.[2] From the two said parts of the body this deadly *gavocciolo* soon began to propagate and spread itself in all directions indifferently; after which the form of the malady began to change, black spots or livid making their appearance in many cases on the arm or the thigh or elsewhere, now few and large, now minute and numerous. And as

---

1   *Celestial bodies*: Astrological medicine proposed that diseases and their spread could be influenced by the movement of the planets and stars.
2   *Gavoccioli*: In English, these swellings are known as buboes and lend their name to the bubonic plague.

the *gavocciolo* had been and still was an infallible token of approaching death, such also were these spots on whomsoever they shewed themselves. Which maladies seemed to set entirely at naught both the art of the physician and the virtues of physic;[3] indeed, whether it was that the disorder was of a nature to defy such treatment, or that the physicians were at fault—besides the qualified there was now a multitude both of men and of women who practiced without having received the slightest tincture of medical science—and, being in ignorance of its source, failed to apply the proper remedies; in either case, not merely were those that recovered few, but almost all within three days from the appearance of the said symptoms, sooner or later, died, and in most cases without any fever or other attendant malady.

Moreover, the virulence of the pest was the greater by reason that intercourse was apt to convey it from the sick to the whole, just as fire devours things dry or greasy when they are brought close to it. Nay, the evil went yet further, for not merely by speech or association with the sick was the malady communicated to the healthy with consequent peril of common death; but any that touched the cloth of the sick or aught else that had been touched or used by them, seemed thereby to contract the disease.

So marvelous sounds that which I have now to relate, that, had not many, and I among them, observed it with their own eyes, I had hardly dared to credit it, much less to set it down in writing, though I had had it from the lips of a credible witness.

I say, then, that such was the energy of the contagion of the said pestilence, that it was not merely propagated from man to man but, what is much more startling, it was frequently observed, that things which had belonged to one sick or dead of the disease, if touched by some other living creature, not of the human species, were the occasion, not merely of sickening, but of an almost instantaneous death. Whereof my own eyes (as I said a little before) had cognizance, one day among others, by the following experience. The rags of a poor man who had died of the disease being strewn about the open street, two hogs came thither, and after, as is their wont, no little trifling with their snouts, took the

---

3   *Physic*: Medicine. "Physician" means "one who practices physic."

rags between their teeth and tossed them to and fro about their chaps; whereupon, almost immediately, they gave a few turns, and fell down dead, as if by poison, upon the rags which in an evil hour they had disturbed.

In which circumstances, not to speak of many others of a similar or even graver complexion, diverse apprehensions and imaginations were engendered in the minds of such as were left alive, inclining almost all of them to the same harsh resolution, to wit, to shun and abhor all contact with the sick and all that belonged to them, thinking thereby to make each his own health secure. Among whom there were those who thought that to live temperately and avoid all excess would count for much as a preservative against seizures of this kind. Wherefore they banded together, and, dissociating themselves from all others, formed communities in houses where there were no sick, and lived a separate and secluded life, which they regulated with the utmost care, avoiding every kind of luxury, but eating and drinking very moderately of the most delicate viands and the finest wines, holding converse with none but one another, lest tidings of sickness or death should reach them, and diverting their minds with music and such other delights as they could devise. Others, the bias of whose minds was in the opposite direction, maintained, that to drink freely, frequent places of public resort, and take their pleasure with song and revel, sparing to satisfy no appetite, and to laugh and mock at no event, was the sovereign remedy for so great an evil: and that which they affirmed they also put in practice, so far as they were able, resorting day and night, now to this tavern, now to that, drinking with an entire disregard of rule or measure, and by preference making the houses of others, as it were, their inns, if they but saw in them aught that was particularly to their taste or liking; which they were readily able to do, because the owners, seeing death imminent, had become as reckless of their property as of their lives; so that most of the houses were open to all comers, and no distinction was observed between the stranger who presented himself and the rightful lord. Thus, adhering ever to their inhuman determination to shun the sick, as far as possible, they ordered their life. In this extremity of our city's suffering and tribulation the venerable authority of laws, human and divine, was abased and all but totally dissolved, for lack of those who should have administered and enforced them, most of whom, like the rest of the citizens, were either dead or sick, or so hard bested for servants that they were unable to execute any office; whereby every man was free to do what was right in his own eyes.

Not a few there were who belonged to neither of the two said parties, but kept a middle course between them, neither laying the same restraint upon their diet as the former, nor allowing themselves the same license in drinking and other dissipations as the latter, but living with a degree of freedom sufficient to satisfy their appetites, and not as recluses. They therefore walked abroad, carrying in their hands flowers or fragrant herbs or divers sorts of spices, which they frequently raised to their noses, deeming it an excellent thing thus to comfort the brain with such perfumes, because the air seemed to be everywhere laden and reeking with the stench emitted by the dead and the dying and the odors of drugs.

Some again, the most sound, perhaps, in judgment, as they we also the most harsh in temper, of all, affirmed that there was no medicine for the disease superior or equal in efficacy to flight; following which prescription a multitude of men and women, negligent of all but themselves, deserted their city, their houses, their estate, their kinsfolk, their goods, and went into voluntary exile, or migrated to the country parts, as if God in visiting men with this pestilence in requital of their iniquities would not pursue them with His wrath, wherever they might be, but intended the destruction of such alone as remained within the circuit of the walls of the city; or deeming, perchance, that it was now time for all to flee from it, and that its last hour was come.

Of the adherents of these diverse opinions not all died, neither did all escape; but rather there were, of each sort and in every place, many that sickened, and by those who retained their health were treated after the example which they themselves, while whole, had set, being everywhere left to languish in almost total neglect. Tedious were it to recount, how citizen avoided citizen, how among neighbors was scarce found any that shewed fellow-feeling for another, how kinsfolk held aloof, and never met, or but rarely; enough that this sore affliction entered so deep into the minds of men and women, that in the horror thereof brother was forsaken by brother, nephew by uncle, brother by sister, and oftentimes husband by wife; nay, what is more, and scarcely to be believed, fathers and mothers were found to abandon their own children, untended, unvisited, to their fate, as if they had been strangers. Wherefore the sick of both sexes, whose number could not be estimated, were left without resource but in the charity of friends (and few such there were), or the interest of servants, who were hardly to be had at high rates and on unseemly terms, and being, moreover, one and all men and women of gross understanding, and for the most part unused to such offices, concerned themselves no farther than to supply the immediate and expressed wants of the sick, and to watch them die; in which service they themselves not seldom perished with their gains. In consequence of which dearth of servants and dereliction of the sick by neighbors, kinsfolk and friends, it came to pass—a thing, perhaps, never before heard of that no woman, however dainty, fair or well-born she might be, shrank, when stricken with the disease, from the ministrations of a man, no matter whether he were young or no, or scrupled to expose to him every part of her body, with no more shame than if he had been a woman, submitting of necessity to that which her malady required; wherefrom, perchance, there resulted in after time some loss of modesty in such as recovered. Besides which many succumbed, who with proper attendance, would, perhaps, have escaped death; so that, what with the virulence of the plague and the lack of due tendance of the sick, the multitude of the deaths, that daily and nightly took place in the city, was such that those who heard the tale—not to say witnessed the fact—were struck dumb with amazement. Whereby, practices contrary to the former habits of the citizens could hardly fail to grow up among the survivors.

It had been, as to-day it still is, the custom for the women that were neighbors and of kin to the deceased to gather in his house with the women that were most closely connected with him, to wail with them in common, while on the other hand his male kinsfolk and neighbors, with not a few of the other citizens, and a due proportion of the clergy according to his quality, assembled without, in front of the house, to receive the corpse; and so the dead man was borne on the shoulders of his peers, with funeral pomp of taper and dirge, to the church selected by him before his death. Which rites, as the pestilence waxed in fury, were either in whole or in great part disused, and gave way to others of a novel order. For not only did no crowd of women surround the bed of the dying, but many passed from this life unregarded, and few indeed were they to whom were accorded the lamentations and bitter tears of sorrowing relations; nay, for the most part, their place was taken by the laugh, the jest, the festal gathering; observances which the women, domestic piety in large measure set aside, had adopted with very great advantage to their health. Few also there were whose bodies were attended to the church by more than ten or twelve of their neighbors, and those not the honorable and respected citizens; but a sort of corpse-carriers drawn from the baser ranks who called themselves *becchini*[4] and performed such offices for hire, would shoulder the bier, and with hurried steps carry it, not to the church of the dead man's choice, but to that which was nearest at hand, with four or six priests in front and a candle or two, or, perhaps, none; nor did the priests distress themselves with too long and solemn an office, but with the aid of the *becchini* hastily consigned the corpse to the first tomb which they found untenanted. The condition of lower, and, perhaps, in great measure of the middle ranks, of the people shewed even worse and more deplorable; for, deluded by hope or constrained by poverty, they stayed in their quarters, in their houses, where they sickened by thousands a day, and, being without service or help of any kind, were, so to speak, irredeemably devoted to the death which overtook them. Many died daily or nightly in the public streets; of many others, who died at home, the departure was hardly observed by their neighbors, until the stench of their putrefying bodies carried the tidings; and what with their corpses and the corpses of others who died on every hand the whole place was a sepulcher.

It was the common practice of most of the neighbors, moved no less by fear of contamination by the putrefying bodies than by charity towards the deceased, to drag the corpses out of the houses with their own hands, aided, perhaps, by a porter, if a porter was to be had, and to lay them in front of the doors, where any one who made the round might have seen, especially in the morning, more of them than he could count; afterwards they would have biers brought up, or, in default,

---

4   *Becchini*: Literally, grave-diggers.

planks, whereon they laid them. Nor was it once or twice only that one and the same bier carried two or three corpses at once; but quite a considerable number of such cases occurred, one bier sufficing for husband and wife, two or three brothers, father and son, and so forth. And times without number it happened, that, as two priests, bearing the cross, were on their way to perform the last office for some one, three or four biers were brought up by the porters in rear of them, so that, whereas the priests supposed that they had but one corpse to bury, they discovered that there were six or eight, or sometimes more. Nor, for all their number, were their obsequies honored by either tears or lights or crowds of mourners; rather, it was come to this, that a dead man was then of no more account than a dead goat would be to-day. From all which it is abundantly manifest, that that lesson of patient resignation, which the sages were never able to learn from the slight and infrequent mishaps which occur in the natural course of events, was now brought home even to the minds of the simple by the magnitude of their disasters, so that they became indifferent to them.

As consecrated ground there was not in extent sufficient to provide tombs for the vast multitude of corpses which day and night, and almost every hour, were brought in eager haste to the churches for interment, least of all, if ancient custom were to be observed and a separate resting-place assigned to each, they dug, for each graveyard, as soon as it was full, a huge trench, in which they laid the corpses as they arrived by hundreds at a time, piling them up as merchandise is stowed in the hold of a ship, tier upon tier, each covered with a little earth, until the trench would hold no more. But I spare to rehearse with minute particularity each of the woes that came upon our city, and say in brief, that, harsh as was the tenor of her fortunes, the surrounding country knew no mitigation, for there—not to speak of the castles, each, as it were, a little city in itself—in sequestered village, or on the open champaign,[5] by the wayside, on the farm, in the homestead, the poor hapless husbandmen and their families, forlorn of physicians' care or servants' tendance, perished day and night alike, not as men, but rather as beasts. Wherefore, they too, like the citizens, abandoned all rule of life, all habit of industry, all

---

5 *Champaign*: Expanse of open countryside.

counsel of prudence; nay, one and all, as if expecting each day to be their last, not merely ceased to aid Nature to yield her fruit in due season of their beasts and their lands and their past labors, but left no means unused, which ingenuity could devise, to waste their accumulated store; denying shelter to their oxen, asses, sheep, goats, pigs, fowls, nay, even to their dogs, man's most faithful companions, and driving them out into the fields to roam at large amid the unsheaved, nay, unreaped corn. Many of which, as if endowed with reason, took their fill during the day, and returned home at night without any guidance of herdsman. But enough of the country! What need we add, but (reverting to the city) that such and so grievous was the harshness of heaven, and perhaps in some degree of man, that, what with the fury of the pestilence, the panic of those whom it spared, and their consequent neglect or desertion of not a few of the stricken in their need, it is believed without any manner of doubt, that between March and the ensuing July upwards of a hundred thousand human beings lost their lives within the walls of the city of Florence, which before the deadly visitation would not have been supposed to contain so many people! How many grand palaces, how many stately homes, how many splendid residences, once full of retainers, of lords, of ladies, were now left desolate of all, even to the meanest servant! How many families of historic fame, of vast ancestral domains, and wealth proverbial, found now no scion to continue the succession! How many brave men, how many fair ladies, how many gallant youths, whom any physician, were he Galen, Hippocrates, or Asclepius himself,[6] would have pronounced in the soundest of health, broke fast with their kinsfolk, comrades and friends in the morning, and when evening came, supped with their forefathers in the other world.

---

6   *Galen, Hippocrates, or Asclepius himself*: The most famous ancient physicians; Galen (see pp. 41–46) popularized the humoral system of medicine that was dominant during Boccaccio's time and for centuries after; Hippocrates (see pp. 26–30) is known as the "father of medicine" for his contributions to medical knowledge and ethics; and Asclepius (see pp. 377–382) is the Greek god of medicine.

An Order of the Lords, for the better direction of the Overseers appointed in the several Parishes of the City of Oxford, against the spreading of the Infection of the Plague*

CITY OF OXFORD
(English, ca. mid-seventeenth century)

This document is a legal decree from the city of Oxford in England, and comes from the latter end of the second pandemic in 1645. This was the most devastating wave in the British Isles, and there were ten major outbreaks in the sixteenth and seventeenth centuries alone, some lasting as long as fifteen years each. In the Order, we have a record of the attempts made to slow the spread of the disease in the city.

---

* City of Oxford, *An Order of the Lords* [...] *against the spreading of the Infection of the Plague*. (Oxford: Leonard Lichfield, 1645).

The infection of the plague being much dispersed in several Parishes and places within this city, to the end that all possible care may be taken to provide for the sick, and to keep the sick from the whole, which, by Gods blessing, may be a great means to stay the infection; it is ordered, that the persons hereafter mentioned, be the overseers for this important service, and take special care in the several parishes and precincts commended to their charge, that these directions here under given be punctually and strictly observed.

1. That when they shall understand that any person is fallen sick in any house, that there be no resort thither by strangers, till it be discerned whether the sickness be infectious or not.

2. That these overseers use their best care, as soon as they understand who are fallen sick, to inform themselves what the nature of the disease is, and the symptoms thereof, and then give farther directions.

3. That as soon as any house is infected, or probably suspected to be infected, that it be shut up, and the persons in the house commanded to keep in the house, till farther order given for opening the house again.

4. That a watch-man be set at the fore-door of the house, both to keep in the persons within the house, and also to fetch them such necessaries as they want, to be delivered to them so discreetly and warily as may not endanger themselves, or those to whom they shall resort.

5. That when the house shall be known to be infected with the plague, forthwith a red-cross be set on the outward door of the house, with an inscription in capital letters, with these words, LORD HAVE MERCY UPON US, and this cross, and the inscription be taken off again. when the house is appointed to be opened, and not before.

6. That the watch-men appointed take an oath for their faithful performance of that service.

7. That every such watch-man, when he sits or goes in the streets, carry a white stick in his hat, that so others may be admonished not to press too near into his company.

8. That if there be a back-door or gate to the house shut up, that that back-door be fast shut, that no passage be that way, and also a padlock hanged upon the fore-door, whereof the watch-man to keep the key.

9. That these overseers appoint searchers and tenders for the sick

persons, and bearers and buriers when any shall die, and give oaths to them also, to observe their several employments faithfully.

10. If any appointed to any of those places or services, being fit for the same, shall refuse to undertake the employment, or neglect it when it is once undertaken, or deal unfaithfully therein, they must know, that they shall be proceeded against with all strictnesses and severity, according to the quality of their faults.

11. That all burials of persons dying of the plague be in the night time, after ten of the clock at the soonest, and without concourse of the people, and that the corpse be laid at least four-foot deep under the ground, and be bestowed in such burying places, as to that purpose shall be appointed.

12. That the church-yards within the city be spared from these burials, they being for the most part small, and how very inconvenient to receive the bodies of these infected persons.

13. That all dogs and cats in the town be forthwith sent away out of town, or such as are found in the streets, or courts of the colleges, to be knocked on the head and their carcasses carried away and buried without the works at a convenient distance.

14. That if any colleges or halls be infected or suspected, that the governors of those houses give speedy notice thereof to the overseers of that parish or precinct within which such college or hall lies, and then those overseers by the advice and approbation of those Governors of the colleges and halls for the time being, send such officers as shall be so thought fit to perform those offices to the sick or infected persons which shall be fit and necessary.

And in such cases so much to be shut up as the overseers, by the advice of the governor of that house, shall think fit.

Diary of Samuel Pepys[*]

SAMUEL PEPYS
(English, 1633–1703)

London-born Samuel Pepys had a storied life in English society: he was instrumental in establishing the British Royal Navy, served in Parliament, and was a Fellow of the Royal Society (England's oldest scientific institution), acting as its president for two years. He is, however, most famous for his personal diary, in which he recorded daily entries for nearly ten years. This work is a remarkable document of the life of a relatively well-to-do resident of London during the seventeenth century, a time of English colonial expansion, civil turmoil, and devastation for London in the form of the Great Plague of 1665 and the Great Fire of 1666. Excerpted here are a small selection of Pepys's entries recording the Plague outbreak in the summer of 1665.

---

[*] Reprinted from Samuel Pepys, *The Diary of Samuel Pepys, M.A., F.R.S.*, ed. Henry B. Wheatley (London: George Bell & Sons, 1893; Project Gutenberg, 2016).

24 May 1665

Up, and by 4 o'clock in the morning, and with W. Hewer, there till 12 without intermission putting some papers in order. Thence to the Coffee-house[1] with Creed, where I have not been a great while, where all the news is of the Dutch being gone out, and of the plague growing upon us in this town; and of remedies against it: some saying one thing, some another. So home to dinner, and after dinner Creed and I to Colvill's, thinking to shew him all the respect we could by obliging him in carrying him 5 tallies[2] of £5000 to secure him for so much credit he has formerly given Povy to Tangier, but he, like an impertinent fool, cavils at it, but most ignorantly that ever I heard man in my life. At last Mr. Viner by chance comes, who I find a very moderate man, but could not persuade the fool to reason, but brought away the tallies again, and so vexed to my office, where late, and then home to my supper and to bed.

10 June

Lay long in bed, and then up and at the office all the morning. At noon dined at home, and then to the office busy all the afternoon. In the evening home to supper; and there, to my great trouble, hear that the plague is come into the City (though it has these three or four weeks since its beginning been wholly out of the City); but where should it begin but in my good friend and neighbor's, Dr. Burnett, in Fenchurch Street: which in both points troubles me mightily. To the office to finish my letters and then home to bed, being troubled at the sickness,[3] and my head filled also with other business enough, and particularly how to put my things and estate in order, in case it should please God to call me away, which God dispose of to his glory!

---

1 Coffee-houses came to England in the 1650s and quickly became important social centers for men. They were common places to trade gossip, read newspapers, and have conversations and debates.
2 *Tallies*: Records of debt and payment.
3 *Troubled at the sickness*: Worried about the plague.

29 June

Up and by water to Whitehall, where the Court full of wagons and people ready to go out of town. To the Harp and Ball, and there drank and talked with Mary, she telling me in discourse that she lived lately at my neighbor's, Mr. Knightly, which made me forbear further discourse. This end of the town every day grows very bad of the plague. The Mortality Bill is come to 267;[4] which is about ninety more than the last: and of these but four in the City, which is a great blessing to us. Thence to Creed, and with him up and down about Tangier business, to no purpose. Took leave again of Mr. Coventry; though I hope the Duke has not gone to stay, and so do others too. So home, calling at Somerset House, where all are packing up too: the Queen-Mother setting out for France this day to drink Bourbon waters[5] this year, she being in a consumption; and intends not to come till winter come twelvemonths. So by coach home, where at the office all the morning, and at noon Mrs. Hunt dined with us. Very merry, and she a very good woman. To the office, where busy a while putting some things in my office in order, and then to letters till night. About 10 o'clock home, the days being sensibly shorter before I have once kept a summer's day by shutting up office by daylight; but my life has been still as it was in winter almost. But I will for a month try what I can do by daylight. So home to supper and to bed.

---

4 [Editor Henry D. Wheatley's note: According to the Bills of Mortality, the total number of deaths in London for the week ending June 27th was 684, of which number 267 were deaths from the plague. The number of deaths rose week by week until September 19th, when the total was 8,297, and the deaths from the plague 7,165. On September 26th the total had fallen to 6,460, and deaths from the plague to 5,533. The number fell gradually, week by week, till October 31st, when the total was 1,388, and deaths from the plague 1,031. On November 7th there was a rise to 1,787 and 1,414 respectively. On November 14th the numbers had gone down to 1,359 and 1,050 respectively. On December 12th the total had fallen to 442, and deaths from the plague to 243. On December 19th there was a rise to 525 and 281 respectively. The total of burials in 1665 was 97,506, of which number the plague claimed 68,596 victims.]

5 *Bourbon waters*: Bourbon-l'Archambault is a town in central France that is set on a mineral spa, the waters of which are used in the promotion of health.

20 July

Up, in a boat among other people to the Tower, and there to the office, where we sat all the morning. So down to Deptford and there dined, and after dinner saw my Lady Sandwich and Mr. Carteret and his two sisters over the water, going to Dagenhams, and my Lady Carteret towards Cranbourne. So all the company broke up in most extraordinary joy, wherein I am mighty contented that I have had the good fortune to be so instrumental, and I think it will be of good use to me. So walked to Redriffe, where I hear the sickness is, and indeed is scattered almost every where, there dying 1089 of the plague this week. My Lady Carteret did this day give me a bottle of plague-water home with me. So home to write letters late, and then home to bed, where I have not lain these 3 or 4 nights. I received yesterday a letter from my Lord Sandwich, giving me thanks for my care about their marriage business, and desiring it to be dispatched, that no disappointment may happen therein, which I will help on all I can. This afternoon I waited on the Duke of Albemarle, and so to Mrs. Croft's, where I found and saluted Mrs. Burrows, who is a very pretty woman for a mother of so many children. But, Lord! to see how the plague spreads. It being now all over King's Street, at the Axe, and next door to it, and in other places.

3 August

Up, and betimes to Deptford to Sir G. Carteret's, where, not liking the horse that had been hired by Mr. Uthwayt for me, I did desire Sir G. Carteret to let me ride his new L40 horse, which he did, and so I left my "hacquenee"[6]—behind, and so after staying a good while in their bedchamber while they were dressing themselves, discoursing merrily, I parted and to the ferry, where I was forced to stay a great while before I could get my horse brought over, and then mounted and rode very finely to Dagenhams; all the way people, citizens, walking to and again to inquire how the plague is in the City this week by the Bill; which by

---

6 [Wheatley's note: Haquenee = an ambling nag fitted for ladies' riding.]

chance, at Greenwich, I had heard was 2,020 of the plague, and 3,000 and odd of all diseases; but methought it was a sad question to be so often asked me. Coming to Dagenhams, I there met our company coming out of the house, having staid as long as they could for me; so I let them go a little before, and went and took leave of my Lady Sandwich, good woman, who seems very sensible of my service in this late business, and having her directions in some things, among others, to get Sir G. Carteret and my Lord to settle the portion, and what Sir G. Carteret is to settle, into land, soon as may be, she not liking that it should lie long undone, for fear of death on either side. So took leave of her, and then down to the buttery, and eat a piece of cold venison pie, and drank and took some bread and cheese in my hand; and so mounted after them, Mr. Marr very kindly staying to lead me the way. By and by met my Lord Crew returning, after having accompanied them a little way, and so after them, Mr. Marr telling me by the way how a maid servant of Mr. John Wright's (who lives thereabouts) falling sick of the plague, she was removed to an out-house, and a nurse appointed to look to her; who, being once absent, the maid got out of the house at the window, and run away. The nurse coming and knocking, and having no answer, believed she was dead, and went and told Mr. Wright so; who and his lady were in great strait what to do to get her buried. At last resolved to go to Burntwood hard by, being in the parish, and there get people to do it. But they would not; so he went home full of trouble, and in the way met the wench walking over the common, which frighted him worse than before; and was forced to send people to take her, which he did; and they got one of the pest coaches and put her into it to carry her to a pest house. And passing in a narrow lane, Sir Anthony Browne, with his brother and some friends in the coach, met this coach with the curtains drawn close. The brother being a young man, and believing there might be some lady in it that would not be seen, and the way being narrow, he thrust his head out of his own into her coach, and to look, and there saw somebody look very ill, and in a sick dress, and stunk mightily; which the coachman also cried out upon. And presently they come up to some people that stood looking after it, and told our gallants that it was a maid of Mr. Wright's carried away sick of the plague; which put the young gentleman into a fright had almost cost him his life, but

Diary of Samuel Pepys

is now well again. I, overtaking our young people, 'light, and into the coach to them, where mighty merry all the way; and anon come to the Blockehouse, over against Gravesend, where we staid a great while, in a little drinking-house. Sent back our coaches to Dagenhams. I, by and by, by boat to Gravesend, where no news of Sir G. Carteret come yet; so back again, and fetched them all over, but the two saddle-horses that were to go with us, which could not be brought over in the horse-boat, the wind and tide being against us, without towing; so we had some difference with some watermen, who would not tow them over under 20s., whereupon I swore to send one of them to sea and will do it. Anon some others come to me and did it for 10s. By and by comes Sir G. Carteret, and so we set out for Chatham: in my way overtaking some company, wherein was a lady, very pretty, riding singly, her husband in company with her. We fell into talk, and I read a copy of verses which her husband showed me, and he discommended, but the lady commended: and I read them, so as to make the husband turn to commend them. By and by he and I fell into acquaintance, having known me formerly at the Exchequer. His name is Nokes, over against Bow Church. He was servant to Alderman Dashwood. We promised to meet, if ever we come both to London again; and, at parting, I had a fair salute on horseback, in Rochester streets, of the lady, and so parted. Come to Chatham mighty merry, and anon to supper, it being near 9 o'clock ere we come thither. My Lady Carteret come thither in a coach, by herself, before us. Great mind they have to buy a little "hacquenee" that I rode on from Greenwich, for a woman's horse. Mighty merry, and after supper, all being withdrawn, Sir G. Carteret did take an opportunity to speak with much value and kindness to me, which is of great joy to me. So anon to bed. Mr. Brisband and I together to my content.

10 August

Up betimes, and called upon early by my she-cozen Porter, the turner's wife, to tell me that her husband was carried to the Tower, for buying of some of the King's powder,[7] and would have my help, but I could give her none, not daring any more to appear in the business, having too much trouble lately therein. By and by to the office, where we sat all the morning; in great trouble to see the Bill this week rise so high, to above 4,000 in all, and of them above 3,000 of the plague. And an odd story of Alderman Bence's stumbling at night over a dead corpse in the street, and going home and telling his wife, she at the fright, being with child, fell sick and died of the plague. We sat late, and then by invitation my Lord Brunker, Sir J. Minnes, Sir W. Batten and I to Sir G. Smith's to dinner, where very good company and good cheer. Captain Cocke was there and Jacke Fenn, but to our great wonder Alderman Bence, and tells us that not a word of all this is true, and others said so too, but by his own story his wife hath been ill, and he fain to leave his house and comes not to her, which continuing a trouble to me all the time I was there. Thence to the office and, after writing letters, home, to draw-over anew my will, which I had bound myself by oath to dispatch by to-morrow night; the town growing so unhealthy, that a man cannot depend upon living two days to an end. So having done something of it, I to bed.

15 August

Up by 4 o'clock and walked to Greenwich, where called at Captain Cocke's and to his chamber, he being in bed, where something put my last night's dream into my head, which I think is the best that ever was dreamt, which was that I had my Lady Castlemayne in my armes and was admitted to use all the dalliance I desired with her, and then dreamt that this could not be awake, but that it was only a dream; but that since it was a dream, and that I took so much real pleasure in it, what a happy thing it would be if when we are in our graves (as Shakespeare resembles it) we could dream, and dream but such dreams as this, that then we should not need to be so fearful of death, as we are this plague time. Here I hear that news is brought Sir G. Carteret that my Lord

---

7   *The King's Powder*: Gunpowder, the sale of which was heavily regulated following the attempt to blow up the House of Lords during the 1605 Gunpowder Plot.

Hinchingbrooke is not well, and so cannot meet us at Cranbourne tonight. So I to Sir G. Carteret's; and there was sorry with him for our disappointment. So we have put off our meeting there till Saturday next. Here I staid talking with Sir G. Carteret, he being mighty free with me in his business, and among other things hath ordered Rider and Cutler to put into my hands copper to the value of £5,000 (which Sir G. Carteret's share it seems come to in it), which is to raise part of the money he is to layout for a purchase for my Lady Jemimah. Thence he and I to Sir J. Minnes's by invitation, where Sir W. Batten and my Lady, and my Lord Bruncker, and all of us dined upon a venison pasty and other good meat, but nothing well dressed. But my pleasure lay in getting some bills signed by Sir G. Carteret, and promise of present payment from Mr. Fenn, which do rejoice my heart, it being one of the heaviest things I had upon me, that so much of the little I have should lie (viz. near £1000) in the King's hands. Here very merry and (Sir G. Carteret being gone presently after dinner) to Captain Cocke's, and there merry, and so broke up and I by water to the Duke of Albemarle, with whom I spoke a great deal in private, they being designed to send a fleet of ships privately to the Streights. No news yet from our fleet, which is much wondered at, but the Duke says for certain guns have been heard to the northward very much. It was dark before I could get home, and so land at Church-yard stairs, where, to my great trouble, I met a dead corpse of the plague, in the narrow ally just bringing down a little pair of stairs. But I thank God I was not much disturbed at it. However, I shall beware of being late abroad again.

30 August

Up betimes and to my business of settling my house and papers, and then abroad and met with Hadley, our clerk, who, upon my asking how the plague goes, he told me it increases much, and much in our parish; for, says he, there died nine this week, though I have returned but six: which is a very ill practice, and makes me think it is so in other places; and therefore the plague much greater than people take it to be. Thence, as I intended, to Sir R. Viner's, and there found not Mr. Lewes ready for me, so I went forth and walked towards Moorefields to see (God forbid my presumption!) whether I could see any dead corpse going to the grave; but, as God would have it, did not. But, Lord! how every body's looks, and discourse in the street is of death, and nothing else, and few people going up and down, that the town is like a place distressed and forsaken. After one turn there back to Viner's, and there found my business ready for me, and evened all reckonings with them to this day to my great content. So home, and all day till very late at night setting my Tangier and private accounts in order, which I did in both, and in the latter to my great joy do find myself yet in the much best condition that ever I was in, finding myself worth £2180 and odd, besides plate and goods, which I value at £250 more, which is a very great blessing to me. The Lord make me thankful! and of this at this day above £1800 in cash in my house, which speaks but little out of my hands in desperate condition, but this is very troublesome to have in my house at this time. So late to bed, well pleased with my accounts, but weary of being so long at them.

31 August

Up and, after putting several things in order to my removal, to Woolwich; the plague having a great increase this week, beyond all expectation of almost 2,000, making the general Bill 7,000, odd 100; and the plague above 6,000. I down by appointment to Greenwich, to our office, where I did some business, and there dined with our company and Sir W. Boreman, and Sir The.[8] Biddulph, at Mr. Boreman's, where a good venison pasty, and after a good merry dinner I to my office, and there late writing letters, and then to Woolwich by water, where pleasant with my wife and people, and after supper to bed. Thus this month ends with great sadness upon the public, through the greatness of the plague every where through the kingdom almost. Every day sadder and sadder news of its increase. In the City died this week 7,496 and of them 6,102 of the plague. But it is feared that the true number of the dead, this

---

8   *The*.: Theodophilus.

week is near 10,000; partly from the poor that cannot be taken notice of, through the greatness of the number, and partly from the Quakers and others that will not have any bell ring for them. Our fleet gone out to find the Dutch, we having about 100 sail in our fleet, and in them the Sovereign one; so that it is a better fleet than the former with the Duke was. All our fear is that the Dutch should be got in before them; which would be a very great sorrow to the public, and to me particularly, for my Lord Sandwich's sake. A great deal of money being spent, and the kingdom not in a condition to spare, nor a parliament without much difficulty to meet to give more. And to that; to have it said, what hath been done by our late fleets? As to myself I am very well, only in fear of the plague, and as much of an ague by being forced to go early and late to Woolwich, and my family to lie there continually. My late gettings have been very great to my great content, and am likely to have yet a few more profitable jobs in a little while; for which Tangier, and Sir W. Warren I am wholly obliged to.

3 September—(Lord's day)

Up; and put on my colored silk suit very fine, and my new periwig, bought a good while since, but durst not wear, because the plague was in Westminster when I bought it; and it is a wonder what will be the fashion after the plague is done, as to periwigs, for nobody will dare to buy any hair, for fear of the infection, that it had been cut off of the heads of people dead of the plague. Before church time comes Mr. Hill (Mr. Andrews failing because he was to receive the Sacrament), and to church, where a sorry dull parson, and so home and most excellent company with Mr. Hill and discourse of music. I took my Lady Pen home, and her daughter Pegg, and merry we were; and after dinner I made my wife show them her pictures, which did mad Pegg Pen, who learns of the same man and cannot do so well. After dinner left them and I by water to Greenwich, where much ado to be suffered to come into the town because of the sickness, for fear I should come from London, till I told them who I was. So up to the church, where at the door I find Captain Cocke in my Lord Brunker's coach, and he come out and walked with me in the church-yard till the church was done, talking of the ill government of our Kingdom, nobody setting to heart the business of the Kingdom, but every body minding their particular profit or pleasures, the King himself minding nothing but his ease, and so we let things go to wrack. This arose upon considering what we shall do for money when the fleet comes in, and more if the fleet should not meet with the Dutch, which will put a disgrace upon the King's actions, so as the Parliament and Kingdom will have the less mind to give more money, besides so bad an account of the last money, we fear, will be given, not half of it being spent, as it ought to be, upon the Navy. Besides, it is said that at this day our Lord Treasurer cannot tell what the profit of Chimney money is, what it comes to per annum, nor looks whether that or any other part of the revenue be duly gathered as it ought; the very money that should pay the City the £200,000 they lent the King, being all gathered and in the hands of the Receiver and hath been long and yet not brought up to pay the City, whereas we are coming to borrow 4 or £500,000 more of the City, which will never be lent as is to be feared. Church being done, my Lord Bruncker, Sir J. Minnes, and I up to the Vestry at the desire of the justices of the Peace, Sir Theo. Biddulph and Sir W. Boreman and Alderman Hooker, in order to the doing something for the keeping of the plague from growing; but Lord! to consider the madness of the people of the town, who will (because they are forbid) come in crowds along with the dead corps to see them buried; but we agreed on some orders for the prevention thereof. Among other stories, one was very passionate, methought, of a complaint brought against a man in the town for taking a child from London from an infected house. Alderman Hooker told us it was the child of a very able citizen in Gracious Street, a saddler, who had buried all the rest of his children of the plague, and himself and wife now being shut up and in despair of escaping, did desire only to save the life of this little child; and so prevailed to have it received stark-naked into the arms of a friend, who brought it (having put it into new fresh clothes) to Greenwich; where upon hearing the story, we did agree it should be permitted to be received and kept in the town. Thence with my Lord Bruncker to Captain Cocke's, where we mighty merry and supped, and very late I by water to Woolwich, in great apprehensions of an ague.

Here was my Lord Bruncker's lady of pleasure, who, I perceive, goes every where with him; and he, I find, is obliged to carry her, and make all the courtship to her that can be.

4 September

Writing letters all the morning, among others to my Lady Carteret, the first I have wrote to her, telling her the state of the city as to health and other sorrowful stories, and thence after dinner to Greenwich, to Sir J. Minnes, where I found my Lord Bruncker, and having staid our hour for the justices by agreement, the time being past we to walk in the Park with Mr. Hammond and Turner, and there eat some fruit out of the King's garden and walked in the Parke, and so back to Sir J. Minnes, and thence walked home, my Lord Bruncker giving me a very neat cane to walk with; but it troubled me to pass by Coombe farm where about twenty-one people have died of the plague, and three or four days since I saw a dead corpse in a coffin lie in the Close unburied, and a watch is constantly kept there night and day to keep the people in, the plague making us cruel, as dogs, one to another.

A Journal of the Plague Year*

DANIEL DEFOE
(English, 1660–1731)

English author Daniel Defoe, author of the early adventure novel *Robinson Crusoe*, was only five years old when the Great Plague hit London in 1665. However, in 1722, he published *A Journal of the Plague Year*—a historically informed novel about a man who lives through the epidemic. Although this is fiction, it is founded on a great deal of historical data. The selections included here come from the opening of the novel.

---

* Reprinted from Daniel Defoe, *A Journal of the Plague Year: Being Observations or Memorials, or the most Remarkable Occurrences [...] Which happened in London During the Great Visitation in 1665* (London, 1722; Project Gutenberg, 2020), 1–40.

It was about the beginning of September, 1664, that I, among the rest of my neighbors, heard in ordinary discourse that the plague was returned again in Holland; for it had been very violent there, and particularly at Amsterdam and Rotterdam, in the year 1663, whither, they say, it was brought, some said from Italy, others from the Levant, among some goods which were brought home by their Turkey fleet; others said it was brought from Candia;[1] others from Cyprus. It mattered not from whence it came; but all agreed it was come into Holland again.

We had no such thing as printed newspapers in those days to spread rumors and reports of things, and to improve them by the invention of men, as I have lived to see practiced since. But such things as these were gathered from the letters of merchants and others who corresponded abroad, and from them was handed about by word of mouth only; so that things did not spread instantly over the whole nation, as they do now. But it seems that the Government had a true account of it, and several councils were held about ways to prevent its coming over; but all was kept very private. Hence it was that this rumor died off again, and people began to forget it as a thing we were very little concerned in, and that we hoped was not true; till the latter end of November or the beginning of December 1664 when two men, said to be Frenchmen, died of the plague in Long Acre, or rather at the upper end of Drury Lane. The family they were in endeavored to conceal it as much as possible, but as it had gotten some vent in the discourse of the neighborhood, the Secretaries of State got knowledge of it; and concerning themselves to inquire about it, in order to be certain of the truth, two physicians and a surgeon were ordered to go to the house and make inspection. This they did; and finding evident tokens of the sickness upon both the bodies that were dead, they gave their opinions publicly that they died of the plague. Whereupon it was given in to the parish clerk, and he also returned them to the Hall; and it was printed in the weekly bill of mortality[2] in the usual manner, thus—

Plague, 2. Parishes infected, 1.

---

1 *Candia*: The Island of Crete, which was at the time part of the Republic of Venice.
2 *Weekly bill of mortality*: Like an anonymous obituary, mortality bills listed the number of people lost in an area of town (called a "parish") each week.

The people showed a great concern at this, and began to be alarmed all over the town, and the more, because in the last week in December 1664 another man died in the same house, and of the same distemper. And then we were easy again for about six weeks, when none having died with any marks of infection, it was said the distemper was gone; but after that, I think it was about the 12th of February, another died in another house, but in the same parish and in the same manner.

This turned the people's eyes pretty much towards that end of the town, and the weekly bills showing an increase of burials in St Giles's parish more than usual, it began to be suspected that the plague was among the people at that end of the town, and that many had died of it, though they had taken care to keep it as much from the knowledge of the public as possible. This possessed the heads of the people very much, and few cared to go through Drury Lane, or the other streets suspected, unless they had extraordinary business that obliged them to it.

This increase of the bills stood thus: the usual number of burials in a week, in the parishes of St Giles-in-the-Fields and St Andrew's, Holborn, were from twelve to seventeen or nineteen each, few more or less; but from the time that the plague first began in St Giles's parish, it was observed that the ordinary burials increased in number considerably. For example:—

From	December 27	to	January	3	{ St Giles's	16
					{ St Andrew's	17
"	January 3	"	"	10	{ St Giles's	12
"					{ St Andrew's	25
"	January 10	"	"	17	{ St Giles's	18
"					{ St Andrew's	28
"	January 17	"	"	24	{ St Giles's	23
"					{ St Andrew's	16
"	January 24	"	"	31	{ St Giles's	24
"					{ St Andrew's	15

"	January 30	"	February 7	{ St Giles's	21
"				{ St Andrew's	23
"	February 7	"	" 14	{ St Giles's	24

The like increase of the bills was observed in the parishes of St Bride's, adjoining on one side of Holborn parish, and in the parish of St James, Clerkenwell, adjoining on the other side of Holborn; in both which parishes the usual numbers that died weekly were from four to six or eight, whereas at that time they were increased as follows:—

From	December 20	to	December 27	{ St Bride's	0
"				{ St James's	8
"	December 27	to	January 3	{ St Bride's	6
"				{ St James's	9
"	January 3	"	" 10	{ St Bride's	11
"				{ St James's	7
"	January 10	"	" 17	{ St Bride's	12
"				{ St James's	9
"	January 17	"	" 24	{ St Bride's	9
"				{ St James's	15
"	January 24	"	" 31	{ St Bride's	8
"				{ St James's	12
"	January 31	"	February 7	{ St Bride's	13
"				{ St James's	5
"	February 7	"	" 14	{ St Bride's	12
"				{ St James's	6

Besides this, it was observed with great uneasiness by the people that the weekly bills in general increased very much during these weeks, although it was at a time of the year when usually the bills are very moderate.

The usual number of burials within the bills of mortality for a week was from about 240 or thereabouts to 300. The last was esteemed a pretty high bill; but after this we found the bills successively increasing as follows:—

					Buried.	Increased.
December	the 20th	to the	27th		291	...
"	27th	"	3rd	January	349	58
January	the 3rd	"	10th	"	394	45
"	" 10th	"	17th	"	415	21
"	" 17th	"	24th	"	474	59

This last bill was really frightful, being a higher number than had been known to have been buried in one week since the preceding visitation of 1656.

However, all this went off again, and the weather proving cold, and the frost, which began in December, still continuing very severe even till near the end of February, attended with sharp though moderate winds, the bills decreased again, and the city grew healthy, and everybody began to look upon the danger as good as over; only that still the burials in St Giles's continued high. From the beginning of April especially they stood at twenty-five each week, till the week from the 18th to the 25th, when there was buried in St Giles's parish thirty, whereof two of the plague and eight of the spotted-fever, which was looked upon as the same thing; likewise the number that died of the spotted-fever in the whole increased, being eight the week before, and twelve the week above-named.

This alarmed us all again, and terrible apprehensions were among the people, especially the weather being now changed and growing warm, and the summer being at hand. However, the next week there seemed to be some hopes again; the bills were low, the number of the dead in all was but 388, there was none of the plague, and but four of the spotted-fever.

But the following week it returned again, and the distemper was spread into two or three other parishes, viz., St Andrew's, Holborn; St Clement Danes; and, to the great affliction of the city, one died within the walls, in the parish of St Mary Woolchurch, that is to say, in Bearbinder Lane, near Stocks Market; in all there were nine of the plague and six of the spotted-fever. It was, however, upon inquiry found that this Frenchman who died in Bearbinder Lane was one who, having lived in Long Acre, near the infected houses, had removed for fear of the distemper, not knowing that he was already infected.

This was the beginning of May, yet the weather was temperate, variable, and cool enough, and people had still some hopes. That which encouraged them was that the city was healthy: the whole ninety-seven parishes buried but fifty-four, and we began to hope that, as it was chiefly among the people at that end of the town, it might go no farther; and the rather, because the next week, which was from the 9th of May to the 16th, there died but three, of which not one within the whole city or liberties;[3] and St Andrew's buried but fifteen, which was very low. 'Tis true St Giles's buried two-and-thirty, but still, as there was but one of the plague, people began to be easy. The whole bill also was very low, for the week before the bill was but 347, and the week above mentioned but 343. We continued in these hopes for a few days, but it was but for a few, for the people were no more to be deceived thus; they searched the houses and found that the plague was really spread every way, and that many died of it every day. So that now all our extenuations abated, and it was no more to be concealed; nay, it quickly appeared that the infection had spread itself beyond all hopes of abatement. That in the parish of St Giles it was gotten into several streets, and several families lay all sick together; and, accordingly, in the weekly bill for the next week the thing began to show itself. There was indeed but fourteen set down of the plague, but this was all knavery and collusion, for in St Giles's parish they buried forty in all, whereof it was certain most of them died of the plague, though they were set down of other distempers; and though the number of all the burials were not increased above thirty-two, and

---

3 *Liberties*: Areas geographically within the city that were not subject to city jurisdiction.

the whole bill being but 385, yet there was fourteen of the spotted-fever, as well as fourteen of the plague; and we took it for granted upon the whole that there were fifty died that week of the plague.

The next bill was from the 23rd of May to the 30th, when the number of the plague was seventeen. But the burials in St Giles's were fifty-three—a frightful number!—of whom they set down but nine of the plague; but on an examination more strictly by the justices of peace, and at the Lord Mayor's request, it was found there were twenty more who were really dead of the plague in that parish, but had been set down of the spotted-fever or other distempers, besides others concealed.

But those were trifling things to what followed immediately after; for now the weather set in hot, and from the first week in June the infection spread in a dreadful manner, and the bills rose high; the articles of the fever, spotted-fever, and teeth began to swell;[4] for all that could conceal their distempers did it, to prevent their neighbors shunning and refusing to converse with them, and also to prevent authority shutting up their houses; which, though it was not yet practiced, yet was threatened, and people were extremely terrified at the thoughts of it.

The second week in June, the parish of St Giles, where still the weight of the infection lay, buried 120, whereof though the bills said but sixty-eight of the plague, everybody said there had been 100 at least, calculating it from the usual number of funerals in that parish, as above.

Till this week the city continued free, there having never any died, except that one Frenchman whom I mentioned before, within the whole ninety-seven parishes. Now there died four within the city, one in Wood Street, one in Fenchurch Street, and two in Crooked Lane. Southwark was entirely free, having not one yet died on that side of the water.

I lived without Aldgate[5], about midway between Aldgate Church and Whitechapel Bars, on the left hand or north side of the street; and as the distemper had not reached to that side of the city, our neighborhood continued very easy. But at the other end of the town their

---

4   *Articles of the fever, spotted fever, and teeth began to swell*: These are listings of other possible causes of death; at the time, "bad teeth" was among the leading causes of death in Europe.
5   *Without Aldgate*: Outside of Aldgate.

consternation was very great: and the richer sort of people, especially the nobility and gentry from the west part of the city, thronged out of town with their families and servants in an unusual manner; and this was more particularly seen in Whitechapel; that is to say, the Broad Street where I lived; indeed, nothing was to be seen but wagons and carts, with goods, women, servants, children, &c.; coaches filled with people of the better sort and horsemen attending them, and all hurrying away; then empty wagons and carts appeared, and spare horses with servants, who, it was apparent, were returning or sent from the countries to fetch more people; besides innumerable numbers of men on horseback, some alone, others with servants, and, generally speaking, all loaded with baggage and fitted out for traveling, as anyone might perceive by their appearance.

This was a very terrible and melancholy thing to see, and as it was a sight which I could not but look on from morning to night (for indeed there was nothing else of moment to be seen), it filled me with very serious thoughts of the misery that was coming upon the city, and the unhappy condition of those that would be left in it.

This hurry of the people was such for some weeks that there was no getting at the Lord Mayor's door without exceeding difficulty; there were such pressing and crowding there to get passes and certificates of health for such as traveled abroad, for without these there was no being admitted to pass through the towns upon the road, or to lodge in any inn. Now, as there had none died in the city for all this time, my Lord Mayor gave certificates of health without any difficulty to all those who lived in the ninety-seven parishes, and to those within the liberties too for a while.

This hurry, I say, continued some weeks, that is to say, all the month of May and June, and the more because it was rumored that an order of the Government was to be issued out to place turnpikes and barriers on the road to prevent people traveling, and that the towns on the road would not suffer people from London to pass for fear of bringing the infection along with them, though neither of these rumors had any foundation but in the imagination, especially at-first.

*

It was a very ill time to be sick in, for if any one complained, it was immediately said he had the plague; and though I had indeed no symptom of that distemper, yet being very ill, both in my head and in my stomach, I was not without apprehension that I really was infected; but in about three days I grew better; the third night I rested well, sweated a little, and was much refreshed. The apprehensions of its being the infection went also quite away with my illness, and I went about my business as usual.

These things, however, put off all my thoughts of going into the country; and my brother also being gone, I had no more debate either with him or with myself on that subject.

It was now mid-July, and the plague, which had chiefly raged at the other end of the town, and, as I said before, in the parishes of St Giles, St Andrew's, Holborn, and towards Westminster, began to now come eastward towards the part where I lived. It was to be observed, indeed, that it did not come straight on towards us; for the city, that is to say, within the walls, was indifferently healthy still; nor was it got then very much over the water into Southwark; for though there died that week 1268 of all distempers, whereof it might be supposed above 600 died of the plague, yet there was but twenty-eight in the whole city, within the walls, and but nineteen in Southwark, Lambeth parish included; whereas in the parishes of St Giles and St Martin-in-the-Fields alone there died 421.

But we perceived the infection kept chiefly in the out-parishes, which being very populous, and fuller also of poor, the distemper found more to prey upon than in the city, as I shall observe afterwards. We perceived, I say, the distemper to draw our way, viz., by the parishes of Clerkenwell, Cripplegate, Shoreditch, and Bishopsgate; which last two parishes joining to Aldgate, Whitechapel, and Stepney, the infection came at length to spread its utmost rage and violence in those parts, even when it abated at the western parishes where it began.

It was very strange to observe that in this particular week, from the 4th to the 11th of July, when, as I have observed, there died near 400 of the plague in the two parishes of St Martin and St Giles-in-the-Fields only, there died in the parish of Aldgate but four, in the parish of Whitechapel three, in the parish of Stepney but one.

Likewise in the next week, from the 11th of July to the 18th, when the week's bill was 1761, yet there died no more of the plague, on the whole

Southwark side of the water, than sixteen. But this face of things soon changed, and it began to thicken in Cripplegate parish especially, and in Clerkenwell; so that by the second week in August, Cripplegate parish alone buried 886, and Clarkenwell 155. Of the first, 850 might well be reckoned to die of the plague; and of the last, the bill itself said 145 were of the plague.

During the month of July, and while, as I have observed, our part of the town seemed to be spared in comparison of the west part, I went ordinarily about the streets, as my business required, and particularly went generally once in a day, or in two days, into the city, to my brother's house, which he had given me charge of, and to see if it was safe; and having the key in my pocket, I used to go into the house, and over most of the rooms, to see that all was well; for though it be something wonderful to tell, that any should have hearts so hardened in the midst of such a calamity as to rob and steal, yet certain it is that all sorts of villainies, and even levities and debaucheries, were then practiced in the town as openly as ever—I will not say quite as frequently, because the numbers of people were many ways lessened.

But the city itself began now to be visited too, I mean within the walls; but the number of people there were indeed extremely lessened by so great a multitude having been gone into the country; and even all this month of July they continued to flee, though not in such multitudes as formerly. In August, indeed, they fled in such a manner that I began to think there would be really none but magistrates and servants left in the city.

As they fled now out of the city, so I should observe that the Court removed early, viz., in the month of June, and went to Oxford, where it pleased God to preserve them; and the distemper did not, as I heard of, so much as touch them, for which I cannot say that I ever saw they showed any great token of thankfulness, and hardly anything of reformation, though they did not want being told that their crying vices might without breach of charity be said to have gone far in bringing that terrible judgment upon the whole nation.

The face of London was—now indeed strangely altered: I mean the whole mass of buildings, city, liberties, suburbs, Westminster, Southwark, and altogether; for as to the particular part called the city, or within the walls, that was not yet much infected. But in the whole the face of things, I say, was much altered; sorrow and sadness sat upon every face; and though some parts were not yet overwhelmed, yet all looked deeply concerned; and, as we saw it apparently coming on, so every one looked on himself and his family as in the utmost danger. Were it possible to represent those times exactly to those that did not see them, and give the reader due ideas of the horror that everywhere presented itself, it must make just impressions upon their minds and fill them with surprise. London might well be said to be all in tears; the mourners did not go about the streets indeed, for nobody put on black or made a formal dress of mourning for their nearest friends; but the voice of mourners was truly heard in the streets. The shrieks of women and children at the windows and doors of their houses, where their dearest relations were perhaps dying, or just dead, were so frequent to be heard as we passed the streets, that it was enough to pierce the stoutest heart in the world to hear them. Tears and lamentations were seen almost in every house, especially in the first part of the visitation; for towards the latter end men's hearts were hardened, and death was so always before their eyes, that they did not so much concern themselves for the loss of their friends, expecting that themselves should be summoned the next hour.

Business led me out sometimes to the other end of the town, even when the sickness was chiefly there; and as the thing was new to me, as well as to everybody else, it was a most surprising thing to see those streets which were usually so thronged now grown desolate, and so few people to be seen in them, that if I had been a stranger and at a loss for my way, I might sometimes have gone the length of a whole street (I mean of the by-streets), and seen nobody to direct me except watchmen set at the doors of such houses as were shut up, of which I shall speak presently.

One day, being at that part of the town on some special business, curiosity led me to observe things more than usually, and indeed I walked a great way where I had no business. I went up Holborn, and there the street was full of people, but they walked in the middle of the great street, neither on one side or other, because, as I suppose, they would not mingle with anybody that came out of houses, or meet with smells and scent from houses that might be infected.

The Inns of Court were all shut up; nor were very many of the lawyers in the Temple, or Lincoln's Inn, or Gray's Inn, to be seen there. Everybody was at peace; there was no occasion for lawyers; besides, it being in the time of the vacation too, they were generally gone into the country. Whole rows of houses in some places were shut close up, the inhabitants all fled, and only a watchman or two left.

*

[A]s I have said before, that they ran to conjurers and witches, and all sorts of deceivers, to know what should become of them (who fed their fears, and kept them always alarmed and awake on purpose to delude them and pick their pockets), so they were as mad upon their running after quacks and mountebanks, and every practicing old woman,[6] for medicines and remedies; storing themselves with such multitudes of pills, potions, and preservatives, as they were called, that they not only spent their money but even poisoned themselves beforehand for fear of the poison of the infection; and prepared their bodies for the plague, instead of preserving them against it. On the other hand it is incredible and scarce to be imagined, how the posts of houses and corners of streets were plastered over with doctors' bills and papers of ignorant fellows, quacking and tampering in physic, and inviting the people to come to them for remedies, which was generally set off with such flourishes as these, viz.: "Infallible preventive pills against the plague." "Neverfailing preservatives against the infection." "Sovereign cordials against the corruption of the air." "Exact regulations for the conduct of the body in case of an infection." "Anti-pestilential pills." "Incomparable drink against the plague, never found out before." "An universal remedy for the plague." "The only true plague water." "The royal antidote against all kinds of infection";—and such a number more that I cannot

---

6   *Quacks and mountebanks, and every practising old woman*: Practitioners of medicine in London were either licensed (as learned physicians, or as surgeons or apothecaries who learned their trade via guilds and official channels) or unlicensed—unlicensed practitioners included midwives, "cunning women" (women with extensive knowledge of practical remedies), and those who sought to defraud patients: quacks and mountebanks fall into this latter category.

reckon up; and if I could, would fill a book of themselves to set them down.

Others set up bills to summon people to their lodgings for directions and advice in the case of infection. These had specious titles also, such as these:—

> "An eminent High Dutch physician, newly come over from Holland, where he resided during all the time of the great plague last year in Amsterdam, and cured multitudes of people that actually had the plague upon them."
>
> "An Italian gentlewoman just arrived from Naples, having a choice secret to prevent infection, which she found out by her great experience, and did wonderful cures with it in the late plague there, wherein there died 20,000 in one day."
>
> "An ancient gentlewoman, having practiced with great success in the late plague in this city, anno 1636, gives her advice only to the female sex. To be spoken with," &c.
>
> "An experienced physician, who has long studied the doctrine of antidotes against all sorts of poison and infection, has, after forty years' practice, arrived to such skill as may, with God's blessing, direct persons how to prevent their being touched by any contagious distemper whatsoever. He directs the poor gratis."

I take notice of these by way of specimen. I could give you two or three dozen of the like and yet have abundance left behind. 'Tis sufficient from these to apprise any one of the humor of those times, and how a set of thieves and pickpockets not only robbed and cheated the poor people of their money, but poisoned their bodies with odious and fatal preparations; some with mercury, and some with other things as bad, perfectly remote from the thing pretended to, and rather hurtful than serviceable to the body in case an infection followed.

I cannot omit a subtlety of one of those quack operators, with which he gulled the poor people to crowd about him, but did nothing for them without money. He had, it seems, added to his bills, which he gave about the streets, this advertisement in capital letters, viz., "He gives advice to the poor for nothing."

Abundance of poor people came to him accordingly, to whom he made a great many fine speeches, examined them of the state of their health and of the constitution of their bodies, and told them many good things for them to do, which were of no great moment. But the issue and conclusion of all was, that he had a preparation which if they took such a quantity of every morning, he would pawn his life they should never have the plague; no, though they lived in the house with people that were infected. This made the people all resolve to have it; but then the price of that was so much, I think 'twas half-a-crown. "But, sir," says one poor woman, "I am a poor almswoman and am kept by the parish, and your bills say you give the poor your help for nothing." "Ay, good woman," says the doctor, "so I do, as I published there. I give my advice to the poor for nothing, but not my physic." "Alas, sir!" says she, "that is a snare laid for the poor, then; for you give them advice for nothing; that is to say, you advise them gratis, to buy your physic for their money; so does every shop-keeper with his wares." Here the woman began to give him ill words, and stood at his door all that day, telling her tale to all the people that came, till the doctor finding she turned away his customers, was obliged to call her upstairs again, and give her his box of physic for nothing, which perhaps, too, was good for nothing when she had it.

But to return to the people, whose confusions fitted them to be imposed upon by all sorts of pretenders and by every mountebank. There is no doubt but these quacking sort of fellows raised great gains out of the miserable people, for we daily found the crowds that ran after them were infinitely greater, and their doors were more thronged than those of Dr Brooks, Dr Upton, Dr Hodges, Dr Berwick, or any, though the most famous men of the time. And I was told that some of them got five pounds a day by their physic.

But there was still another madness beyond all this, which may serve to give an idea of the distracted humor of the poor people at that time: and this was their following a worse sort of deceivers than any of these; for these petty thieves only deluded them to pick their pockets and get their money, in which their wickedness, whatever it was, lay chiefly on the side of the deceivers, not upon the deceived. But in this part I am going to mention, it lay chiefly in the people deceived, or equally in both; and this was in wearing charms, philtres,[7] exorcisms, amulets, and I know not what preparations, to fortify the body with them against the plague; as if the plague was not the hand of God, but a kind of possession of an evil spirit, and that it was to be kept off with crossings, signs of the zodiac, papers tied up with so many knots, and certain words or figures written on them, as particularly the word Abracadabra, formed in triangle or pyramid, thus:—

```
ABRACADABRA
ABRACADABR    Others had the Jesuits'
ABRACADAB     mark in a cross:
ABRACADA         I H
ABRACAD          S.
ABRACA
ABRAC         Others nothing but this
ABRA          mark, thus:
ABR
AB               * *
A                {*}
```

I might spend a great deal of time in my exclamations against the follies, and indeed the wickedness, of those things, in a time of such danger, in a matter of such consequences as this, of a national infection. But my memorandums of these things relate rather to take notice only of the fact, and mention only that it was so. How the poor people found the insufficiency of those things, and how many of them were afterwards carried away in the dead-carts and thrown into the common graves of every parish with these hellish charms and trumpery hanging about their necks, remains to be spoken of as we go along.

---

7   *Philtres*: Drugs or potions meant to induce love or libido.

Compare & Consider

COMPARE

Compare the works concerned with the bubonic plague, presented here, to those concerned with other epidemics, including those by Thucydides (pp. 20–25), Rhazes (pp. 47–56), Girolamo Fracastoro (pp. 75–83), Lady Mary Wortley Montagu (pp. 163–166), Zabdiel Boylston (pp. 167–171), Mary Jones (pp. 172–173), and Edward Jenner (pp. 187–194).

CONSIDER

What do these texts show us about the social response to disease as opposed to a medical response? How do individuals and communities act and react when faced with contagion? How does the reaction to epidemic outbreak in these texts compare to that of more recent outbreaks? What are the ethical implications of the restrictions and/or behaviors described in these works?

Doing Battle
HEALTH AND MEDICINE ON THE FRONT LINES

Among the vast network of consequences arising from war are medical needs: the treatment of wounds on the field, the long-term impact of trauma (on soldiers, practitioners, and civilians alike), and the health of individuals and societies during and in the aftermath of conflict. The health-related impacts of war have been documented across many media. Included here are a few examples illustrating just some of the many ways individuals and cultures have presented these impacts [See Illustration 19].

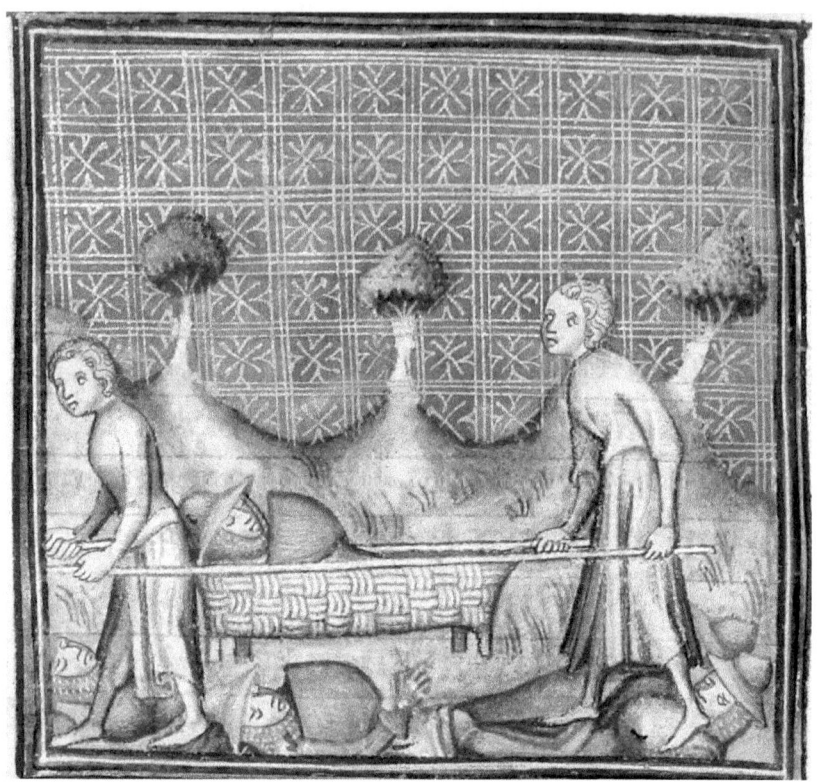

Illustration 19. An early stretcher, ca. 1364–1373. Valerius Maximus's *Facta et Dicta Memorabilia* (Memorable Facts and Deeds), trans. Simon de Hesdin. Bibliothèque nationale de France, Français 9749, f.67v. A manuscript illustration depicting a wounded soldier being carried off in an early example of a stretcher, from a medieval manuscript translation of historical anecdotes by first century author Valerius Maximus. Source: gallica.bnf.fr / BnF.

The Iliad*

HOMER
(Greek, ca. ninth or eighth century BCE)

The poet Homer is credited with the two most important and influential works of ancient Greek literature: the epic poems the *Iliad* and the *Odyssey*. The genre of epic poetry tells of some of the major historical events, legends, and figures in a culture. This excerpt, from a popular and readable prose translation by Samuel Butler, is set during the ten-year siege of Ilium, commonly known as the Trojan War. According to recorded stories of the Trojan War, the famed heroes Achilles and Patroclus (who were close friends and likely also lovers) were both skilled in treating the wounds of fellow soldiers; this is apparent in examples from both art and literature [See Illustration 20].

---

* Reprinted from Samuel Butler, trans., *The Iliad of Homer, Rendered into English Prose* (London: Longmans, Green, 1898), book 11, Internet Classics Archive.

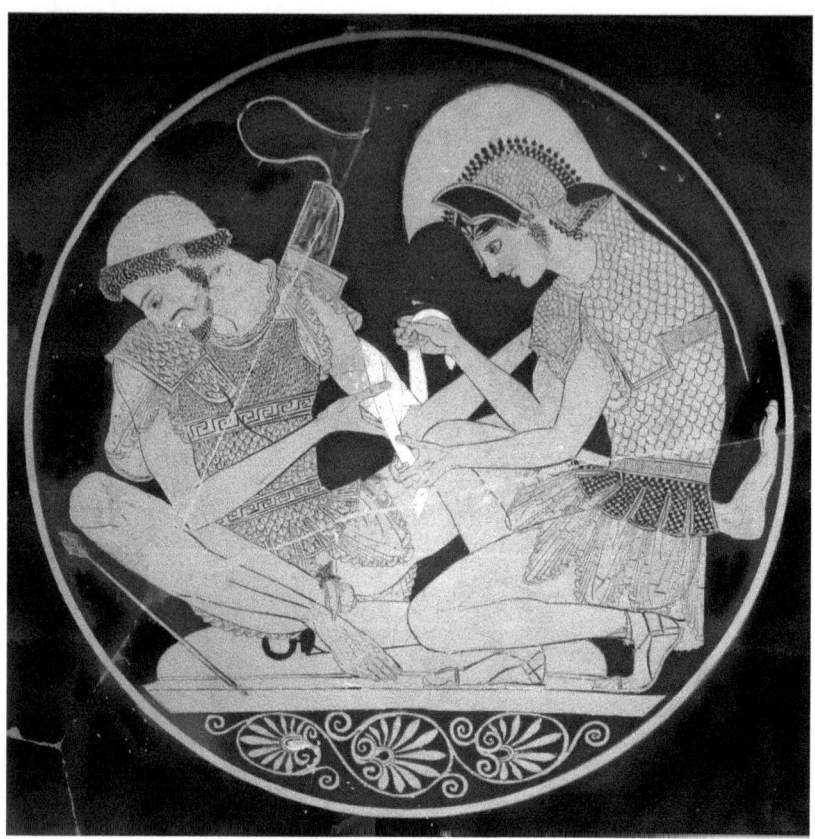

Illustration 20. Achilles Tending Patroclus, ca. 500 BCE. Tondo of an Attic vase from Vulci, attributed to Sosias. Altes Museum, Berlin. This image depicts a scene from the account of the Trojan War, in which Achilles tends to an arrow wound in the Patroclus's arm.

Patroclus Tends to Eurypylus

When he had got as far as the ships of Ulysses, where was their place of assembly and court of justice, with their altars dedicated to the gods, Eurypylus son of Euaemon met him, wounded in the thigh with an arrow, and limping out of the fight. Sweat rained from his head and shoulders, and black blood welled from his cruel wound, but his mind did not wander. The son of Menoetius when he saw him had compassion upon him and spoke piteously saying, "O unhappy princes and counsellors of the Danaans, are you then doomed to feed the hounds of Troy with your fat, far from your friends and your native land? say, noble Eurypylus, will the Achaeans be able to hold great Hector in check, or will they fall now before his spear?"

Wounded Eurypylus made answer, "Noble Patroclus, there is no hope left for the Achaeans but they will perish at their ships. All they that were princes among us are lying struck down and wounded at the hands of the Trojans, who are waxing stronger and stronger. But save me and take me to your ship; cut out the arrow from my thigh; wash the black blood from off it with warm water, and lay upon it those gracious herbs which, so they say, have been shown you by Achilles, who was himself shown them by Chiron,[1] most righteous of all the centaurs. For of the physicians Podalirius and Machaon, I hear that the one is lying wounded in his tent and is himself in need of healing, while the other is fighting the Trojans upon the plain."

"Hero Eurypylus," replied the brave son of Menoetius, "how may these things be? What can I do? I am on my way to bear a message to noble Achilles from Nestor of Gerene, bulwark of the Achaeans, but even so I will not be unmindful your distress."

With this he clasped him round the middle and led him into the tent, and a servant, when he saw him, spread bullock-skins on the ground for him to lie on. He laid him at full length and cut out the sharp arrow from his thigh; he washed the black blood from the wound with warm water; he then crushed a bitter herb, rubbing it between his hands, and spread it upon the wound; this was a virtuous herb which killed all pain; so the wound presently dried and the blood left off flowing.

---

1 *Chiron*: The most respected of all the centaurs, proficient in medicine, and teacher of Asclepius, the Greek god of medicine (see pp. 377–382).

Photography from the American Civil War

VARIOUS ARTISTS
1861–1865

The American Civil War was the most widely documented conflict of the nineteenth century, and pioneering photographers like Matthew Brady and Alexander Gardner likewise made it the first war to be extensively documented in photographs. (The first war ever recorded in photos was the Mexican-American War of 1846–1848). These pictures, many of which were created with twin lenses for viewing in stereoscopes (an early form of 3D), brought the terrible realities of war more clearly into focus for those who were not near the front lines. Included here are some of these documentary efforts [See Illustrations 21 and 22].

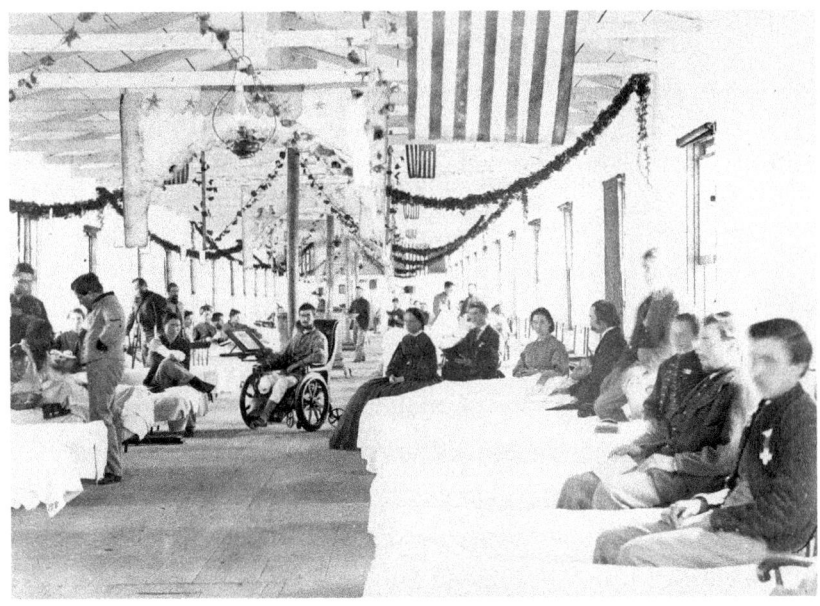

Illustration 21. A photograph depicting the conditions inside a hospital ward by an unknown photographer. A Ward in Armory Square Hospital, Washington, D.C., ca. 1862–1865. Library of Congress Prints and Photographs Division, Washington, D.C.

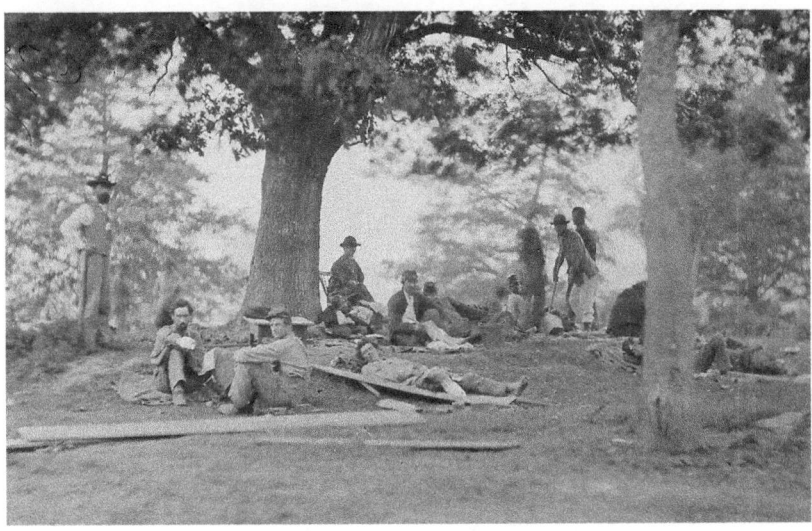

Illustration 22. A photograph depicting wounded soldiers lying under tree cover following the Battle of Spotsylvania on May 19 or 20, 1864, by Matthew Brady. Wounded Soldiers Under Trees, Marye's Heights, Fredericksburg, 1864. War Department. Office of the Chief Signal Officer. The National Archives.

Reminiscences of My Life in Camp with the 33d United States Colored Troops*

SUSIE KING TAYLOR
(American, 1848–1912)

Susie King Taylor was an army nurse with the 33rd US Colored Infantry Regiment [See Illustration 23]. Born into slavery in Georgia in 1848, she learned to read and write in an illegal school. In 1862, she fled to an island off the coast of Georgia, and ran a school for newly freed slaves. The Civil War raged on, however, and she traveled with her husband's regiment for three years. Even though she signed on as a laundry-woman, she largely worked as a nurse (a position for which no formal training was required or available at the time). The excerpts here are drawn from her memoir, published in 1902.

---

* Reprinted from Susie King Taylor, *Reminiscences of My Life in Camp with the 33d United States Colored Troops Late 1st S.C. Volunteers* (Boston: 1902; University of North Carolina at Chapel Hill, 1999), 31–35.

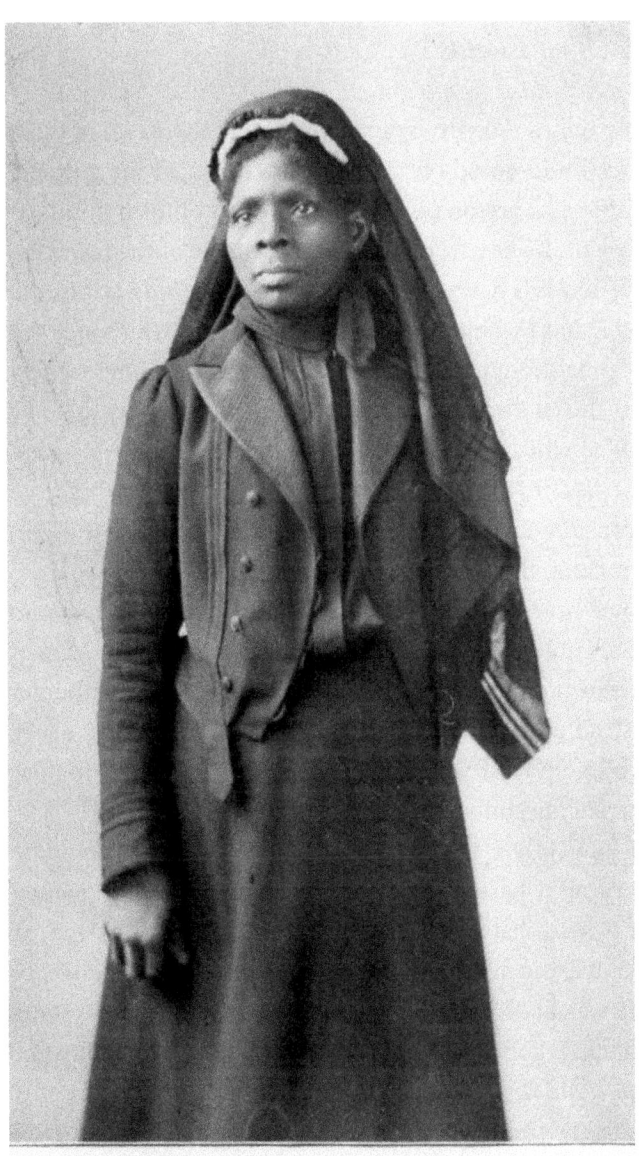

Illustration 23. A photograph of Susie King Taylor, known as the first African American Army Nurse, ca. 1862–1866, published in her memoir in 1902. 7.5 × 5.1 in. (19 × 13 cm). Library of Congress Prints and Photographs Division, Washington, D.C.

On Morris and Other Islands

Fort Wagner being only a mile from our camp, I went there two or three times a week, and would go up on the ramparts to watch the gunners send their shells into Charleston (which they did every fifteen minutes), and had a full view of the city from that point. Outside of the fort were many skulls lying about; I have often moved them one side out of the path. The comrades and I would have quite a debate as to which side the men fought on. Some thought they were the skulls of our boys; others thought they were the enemy's; but as there was no definite way to know, it was never decided which could lay claim to them. They were a gruesome sight, those fleshless heads and grinning jaws, but by this time I had become accustomed to worse things and did not feel as I might have earlier in my camp life.

It seems strange how our aversion to seeing suffering is overcome in war,– how we are able to see the most sickening sights, such as men with their limbs blown off and mangled by the deadly shells, without a shudder; and instead of turning away, how we hurry to assist in alleviating their pain, bind up their wounds, and press the cool water to their parched lips, with feelings only of sympathy and pity....

About four o'clock, July 2, the charge was made. The firing could be plainly heard in camp. I hastened down to the landing and remained there until eight o'clock that morning. When the wounded arrived, or rather began to arrive, the first one brought in was Samuel Anderson of our company. He was badly wounded. Then others of our boys, some with their legs off, arm gone, foot off, and wounds of all kinds imaginable. They had to wade through creeks and marshes, as they were discovered by the enemy and shelled very badly. A number of the men were lost, some got fastened in the mud and had to cut off the legs of their pants, to free themselves. The 103d New York suffered the most, as their men were very badly wounded.

My work now began. I gave my assistance to try to alleviate their sufferings. I asked the doctor at the hospital what I could get for them to eat. They wanted soup, but that I could not get; but I had a few cans of condensed milk and some turtle eggs, so I thought I would try to make some custard. I had doubts as to my success, for cooking with turtle eggs was something new to me, but the adage has it, "Nothing ventured, nothing done," so I made a venture and the result was a very delicious custard. This I carried to the men, who enjoyed it very much. My services were given at all times for the comfort of these men. I was on hand to assist whenever needed. I was enrolled as company laundress, but I did very little of it, because I was always busy doing other things through camp, and was employed all the time doing something for the officers and comrades.

The Wound-Dresser*

WALT WHITMAN
(American, 1819–1892)

New York-born Walt Whitman's experiences during the Civil War (see also pp. 262–271) offered inspiration for his poetry collection *Drum-Taps*, which he originally published in 1865. The Civil War poetry sequence underwent several revisions: originally fifty-three poems, Whitman added eighteen more to the volume *Sequel to Drum-Taps: When Lilacs Last in the Dooryard Bloom'd and other poems* (also 1865), and eventually included the full sequence—with some poems revised yet again—in his famous, ever-evolving work *Leaves of Grass*. The poem included here was originally titled "The Dresser" in the first edition of *Drum-Taps*. It is told from the perspective of a veteran Civil War nurse and looks back on the experience of caring for the wounded.

---

* Reprinted from Walt Whitman, *Leaves of Grass* (Philadelphia: Rees Welsh, 1882), 241–44, Internet Archive.

The Wound-Dresser

1.
An old man bending I come among new faces,
Years looking backward resuming in answer to children,
Come tell us old man, as from young men and maidens that love me,
(Arous'd and angry, I'd thought to beat the alarum, and urge relentless war,
But soon my fingers fail'd me, my face droop'd and I resign'd myself, [5]
To sit by the wounded and soothe them, or silently watch the dead;)
Years hence of these scenes, of these furious passions, these chances,
Of unsurpass'd heroes, (was one side so brave? the other was equally brave;)
Now be witness again, paint the mightiest armies of earth,
Of those armies so rapid so wondrous what saw you to tell us? [10]
What stays with you latest and deepest? of curious panics,
Of hard-fought engagements or sieges tremendous what deepest remains?

2.
O maidens and young men I love and that love me,
What you ask of my days those the strangest and sudden your talking recalls,
Soldier alert I arrive after a long march cover'd with sweat and dust, [15]
In the nick of time I come, plunge in the fight, loudly shout in the rush of successful charge,
Enter the captur'd works—yet lo, like a swift running river they fade,
Pass and are gone they fade—I dwell not on soldiers' perils or soldiers' joys,

(Both I remember well—many of the hardships, few the joys, yet
   I was content.)

But in silence, in dreams' projections, [20]
While the world of gain and appearance and mirth goes on,
So soon what is over forgotten, and waves wash the imprints off
   the sand,
With hinged knees returning I enter the doors, (while for you
   up there,
Whoever you are, follow without noise and be of strong heart.)

Bearing the bandages, water and sponge, [25]
Straight and swift to my wounded I go,
Where they lie on the ground after the battle brought in,
Where their priceless blood reddens the grass the ground,
Or to the rows of the hospital tent, or under the roof'd hospital,
To the long rows of cots up and down each side I return, [30]
To each and all one after another I draw near, not one do I miss,
An attendant follows holding a tray, he carries a refuse pail,
Soon to be fill'd with clotted rags and blood, emptied, and fill'd
   again.

I onward go, I stop,
With hinged knees and steady hand to dress wounds, [35]
I am firm with each, the pangs are sharp yet unavoidable,
One turns to me his appealing eyes—poor boy! I never knew
   you,
Yet I think I could not refuse this moment to die for you, if that
   would save you.

3.
On, on I go, (open doors of time! open hospital doors!)
The crush'd head I dress, (poor crazed hand tear not
 the bandage away,) [40]
The neck of the cavalry-man with the bullet through and
 through I examine,
Hard the breathing rattles, quite glazed already the eye, yet life
 struggles hard,
(Come sweet death! be persuaded O beautiful death!
In mercy come quickly.)

From the stump of the arm, the amputated hand, [45]
I undo the clotted lint, remove the slough, wash off the matter
 and blood,
Back on his pillow the soldier bends with curv'd neck and side
 falling head,
His eyes are closed, his face is pale, he dares not look on the
 bloody stump,
And has not yet look'd on it.

I dress a wound in the side, deep, deep, [50]
But a day or two more, for see the frame all wasted and sinking,
And the yellow-blue countenance see.

I dress the perforated shoulder, the foot with the bullet-wound,
Cleanse the one with a gnawing and putrid gangrene, so
 sickening, so offensive,
While the attendant stands behind aside me holding the tray
 and pail. [55]

I am faithful, I do not give out,
The fractur'd thigh, the knee, the wound in the abdomen,
These and more I dress with impassive hand, (yet deep in my
 breast a fire, a burning flame.)

4.
Thus in silence in dreams' projections,
Returning, resuming, I thread my way through
    the hospitals, [60]
The hurt and wounded I pacify with soothing hand,
I sit by the restless all the dark night, some are so young,
Some suffer so much, I recall the experience sweet and sad,
(Many a soldier's loving arms about this neck have cross'd and
    rested,
Many a soldier's kiss dwells on these bearded lips.) [65]

Images of World War I

VARIOUS ARTISTS
1914–1918

Known in its own time as the "Great War," World War I was one of the largest and deadliest wars of all time; one estimate suggests that around 8.5 million military personnel and 13 million civilians were killed over the course of the war, and up to almost 20 million more were wounded. Of these casualties, an estimated 2 million combatants were lost to infections or disease, and many civilians faced malnutrition and disease as well [See Illustrations 24 and 25].

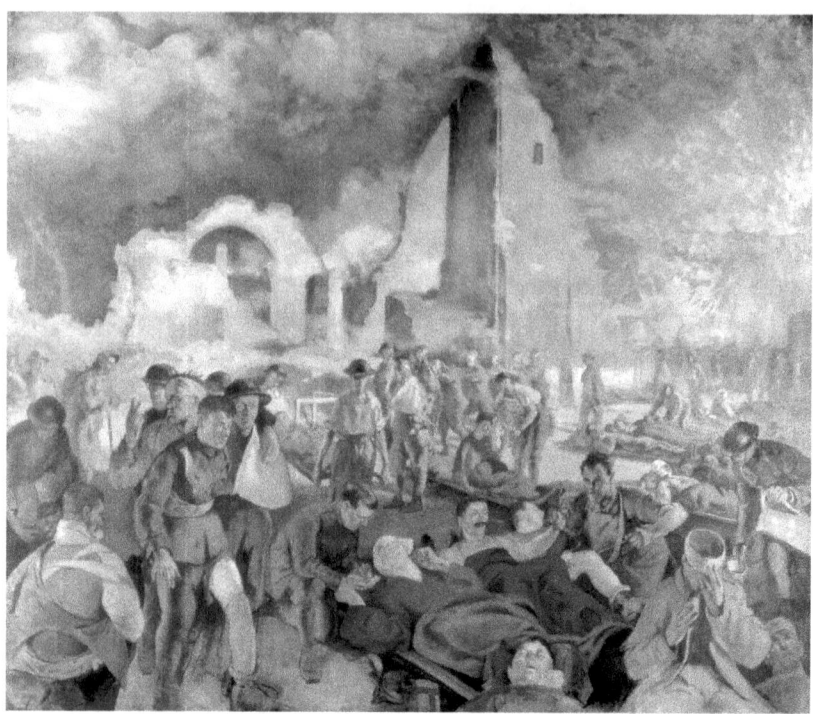

Illustration 24. Henry Tonks (1862–1937), *An Advanced Dressing Station in France, 1918*, 1918. Oil on canvas, 71.96 × 85.98 in. (182 × 218 cm). Imperial War Museum, London. Henry Tonks began his career as a surgeon, but he eventually turned to art, becoming a professor of fine art in London in 1892. During World War I, he served in both capacities, practicing medicine and producing art (like this painting) during tours. Google Art Project.

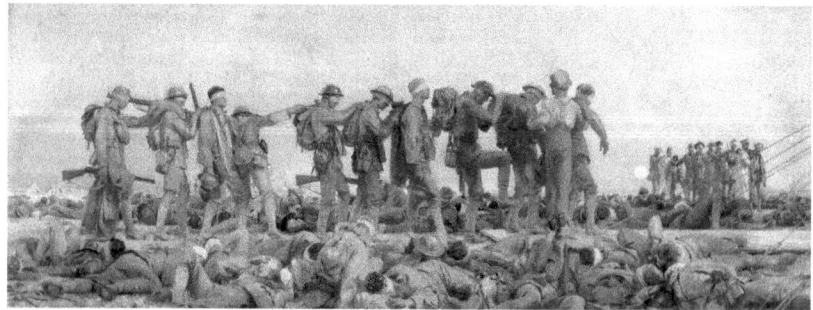

Illustration 25. John Singer Sargent, *Gassed*, 1919. Oil on canvas, 90.9 in. × 20 ft. (2.3 × 6 m). Imperial War Museum, London. In this enormous 20-foot-long oil painting, British painter Sargent depicts blinded solders helping each other across a bleak landscape following a mustard gas attack. Google Art Project.

Food Propaganda: Making Nutrition Patriotic

VARIOUS ARTISTS
American (1917–1918)

While American soldiers fought abroad during World War I, citizens at home were encouraged to change their eating habits in order to support the war effort and to provide more resources for those engaged in Europe. Through poster campaigns, the United Stated Food Administration, The War Garden Commission, and local health departments shaped public consumption in ways that still feel familiar today: promoting home gardens (called "Victory Gardens"); eating less meat, wheat, and sugar; and reducing food waste. Included here are a few examples of the many posters that circulated [See Illustrations 26, 27, and 28].

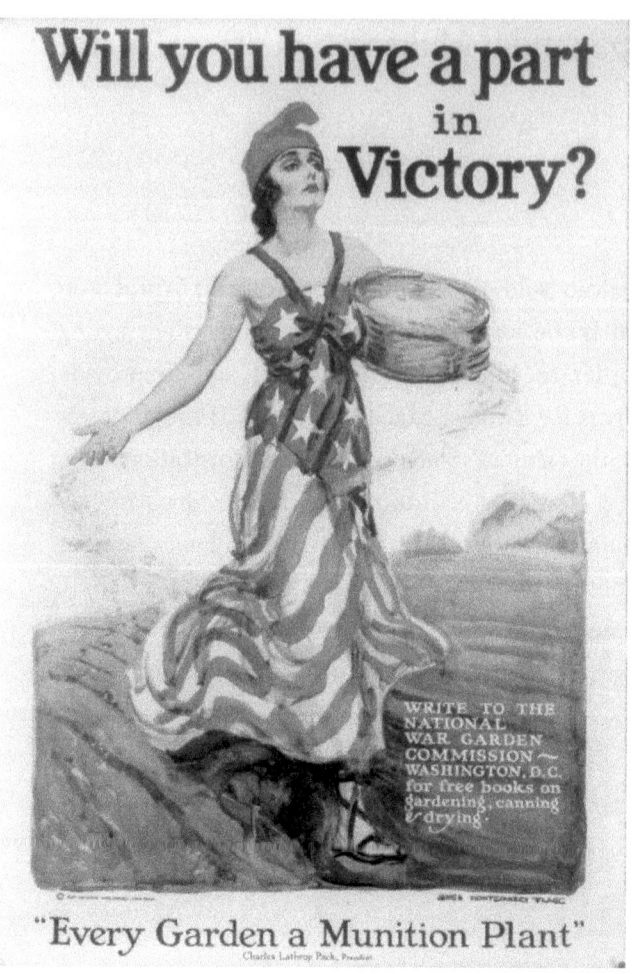

Illustration 26. "Will You Have a Part in Victory?" ca. 1918. Poster, 33 × 22 in. (84 × 56 cm). Library of Congress Prints and Photographs Division, Washington, D.C. This poster by American artist James Montgomery Flagg (1877–1960) and the National War Garden Commission promoted home gardening and food preservation. This was intended to reduce strain on the national food supply and allow individual households to supplement the allowed rations.

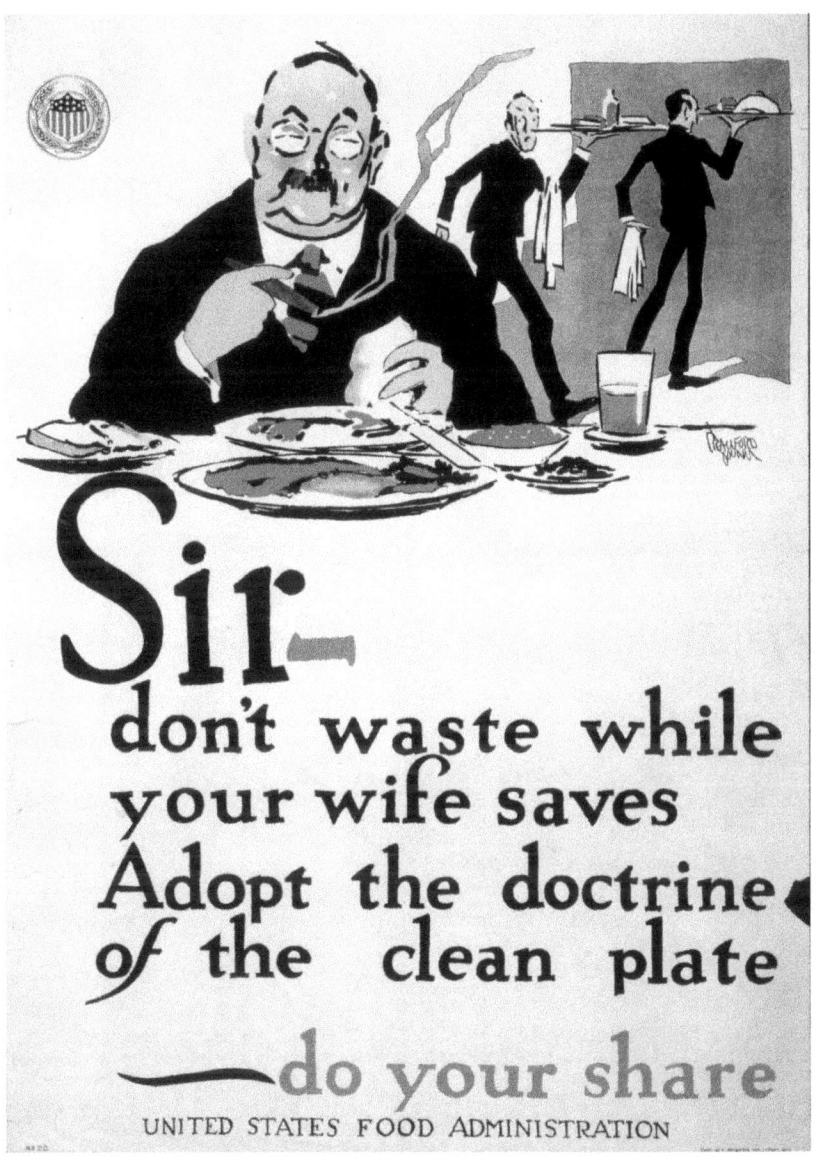

Illustration 27. "Sir—Don't Waste while Your Wife Saves," 1917. Poster, 29.5 × 20.9 in. (74 × 53 cm). Library of Congress Prints and Photographs Division, Washington, D.C. Commissioned from American artist William Crawford Young by the U.S. Food Administration, this poster targeted audiences with money to spend in restaurants or on grand meals and promotes the "doctrine of the clean plate," a rejection of lavish mealtime spreads and culinary excess in favor of thrift and monitoring consumption.

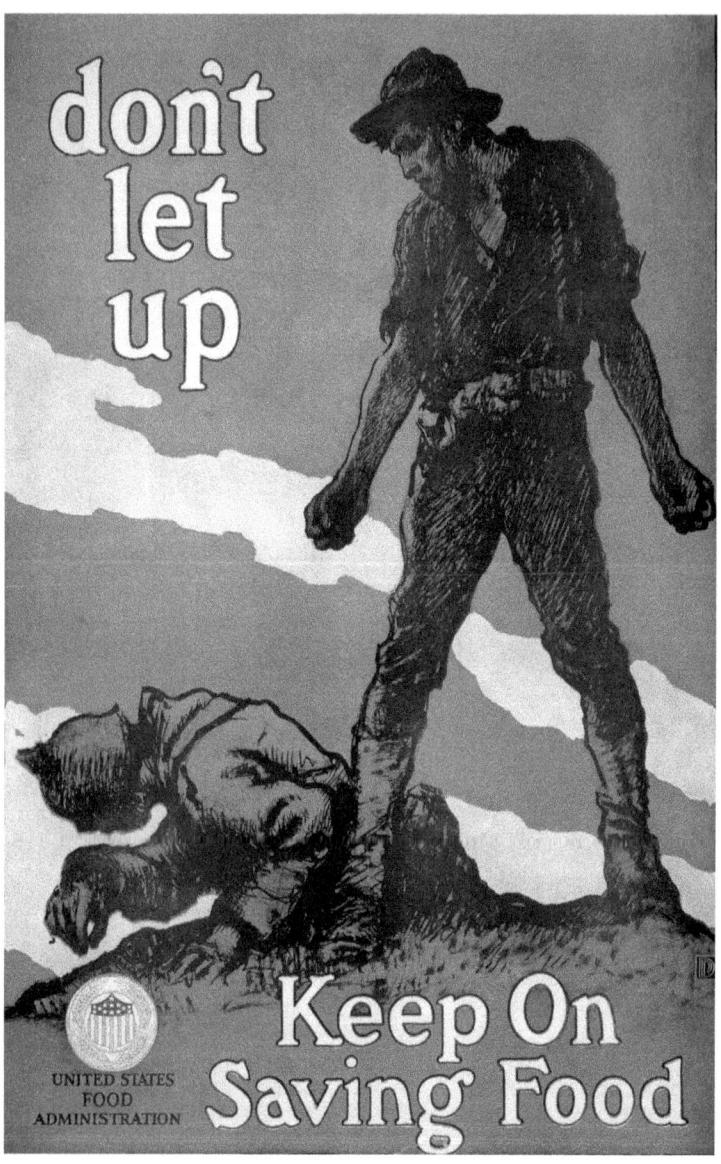

Illustration 28. "Don't Let Up—Keep on Saving Food," 1918. Poster, 21 × 13.8 in. (54 × 35 cm). Library of Congress Prints and Photographs Division, Washington, D.C. Commissioned from American artist Francis Luis Mora (1874–1940) by the U.S. Food Administration, this poster explicitly references the front lines and encourages the American public to prevent food waste at home in order to aid in the war effort abroad.

Compare & Consider

COMPARE

Examine the approaches to health and medicine in wartime in relation to other personal narratives of caretakers during the Civil War (Walt Whitman, pp. 262–271; Emily Elizabeth Parsons, pp. 249–257) and to the reflections on the impact of war on returning veterans (Wilfred Owen, pp. 332–333; W. H. R. Rivers, pp. 334–343; Siegfried Sassoon, pp. 344–346).

CONSIDER

How have attitudes towards the mental health of soldiers changed (or stayed the same) over time? What is the effect of different modes, media, or genres (i.e., visual vs. written, photographs vs. paintings, poetry vs. memoir) on the audience's response to the issues of wartime health and medicine? What values are reflected in the various works and genres here?

Acknowledgments

This book would not have been possible without the support of the folks at Chemeketa Press. In particular, Brian Mosher first got me talking about the idea, Steve Richardson guided me through the project's early development, and Abbey Gaterud provided critical, professional wisdom in pulling all the pieces together. Stephanie Lenox, my editor, helped shape much of this book, and her questions and suggestions improved the work immeasurably.

I am indebted to all those who provided invaluable feedback—formally and informally—at various stages of the development process, especially Matthew Hodgson, Jeremy Trabue, and Dr. Arden Hegele.

My composition students braved early (and often unedited) versions of many selections that eventually landed in this collection; I am grateful for their thoughtful questions and insightful discussions, and their willingness to dive into these works. Special thanks goes out to those students who volunteered to read and provide feedback on additional texts in their own free time, and whose thoughts helped tailor many of the footnotes and introductions.

Finally, the backbone of this (and all) work of mine: Wyant Rowe, as always, offered encouragement and advice, sharpened my thinking, and strengthened my writing, from the project's start to finish. Adventures with our son Cyril kept my spirits high. This work exists only because of them and their support, and words cannot capture the depth of my gratitude and love for them.

Index

A
Addison, Joseph 157
American Civil War 249, 262, 263, 460
anatomy 5, 9, 42, 59, 62, 77, 133, 144, 146, 153, 365
anesthetic 5, 232, 244, 328
    anesthesia 232
animalcules 148–52
antidote 61, 92, 125, 131, 450
apocrypha/ apocryphal 369
Asclepius 77, 129, 159, 169, 179, 377, 378, 379, 423, 459
auscultation 200, 202
autopathography 7, 109, 211
Ayurveda 13, 14, 367, 368

B
Beard, George Miller 258, 285, 287, 313,
Bedlam 204
bezoar 125
Black Death 6, 7, 8, 100, 225, 413–54. *See also* plague/epidemic
blood circulation 135
Boccaccio, Giovanni 415
Boylston, Zabdiel 167, 187
Brady, Matthew 160–61
Brown, Sarah 181
Buchan, William 174

C
children 15, 48, 49, 52, 105, 128, 158, 161, 163, 165, 166, 168, 174, 175, 176, 177, 181, 186, 190, 191, 210, 214, 238, 239, 240, 243–44, 256, 264, 266, 273, 277, 279, 280, 281, 290, 292, 293, 294, 303, 314, 317, 318, 325, 328, 330, 351, 353, 371, 386, 402, 420, 430, 437, 446, 449, 467
    baby 238, 256, 279, 280–84, 291, 296
    childcare 163, 165, 166, 168, 174–77, 181, 186, 190–91, 277–81
Conolly, John 408
cowpox 187
Crumpler, Rebecca Lee 277

D
death 17, 23, 25, 32, 33, 34, 38–40, 57, 76, 90, 100, 102, 110, 114, 116, 117, 123, 124, 129–32, 161, 172, 230, 231, 239, 244, 249, 266, 269, 273, 278, 321, 322, 324, 325, 330, 360, 370, 377, 380, 393, 410, 414, 416, 417, 418, 420, 421, 431, 433, 435, 445, 449, 469
de Chauliac, Guy 67, 194
Defoe, Daniel 439
de Montaigne, Michel 385, 392
Diamond, Hugh Welch 408
Dickinson, Emily 246
Donne, John 7, 109, 114, 122, 308

E
Elyot, Thomas 84, 174
embryology 133, 138, 392–93, 394–95. *See also* generation
enslaved people 167, 211, 358
    slavery 40, 211, 310, 356, 462
ether 232, 233. *See also* anesthesia
ethics 4, 7, 27–29, 47, 67–68, 194, 365, 423

F
female practitioners 143, 157, 235, 249, 272, 277, 462
four humors *See* humors/humoral theory
Fracastoro, Girolamo 75
Freud, Sigmund 9, 313
Frost, Robert 328

G
Galen 26, 41, 48, 62, 88, 126, 138, 142, 423
    Galenism 41, 90. *See also* humors/humoral theory
Gardner, Alexander 460
generation 78, 138, 139, 141, 142, 149, 238, 390, 394
    reproduction 133, 141, 146, 238, 392,
Gerard, John 87
germ theory 4, 34, 75, 126
Gilman, Charlotte Perkins 287
Gould, Hannah Flagg 222

H
Harvey, William 133
hemorrhagic fever 21. *See also* plague/epidemic
Henley, William Ernest 242
herbal 91
Hezekiah 369
Hippocrates 1, 26, 41, 42, 44, 45, 46, 62, 161, 194, 202, 308, 365, 391, 423

Homer 457
homunculus 394
hospitals 194, 202, 204, 237, 239, 240, 262, 266, 268, 270, 271, 335, 470
  hospital management 194, 204, 235
house call 347, 354
humors/humoral theory 4, 15, 17, 26, 29, 30, 41, 42, 44, 45, 46, 48, 52, 58, 61–65, 76–79, 92, 126, 169, 176. *See also* Galenism
  four humors 4, 26, 29, 41, 42, 48, 58, 62, 63, 78, 92, 126
hysteria 103, 106, 259, 313, 334
  suffocation of the mother 103, 106

I
influenza 6, 21, 375, 413. *See also* plague/epidemic
insanity 199, 204, 260
Isaiah 369

J
Jenner, Edward 187
Jones, Mary 172
Jorden, Edward 103

K
Kafka, Franz 347

L
Laënnec, René 200
Li Shizhen 96
Long, Crawford Williamson 232, 249, 328
Lucretius 31, 76

M
man as microcosm 110
manus Dei 365, 371
materia medica 96
maternal impression 182, 388, 392
Mather, Cotton 167, 312
medical humanities 2
  health humanities 2
meditations 229
mental health 6, 7, 69, 204, 246, 285, 287, 332, 334, 344, 383

mental illness 258, 330, 408
Mew, Charlotte Mary 330
miasma 34, 50
midwifery/midwives 143, 159, 160, 182, 318, 326, 398, 450
  man-midwives 159, 160, 183
migraine 57
monsters 323, 383, 387, 388, 390, 393
  monstrum 383
  monstrous birth 384, 385, 388, 392, 396
Montagu, Lady Mary Wortley 163, 167, 187
Mortality Bill/Bills of Mortality 429, 440–45

N
Nashe, Thomas 100
neurasthenia 258, 285, 287, 288, 313, 334, 344
  nervous exhasution 258
  nervousness 258
  Rest Cure 288, 294, 295
Nightingale, Florence 235
nurses/nursing (lactation and children) 15, 143, 146, 174, 181
nurses/nursing (profession) 23, 235, 249, 252, 262, 268, 272, 462, 466

O
Oedipus complex 313
Ohiyesa/Charles Alexander Eastman 318
Owen, Wilfred 332, 344

P
Paracelsus 90, 365, 392, 394
  Paracelsianism 90
Paré, Ambroise 125, 388, 392
Parsons, Emily Elizabeth 249
penis envy / castration complex 313, 317
Pepys, Samuel 427
Percival, Thomas 194
pharmacology/pharmacy 4, 47, 87, 90, 96, 126
Philosophical Transactions 148, 168, 169
phlebotomy/bloodletting 17, 59, 64–66, 134
phrenology 400, 408

physic 85, 106, 120, 126, 158, 159, 161, 175, 280, 417, 450, 452
Pindar 377
plague/epidemic 8, 20, 21, 24, 25, 76, 79, 81, 100, 163, 164, 169, 225, 314, 315, 365, 375, 377, 413–54
    Athenian 20, 34
    bubonic 8, 21, 100, 225, 413–54. *See also* Black Death
Poe, Edgar Allan 225
poison 15, 61, 76, 91–95, 123, 125, 131, 132, 191, 210, 240, 332, 334, 418, 450, 451
pregnancy 27, 52, 127, 181, 183, 206, 388, 392, 396
Prince, Mary 7, 211

Q
quacks/quackery 157–61, 450, 451

R
regimen 17, 27, 50, 53, 54, 59, 84
repression 334, 344
Rhazes 47, 67
rheumatism 211, 212, 214, 215, 216, 270, 361
Rivers, W. H. R. 332, 334, 344
Robinson, Agnes Mary Frances 285, 439
Royal College of Physicians 104, 308

S
Sassoon, Siegfried 330, 332, 334, 344
Seneca 37
Sharp, Jane 143, 160, 183
shell shock 332, 334, 344
    post-traumatic stress disorder/PTSD 332, 334
    war neurosis 335
Sirach 369, 371
smallpox 5, 21, 47, 163, 167, 172, 187, 190, 256, 312, 413. *See also* plague/epidemic
    variola 167, 190
    varioloid 256
Stephen, Julia 272
stethoscope 200
surgery/surgeons 3, 5, 13, 14, 16, 27, 47, 67, 68, 125, 167, 192, 195, 196, 197, 203, 232, 242, 251, 253, 254, 322, 351, 365, 367, 388, 398, 440, 472
Sushruta 13, 16, 194, 367, 368
syphilis 75, 82, 93, 94, 129, 132, 192, 198. *See also* plague/epidemic

T
Tate, Nahum 153
Taylor, Susie King 462
The Royal Society 148, 168, 192, 334, 427
Thucydides 20, 34
Toft, Mary 396
traditional Chinese medicine 96
Tuatha Dé Danann 373
typhoid fever 264, 267, 270, 271
typhus 21. *See also* plague/epidemic
vaccines/vaccination 5, 163, 187, 256. *See also* variolation
van Leeuwenhoek, Antonie 151
variolation 165, 167, 169, 170, 171. *See also* vaccines/vaccination
    inoculation 163, 167, 170, 171, 312
Vaught, L. A. 403
von Bingen, Hildegard 57

W
wandering womb 107
war 20, 249, 262, 277, 332, 334, 344, 347, 455–77
Whitman, Walt 262, 466
Williams, William Carlos 354
willow 87–89, 324
womb 7, 103–108, 127, 128, 138, 139, 383, 390, 392–94
    matrix 103
    mother 103, 104, 106, 107, 108
    uterus 14, 103, 104, 105, 106, 107, 108, 398, 399

www.ingramcontent.com/pod-product-compliance
Ingram Content Group UK Ltd.
Pitfield, Milton Keynes, MK11 3LW, UK
UKHW021045200426
11947UKWH00037B/1512